Principles and Practice of

ASSISTED REPRODUCTIVE TECHNOLOGY

Principles and Practice of
ASSISTED REPRODUCTIVE TECHNOLOGY

VOLUME 3
ATLAS OF HUMAN EMBRYOLOGY

Third Edition

Editor

Kamini A Rao
MBBS DGO MCh FRCOG FNAMS FICOG PGDMLE
Chief Mentor
Former Founder and Medical Director
Milann Group of Fertility Centers
Bengaluru, Karnataka, India

Co-Editors

Mohammed Ashraf C PhD
Associate Director and Senior Embryologist
Milann Fertility Centre
Bengaluru, Karnataka, India

Mir Jaffar PhD
Scientific Director and Chief Embryologist
Valley Fertility Center
Srinagar, Jammu and Kashmir, India

Foreword

Geeta Nargund

JAYPEE

JAYPEE BROTHERS MEDICAL PUBLISHERS
The Health Sciences Publisher
New Delhi | London

Jaypee Brothers Medical Publishers (P) Ltd.

Headquarters
EMCA House, 23/23-B
Ansari Road, Daryaganj
New Delhi 110 002, India
Landline: +91-11-23272143, +91-11-23272703
+91-11-23282021, +91-11-23245672
e-mail: jaypee@jaypeebrothers.com

Corporate Office
4838/24, Ansari Road, Daryaganj
New Delhi 110 002, India
Phone: +91-11-43574357
Fax: +91-11-43574314
e-mail: jaypee@jaypeebrothers.com

Overseas Office
JP Medical Ltd.
83, Victoria Street, London
SW1H 0HW (UK)
Phone: +44-20 3170 8910
e-mail: info@jpmedpub.com

EU GPSR Authorised Representative
Logos Europe, 9 rue Nicolas Poussin
17000, La Rochelle, France
Phone: +33 (0) 6 67 93 73 78
e-mail: contact@logoseurope.eu

Website: www.jaypeebrothers.com
Website: www.jaypeedigital.com

Inquiries for bulk sales may be solicited at: jaypee@jaypeebrothers.com

Principles and Practice of Assisted Reproductive Technology—Vol. 3 (Atlas of Human Embryology)

First Edition: 2014
Second Edition: 2019
Third Edition: 2023, *Reprint:* 2024, 2025, **2026**

ISBN: 978-93-5696-037-4

Printed at: Samrat Offset Pvt. Ltd.

Contents

VOLUME 1: INFERTILITY

SECTION 1: ANATOMY AND PHYSIOLOGY

1. **Anatomy of the Reproductive System** 3
Sonal Agarwal, Mir Jaffar
Female Reproductive System 3; Male Reproductive System 8

2. **Regulation and Physiology of Menstrual Cycle** 16
Arveen Vohra
Reproductive Neuroendocrinology 16; Hormones in Female Reproduction 18;
Multiple Choice Questions with Answers 38

3. **Oogenesis and Folliculogenesis** 42
Suvarna Rathor Zirpe
Formation of Female Gonads 42; Stages of Oogenesis 42; Stages of Folliculogenesis 43;
Prevention of Premature Luteinization 49; Two-cell, Two-gonadotropin Theory 49; Clinical Implications 50

4. **Spermatogenesis** 53
Manishi Mittal
Gonadogenesis 53; The Seminiferous Tubules 53; Spermatogenesis 54

5. **Fertilization and Embryogenesis** 66
Divya Sardana
Egg Transport 66; Sperm Transport 66; Viability of Gametes 66; Capacitation 67; Process of Fertilization 67;
Embryogenesis 68; Genome Activation 69; Blastocyst Formation 69; Clinical Application in Assisted Reproductive
Technology 70

6. **Implantation** 73
Nisha Singh, Divyashree PS
Preimplantation Embryo Development and Genomic Activation 73; Hatching of Blastocyst 74;
Embryo-endometrial Interaction During Implantation 76; Embryo–Maternal Cross-dialogue 86; Immune Acceptance
of Pregnancy 87; Mechanisms at the Trophoblast to Escape Immune Attack 90

7. **Embryo-Endometrial Crosstalk and Endometrial Receptivity** 97
Nalini Mahajan, Anshu Dhar
Implantation 97; Factors Affecting Implantation 101

SECTION 2: REPRODUCTIVE ENDOCRINOLOGY

8. **Synthesis and Metabolism of Steroid Hormones** 107
R Suchindra
Steroid Hormone Synthesis 107; Steroids and Pathophysiology 111

9. **Puberty and Aberrations** 115
Pratibha Saran Malik
Hypothalamic–Pituitary–Gonadal Axis 115; Menstrual Cycle: A Recap of Events 116; Onset of Puberty:
Neuroendocrine Control 117; Genetic Factors Controlling Pubertal Onset 117; Nutritional Factors Determining
Onset of Puberty 118; Stages of Pubertal Development 118; Normal Variants of Puberty 120; Disorders of
Puberty 120; Growth Problems in Normal Adolescents 126

10. Amenorrhea ... 130

Abha Majumdar, Neeti Tiwari

Physiology of Menstruation 130; Classification of Amenorrhea (According to the Etiology List of Conditions) 130; Evaluation of Amenorrhea 131; History and Examination 131; Investigations for Primary and Secondary Amenorrhea 133; Evaluation of Specific Conditions in Amenorrhea 134; Management of Amenorrhea 135; Management of End-organ Disorders 136; Management of Polycystic Ovarian Syndrome with Amenorrhea 137; Management of Gonadal Agenesis and Dysgenesis 137; Management of Premature Ovarian Failure 138; Management of Hypogonadotropic Hypogonadism 138

11. Endocrine Disorders Affecting Reproduction ... 140

Chaitra Narayan Nayak

Hypothalamus–Pituitary Unit 140; Epidemiology 141; Other Disorders of Pituitary 142; Thyroid and Reproduction 143; Thyroid and Subfertility 145; Thyroid and Pregnancy 146; Adrenal Disorders 146 Endocrine-disrupting Compounds 148

12. Hirsutism ... 149

Anjali Sharma

Normal Development and Regulation of Growth 149; Diagnosis of Hirsutism 150; Etiology of Hirsutism 150; Investigations and Management 152; Treatment and Management 152; Follow-up 154

13. Luteal Phase Defect ... 156

Deepti Sharma

Definition 156; Incidence and Prevalence 156; Physiology of Luteal Phase 156; Pathophysiology of Luteal Phase Defect in Natural Cycles 158; Pathophysiology of Luteal Phase Defect in Controlled Ovarian Stimulation Cycles 158; Diagnosis of Luteal Phase Defect 159; Color Doppler in Luteal Phase Defect 160; Treatment of Luteal Phase Defect 160; In Natural Cycles 162; In Intrauterine Insemination Cycles 162; In Controlled Ovarian Stimulation Cycles 162; In Frozen Embryo Transfer Cycles and Donor–Recipient Cycles 162

14. Anovulation ... 167

Ashwini Sidhmalswamy G

Classification 167; Etiopathogenesis 167; Diagnosis 169; Treatment 170

15. Declining Fertility ... 176

Mahesh Koregol, Soumya Mahesh Koregol, Navya N

Total Fertility Rate Trends 176; The Indian Scenario 176; Major Causes of Fertility Decline: Short Term and Long Term 176; Education—"The Most Effective Contraception" 176; Working Women and the Myth of "Having it All" 177; Economy—"Money Makes Many Things"—Does it Hold True for Having Children 177; Changing Relationship Dynamics—it is Simply Complicated 177; Is Assisted Reproductive Technology Genetically Affecting Human Fecundity? Lessons from the Cattle Industry 177; Decline in Male Fertility 178; Role of Fertility Specialists: Increase Awareness and Optimize Natural Fertility 178

SECTION 3: COMBINED TOPICS

16. Evaluation of Infertility ... 183

Dipti Das, Kamini A Rao

Diagnosis of Infertility (Male) 183; Hormonal Evaluation 188; Extended Semen Analysis 189; Recommendations 191; Diagnosis of Infertility (Female) 191

17. Immunology and Infertility ... 201

Tity Chacko, Anupama Patil

Immune System 201; Exploring Treatment Options for Tackling Fetal Rejection 201; Harms and Benefits of Immunotherapy 203

18. Cytogenetics and Subfertility ... 206

CV Kannaki Uthraraj, KS Mangayarkarasi

Role of Genetics in Infertility 206; Basics of Cytogenetics 206; Specific Indications for Cytogenetic Studies in a Subfertile Couple 210; Numerical Abnormalities/Aneuploidies 211; Structural Anomalies of Chromosomes 216

19. Obesity and Infertility 221

Nupur Garg

Obesity and Impaired Reproductive Potential *221*; Fertility Risks in Obesity *221*; Diagnosis and Classification of Obesity *222*; Concept of Normal-weight Obesity *223*; Pathophysiology of Obesity *223*; Role of Gut Microbiome in Origin of Obesity *223*; Endocrine Function of Adipose Tissue—the Role of Adipokines *224*; Obesity and Polycystic Ovary Syndrome *226*; Obesity and Assisted Conception *226*; Response to Gonadotropin Stimulation and Cycle Cancellation *227*; Obesity and Male Infertility *228*; Role of Pre- and Probiotics *231*; Matching Weight-loss Medication to a Patient's Profile *231*; Bariatric Surgery *232*; Obesity and Ethical Dilemmas *233*; Transgenerational Effects *233*; Nutrigenomics *233*

20. Unexplained Infertility 239

Abha Bhat

Incidence *239*; Causes *239*; Unexplained Male Infertility *239*; Female Infertility *241*; Investigations of the Male Partner *243*; Investigations of the Female Partner *243*; Management *245*

21. Fertility Preservation 250

Sonia Malik, Aneesha Grover

Indications of Fertility Preservation *250*; Fertility preservation in Women *250*; Fertility Preservation in Males *251*; Model of Care for Patients Seeking Fertility Preservation *254*; Criteria for Selection of Patients Who can be Offered Fertility Preservation *254*; Interventions for Fertility Preservation *254*; Emerging Technologies *258*; Posthumous Reproduction *261*; Recommendations for Fertility Preservation *264*

22. Counseling in Infertility 270

Prathap Tharyan, Sudeepa Chaparala

Infertility is a Global Problem *270*; Infertility, and its Treatment, is Associated with Considerable Distress *270*; Counseling in Infertility and Assisted Reproductive Technology *271*; Negative Counseling *276*

23. Assisted Reproductive Technology in Patients with Chronic Medical Disorders 278

Anuradha Kumari, Devi R

Preconception Counseling *278*; Assisted Reproduction in Patients at Risk of Thrombosis *278*; Autoimmunity and In Vitro Fertilization *281*; Systemic Lupus Erythematosus *281*; Antiphospholipid Antibody Syndrome *281*; Treatment Strategies to Preserve Fertility *282*; Impact of Assisted Reproduction Technique on Systemic Lupus Erythematosus and Antiphospholipid Syndrome *283*; Effect of Systemic Lupus Erythematosus and Antiphospholipid Syndrome on Pregnancy *283*; Preconception Counseling *283*; Management During In Vitro Fertilization *283*; Fertility and Assisted Reproductive Technology in Women with Chronic Kidney Disease and Renal Transplant Recipients *284*; Factors Affecting Fertility in Women with Chronic Kidney Disease *284*; Management of Infertility in Women with Chronic Kidney Disease *286*; IVF Management *286*; Maternal and Fetal Risks in Pregnancy *287*; Inflammatory Bowel Disease and Assisted Reproductive Technologies *287*; Background *287*; Impact of Inflammatory Bowel Disease on Fertility *287*; Effect of IBD on ART and Pregnancy *287*; Impact of Pregnancy on Inflammatory Bowel Disease *288*; Management During In Vitro Fertilization *288*; ART in Patient with Epilepsy *289*; Pathophysiology of Reproductive and Endocrine Dysfunction in Epilepsy *289*; Effect of Hormones on Epilepsy *289*; Effect of Epilepsy and Antiepileptic Drugs on In Vitro Fertilization *289*; Impact of Epilepsy and Antiepileptic Drugs on Pregnancy *289*; Preconception Counseling *290*; Management During Assisted Reproductive Technology *291*; Management in Early Pregnancy *291*; ART in Women with Hypertension *291*; Impact of Hypertension on In Vitro Fertilization Outcomes *291*; Impact of In Vitro Fertilization on Hypertension *291*; Pre IVF and Preconception Workup and Advice *292*; Antihypertensive Medications *292*; In Vitro Fertilization Management *292*; ART in Women with Diabetes Mellitus *293*; Diabetes and Fertility *293*; Impact of Diabetes on Assisted Reproductive Technology Outcomes *293*; Effect of IVF and Pregnancy on Diabetes *295*; Preconception Care and In Vitro Fertilization Management *295*

SECTION 4: MALE INFERTILITY

24. Etiopathogenesis of Male Infertility 305

Haritha Mannem, Sathya Balasubramanyam

Pretesticular Causes *306*; Testicular Causes *307*; Genetic Causes *308*; Inflammation *314*; Infections—Effect on the Male Reproductive Tract *314*; Reactive Oxygen Species *315*; Effects of Coronavirus Disease 2019 on Male Fertility *315*; Factors that Help in Prognosticating Male Infertility *316*

25. **Clinical and Endocrinological Evaluation of Infertile Male** 322
Radha Pandiyan, S Sowbarnika, D Ramesh Raja, N Pandiyan
Aim of Evaluation of the Infertile Male *322*; Principles of Management of the Male Partner *323*; Part I: Clinical Evaluation of Infertile Male *323*; Part II: Clinical Evaluation of Infertile Male *325*; Investigations for Male Infertility *326*; Genetics in Male Infertility *329*

26. **Sexual Dysfunction in Male Infertility** 332
Vasan SS, Fahim L Rajwate
Biological Basis of Male Sexual Response *332*; Nonconsummation of Marriage *333*; Ejaculatory Disturbances *334*; Vibratory Stimulation *337*; Erectile Dysfunction Introduction *339*; Key Recommendations *345*

27. **Ultrasound in Male Infertility** 350
Kuldeep Jain, Bharti Jain, Maansi Jain
Etiological Distribution *350*; Indications of Scrotal Ultrasound *350*; Clinical Applications *352*; Epididymal Diameters *354*; Scrotal Ultrasound in Varicocele *354*; Indications of Transrectal Ultrasound *355*

28. **Medical Management of Male Infertility** 359
Sonal Agarwal, Vinay Kumar
Medical Therapy *359*; Specific Therapy *359*; Nonspecific Treatment (Empirical Therapy) *368*; Effect on Male Infertility in COVID-19 Era *369*

29. **Azoospermia: Evaluation and Management** 374
Ameya Rangnath Sangle, Tarun Dilip Javali
Terminology *374*; Definition *374*; Classification of Azoospermia *374*; Clinical Classification of Azoospermia *374*; Evaluation of a Male Patient with Azoospermia *374*; Etiology of Azoospermia *376*

30. **Varicocele and Infertility** 385
Ameya Rangnath Sangle, Varun Huilgol, Tarun Dilip Javali
Etiology of Varicocele *385*; Pathogenesis *385*; Oxidative Stress *386*; Impairment of Spermatogenesis by Scrotal Hyperthermia *386*; Deoxyribonucleic Acid Damage and Apoptosis *386*; Clinical Grading *387*; Management *387*

31. **Spinal Cord Injuries and Male Infertility** 392
Yalavarthi Pavan Ganesh, Tarun Dilip Javali, Mahendra V Javali
Spinal Cord Injury *392*; Male Infertility Due to Spinal Cord Injuries *394*; Management of Couples with SCI-related Male Factor Infertility *400*

32. **Algorithms for Genetic Evaluation of Infertile Males** 406
Stacy Colaco, Deepak Modi
Practical Approach for Genetic Testing for Infertile Males and its Applications in Clinical Practice *406*; Multiple Morphological Abnormalities of the Sperm Flagella *409*

SECTION 5: FEMALE FACTOR INFERTILITY

33. **Uterine Factors in Infertility** 413
Mala Arora, Mahesh Koregol, Soumya Mahesh Koregol, Navya N
Congenital Uterine Anomalies *413*; Myomas *420*; Adenomyosis *426*; Endometrial Factors *429*; Asherman's Syndrome *432*; Genitourinary Tuberculosis *432*

34. **Tubal Factors in Infertility** 438
Pratap Kumar, Aswathy Kumaran
Causes for Tubal Subfertility *438*; Evaluation for the Tubal Factor Infertility—Guidelines and Recommendations *439*; Ultrasound Evaluation of Fallopian Tubes *440*; Tubal Assessment Tests *440*; Management of Tubal Infertility *443*; Management of Tubal Ectopic Pregnancy *447*

35. **Infections and Infertility** 450
Chandrika Kulkarni
Chlamydia *450*; Gonorrhea *451*; Nongonococcal–Nonchlamydial Infections *452*; Sexually Transmitted Viral Infections *456*

36. Tuberculosis and Infertility **463**
JB Sharma, Sona Dharmendra, Gowri Rapaka
History 463; Microbiology of Mycobacterium Tuberculosis 463; Epidemiology of Female Genital Tuberculosis 463; Pathogenesis 464; Pathogenesis of Infertility in Genital Tuberculosis 465; Diagnosis 466; Investigations 466; Treatment 468; Drug Treatment of Drug Sensitive FGTB 469; In Vitro Fertilization and Embryo Transfer in FGTB 469; New Tuberculosis Research 470

37. Sonoendocrinology and Cycle Monitoring-Assisted Reproduction Technology **474**
Sonal Panchal, Chaitanya Nagori
Imaging Modalities for Assessment of Reproductive System 474; Preovulatory Period 479; Estrogen Affects Endometrium 480; Secretory Phase Assessment 483; Correlation of Progesterone to Ultrasound Findings 484

38. Transvaginal Ultrasound and Doppler in Infertility **487**
Sonal Panchal, Chaitanya Nagori
Diagnosis of Abnormalities Causing Subfertility 487; Cycle Assessment 507

39. Polycystic Ovary Syndrome **518**
Gotte Jhansi, Vyshnavi A Rao
Diagnosis—Evolution of the Diagnostic Criteria 518; Prevalence 519; Polycystic Ovary Syndrome—Phenotypes 519; At the Peripheral Compartment (Skin and Adipose Tissue) 525; Clinical Presentation 530; Evaluation 532; Management 535; Summary of Evaluation and Management of PCOS 545; Adjuvants to Improve Metabolic and Reproductive Function 546; Polycystic Ovary Syndrome in Adolescents 548; Polycystic Ovary Syndrome and Pregnancy 550; Polycystic Ovary Syndrome and Menopause 551

40. Assessment of Ovarian Reserve **559**
Padma Rekha Jirge
Ovarian Reserve Tests 559; Biological Age 559; Basal Serum Follicle-stimulating Hormone 560; Serum Estradiol 560; Serum Inhibin B 560; Serum Anti-Müllerian Hormone 560; Dynamic Tests 561; Antral Follicle Count 561; Ovarian Volume 561; Ovarian Doppler Assessment 561; Ovarian Biopsy 561; Discussion 561

41. Endometriosis **565**
Nandita Palshetkar, Rohan Palshetkar, Erika Patel
Pathogenesis of Endometriosis 565; Pathogenesis of Endometriosis Causing Infertility 565; Clinical Features 567; Diagnosis of Endometriosis 567; Staging 568; Management Options 568; Treatment of Endometriosis Associated Infertility 572; Ovarian Endometrioma 574; Adolescent Endometriosis 575; Endometriosis and Cancer 576

42. Endoscopy in Infertility **580**
Nutan Jain, Tania G Singh, Vandana Jain, Shayari Jain
Equipment 580; Laparoscopic Surgery on Uterus Myomectomy 580; Laparoscopic Tubal Surgery 584; Endometriosis 591; Laparoscopic Ovarian Drilling 592; Laparoscopy Complications 593; Hysteroscopy 594; Hysteroscopic Myomectomy 594; Hysteroscopic Tubal Cannulation for Proximal Tubal Block 597; Hysteroscopy for Metroplasty 599; Intrauterine Adhesions (Asherman's Syndrome) 601; Hysteroscopy for Retained Fetal Bones 602

43. Reconstructive Surgeries Enhancing Fertility **605**
Yehia Shawki, Osama Shawki, Amr Wahba, Zakiya Ahmed
Reconstruction of Distorted Pelvic Anatomy 605; Endometriosis and Infertility 607; Reconstruction of Blocked Fallopian Tubes 607; Reconstruction of Distorted Uterine Cavity 609; Uterine Septum 609; Intrauterine Adhesions 611; Submucous Myomas 612; Endometrial Polyps 612; Multiple Choice Questions 613

SECTION 6: INTRAUTERINE INSEMINATION

44. Intrauterine Insemination **619**
Natchandra Chimote, Bindu Chimote
Indications for IUI Treatment 619; Contraindications 619; IUI in a Historical Perspective 620; Prognostic Factors Influencing IUI Success 634; Efficacy and Safety of Intrauterine Insemination and Assisted Reproductive Technology in Populations Serodiscordant for Human Immunodeficiency Virus 635; Future Developments 636

45. **Optimizing Success in Intrauterine Insemination** 643
Kamini A Rao, Jampana Pallavi
Patient Selection and Workup 643; Indications of Intrauterine Insemination 644; Patient Preparation 644; Monitoring of Intrauterine Insemination 645; Time and Number of Intrauterine Insemination 645; Site of Insemination 645; Semen 645; Abstinence Duration 645; Semen Parameters 646; DNA Fragmentation Index 646; Paternal Age 646; Collection to Intrauterine Insemination Time Interval 646; Semen Preparation Technique 646; Technique of Intrauterine Insemination 647; European Society of Human Reproduction and Embryology Capri Workshop 2009 648

SECTION 7: OVARIAN STIMULATION

46. **Drugs for Ovarian Stimulation** 653
Duru Shah, Sabahat Rasool
Oral Ovulogens 653

47. **Ovulation Induction and Ovarian Stimulation Protocols** 664
Rutvij Dalal, Sonal Agarwal
Ovulation Induction and Superovulation 664; Category of Patients Benefiting from Ovulation Induction 664; Physiology of Ovulation 665; Management Options for Ovulation Induction 666; Stimulation Protocols in ART 673; Individualizing Approach Toward Patient for COS 673; Individualization of Gonadotropin Preparation and Dosage 675; Different Protocols for Stimulation 676; Gonadotropin-releasing Hormone Agonist 676; Protocols for Agonist 677; Gonadotropin-releasing Hormone Antagonists 679; Protocol for Antagonist Protocol 679; GnRH Agonist Versus Antagonist 680; Trigger 680; Natural Cycle In Vitro Fertilization 681; Modified Natural Cycle In Vitro Fertilization 681; Mild In Vitro Fertilization 681; Kato Protocol 682; Controlled Ovarian Stimulation with Letrozole Supplementation (Cost-less Protocol) 682; Shanghai Protocol 683; Duplex Protocol 683; Ultralong Protocol for Endometriosis (ESHRE 2013 Guidelines) 683; Studies Done in COVID-19 Era 685

48. **Role of Adjuvants in Ovarian Stimulation** 690
Mirudhubashini Govindarajan, Ramya Jayaram
Adjuvants for Ovarian Stimulation in Poor Responders 690; Adjuvants for Hyper-responders 693; Adjuvants to Oral Ovulogens 693

49. **Gonadotropin-releasing Hormone Analogs** 696
Mamta Dighe
Endogenous Gonadotropin-releasing Hormone 696; Gonadotropin-releasing Hormone Agonists 696; Gonadotropin-releasing Hormone Antagonists 697; Clinical Uses of Gonadotropin-releasing Hormone Analogs 698

50. **Monitoring of Ovarian Stimulation** 704
Snehal Dhobale Kohale
Need for Monitoring 704; Methods of Monitoring 704; Stages of Monitoring 704; Choosing Methods of Monitoring 705; Abnormal Responses in Ovarian Stimulation 713; Hormonal Monitoring of Ovarian Stimulation 714

51. **Ovulation Trigger** 721
Vyshnavi A Rao, K Aruna Saradha
Ovulation Trigger 722; Luteal Coasting 727; Freezing of Embryos 727; Predictors of Success after Gonadotropin-releasing Hormone Agonist Trigger 728; Ovarian Hyperstimulation Syndrome in Gonadotropin-releasing Hormone Agonist Trigger 728; Ovulatory Trigger in Breast Cancer Patients 730

52. **Individualized Controlled Ovarian Stimulation** 733
Richa Sharma, Anindita Thakker
Basics 733; Prognostic Factors for Ovarian Response and Protocol Recommended 734; Role of Luteinizing Hormone and Receptor Polymorphism 734; Role of AMH, AFC, and Other Biomarkers in Individualized COS 736; Individualized Controlled Ovarian Stimulation and Different Stimulation Protocols 736; Low Prognosis Groups—POSEIDON (Patient-oriented Strategy Encompassing Individualized Oocyte Number) Classification 738; Role of Luteinizing Hormone 739; Individualization for Time Constraint 739; Individualization for Necessity of Low Estrogen 739

53. In Vitro Fertilization Lite **742**
Adrija Kumar Datta, Stuart Campbell, Geeta Nargund, Anuradha Kumari
What is "In Vitro Fertilization Lite"? 742; Evolution of Ovarian Stimulation—Resurgence of Natural or Mild IVF 742; Why Adopt a Milder Approach? 743; When do We Consider Using a Mild Ovarian Stimulation Protocol? 745; What are the Limiting Factors in MS-IVF? 745; Future Prospects 746

54. Role of Luteinizing Hormone in Ovarian Stimulation **750**
Nivedita Shetty, Shraddha Pol
Physiology of the Role of LH in Folliculogenesis 750

55. Anesthesia in Assisted Reproductive Techniques **757**
Dorothy Dessa, Ravi Kumar IR
Anesthetic Considerations 757; Ideal Features of the Anesthetic Technique for the Procedure of In Vitro Fertilization 757; General Considerations 757; Anesthesia Techniques—Options Available to the Anesthetist 758; Conscious Sedation 758; Anesthesia in Embryo Transfer 759; Anesthesia for Surgical Sperm Retrieval 759; Analgesia for Hysterosalpingography 760; General Anesthesia 760; Regional Anesthesia 760; Key Drugs, Dosage and Side Effect 761

56. Oocyte Retrieval **765**
Sankalp Singh, Nivedita Ananth, Swati Singh, Mohammed Ashraf C
History 765; Vaginal Preparation Before Oocyte Retrieval 765; Role of Prophylactic Antibiotics 766; Anesthesia and Oocyte Retrieval 766; Instruments for Oocyte Retrieval 766; Aspiration Setup 767; Troubleshooting in Oocyte Retrieval 769; Role of Follicular Flushing 770; Oocyte Retrieval in Difficult Cases 770; Complications of Oocyte Retrieval 771

57. Embryo Transfer **774**
Arya Rajendran, Akanksha Gautam Allahbadia, Swati Gautam Allahbadia, Gautam Allahbadia
Definition of Embryo Transfer 774; Types of Embryo Transfer 774; How to Plan a Good Embryo Transfer? 775; Factors Affecting Success of Embryo Transfer 775; Embryo Transfer Catheters 778; Popular Commercially Available Embryo Transfer Catheters 779; Recent Advances 786

58. Troubleshooting in Assisted Reproductive Technology **792**
Harpreet Kaur, Mir Jaffar
Clinical Parameters 792; Laboratory Parameters 794; Strategies to Minimize Infection 795; Troubleshooting a Cryopreservation System 796; Troubleshooting Intracytoplasmic Sperm Injection Procedure 796

59. Luteal Phase Support **799**
Sonal Agarwal, Neha Tyagi, Kamini A Rao
Physiology 799; Luteal Phase Defect 800; Luteal Phase Support in ART: Why is it Needed? 800; Luteal Phase Support 800

SECTION 8: DILEMMA IN ART

60. Poor Responders **809**
Madhuri Milind Patil
Prediction of Poor Responders 810; Management of Poor Responders 812; Change in Protocol 815; Assisted Reproductive Technology Treatment Outcome According to POSEIDON Classification 820; Newer Treatment Modalities 820; Outcome after Assisted Reproductive Technology in Poor Responders 820

61. Recurrent Implantation Failure **829**
Divyashree PS
Definition of Recurrent Implantation Failure 829; Incidence 829; Implantation 830; Assumed Etiologies for Recurrent Implantation Failure 830; Investigations 833; Management 838

62. Empty Follicle Syndrome **855**
Ayesha Gupta, Kamini A Rao
Definition 855; Incidence 855; Classification of Empty Follicle Syndrome 855; Etiopathophysiology 856; Risk Factors for Empty Follicle Syndrome 857; Diagnosis and Prevention 858; Management of EFS in the Current Cycle 858; Management of Subsequent Cycles after Empty Follicle Syndrome 859; Prognosis 859

63. Role of Aneuploidy Screening in Preimplantation Embryos 861
Jwal Banker, Manish Banker, Parul Arora
Origin of Aneuploidy *861*; Proposed Indications for PGT-A *861*; Counseling *862*; Techniques and Limitations *862*; Different Methods for Chromosomal Analysis *863*; Results of Aneuploidy Screening in Various Patient Groups *867*; Concerns with Preimplantation Genetic Testing *869*; Preimplantation Genetic Testing as Universal Screening *869*; Legal Aspects and Regulations with Preimplantation Genetic Testing *871*

64. Preimplantation Genetic Testing of Embryos...... 876
Rohit Gutgutia, Santosh Kumar Jena
Preimplantation Genetic Testing for Aneuploidy *876*; Pre-preimplantation Genetic Testing for Aneuploidy Workup and Counseling *876*; In Vitro Fertilization Cycle *877*; Embryo Biopsy and Tubing *877*; Genetic Analysis *877*; Comparative Genomic Hybridization *877*; Array Comparative Genomic Hybridization *878*; Single Nucleotide Polymorphism Microarrays *878*; Next-generation Sequencing *878*; Interpretation of Result *878*; Mosaic Embryos *878*; Management of Mosaic Embryos *878*; Segmental Aneuploidy *878*; Limitations of Preimplantation Genetic Testing for Aneuploidy Testing *879*; Adverse Effects of Biopsy *879*; Difficult Situations in Preimplantation Genetic Testing *879*; Preimplantation Genetic Testing for Monogenic Disorders or Single Gene Disorders *879*; Indication of Preimplantation Genetic Testing for Monogenic Disorders or Single Gene Disorders *879*; Pre-preimplantation Genetic Testing Work-up *879*; Genetic Analysis in Case of Preimplantation Genetic Testing for Monogenic Disorders or Single Gene Disorders *880*; Preimplantation Genetic Testing for Structural Chromosomal Rearrangements *880*; Human Leukocyte Antigen Typing *880*; Mitochondrial DNA Quantification in Preimplantation Genetic Testing *880*; Noninvasive Preimplantation Genetic Testing *880*; Basis of Noninvasive Preimplantation Genetic Testing *880*; Limitation of Noninvasive Preimplantation Genetic Testing *881*; Current Status of Noninvasive Preimplantation Genetic Testing *881*; Future Perspective *881*

65. Epigenetics and Assisted Reproductive Technology 883
Mandeep Kaur, Ajitabh Shukla
Epigenetics *883*; Genomic Imprinting *884*; Human Phenotypes Associated with Imprinted Genes *884*; Epigenetics in Fetal Origin of Adult Disease *884*; When did the Concern Start? *885*; What is the Most Crucial Period for Imprinting? *885*; Potential Risks in Assisted Reproductive Technology *885*; Specific Imprinting Disorders *886*; Global Imprinting Disorders *887*; What is the Evidence of Association? *887*; Prevention *887*; Imprinting and Assisted Reproductive Technology: Future Considerations *887*; Other Epigenetic Issues *888*

SECTION 9: COMPLICATIONS IN ART

66. Ovarian Hyperstimulation Syndrome...... 893
Surbhi Gupta, Divyashree PS
Classification *893*; Etiology and Pathophysiology *893*; Risk Factors for Ovarian Hyperstimulation Syndrome *898*; Clinical Features *898*; Prevention *899*; Experimental Methods *904*; Management *904*

67. Ectopic Pregnancy 913
Rishma Dhillon Pai, Hrishikesh Pai, Nidhi Shah Gandhi, Navina Singh
Definition *913*; Heterotopic Pregnancy *913*; History of Ectopic Pregnancy *913*; Incidence *913*; Common Sites for Ectopic Pregnancy *913*; Risk Factors *913*; Clinical Features *914*; Diagnosis *914*; Tubal Pregnancy *916*; Nontubal Ectopic Pregnancy *917*; Cesarean Scar Pregnancy *917*; Interstitial Pregnancy *917*; Cornual Pregnancy *917*; Ovarian Pregnancy *918*; Abdominal Pregnancy *918*; Heterotopic Pregnancy *918*; Laparoscopy *919*; Primordial and Primary Prevention of Ectopic Pregnancy During In Vitro Fertilization *919*; Management of Tubal Pregnancy *920*; Management of Nontubal Ectopic Pregnancy *923*; Post-treatment *924*; Long-term Fertility Prospects Following an Ectopic Pregnancy (Royal College of Obstetricians and Gynaecologists, 2016) *924*; Counseling and Psychological Support *924*

68. Multiple-order Births 926
Veronica Irene Yuel
Incidence *926*; Etiology *926*; Pathophysiology *927*; Pathogenesis *928*; Clinical Features *928*; Diagnosis *930*; Complications *931*; Treatment *931*

SECTION 10: THIRD PARTY REPRODUCTION

69. **Oocyte and Sperm Donation** 937

Jaideep Malhotra, Ashwini Mohandas, Narendra Malhotra, Neharika Malhotra

Oocyte Donation *938*; Legalities Pertaining Oocyte Donation as per Assisted Reproductive Technology (Regulation) Act, 2021 *939*; Important Points Regarding Oocyte Donation in the ART Act *940*; Evaluation *941*; Counseling *942*; Sex-selective Assisted Reproductive Technology Practice *943*; Stimulation Protocols in Oocyte Donor In Vitro Fertilization Cycle *943*; Endometrial Preparation of Recipient *943*; Factors Predicting Success of a Donor Program *944*; Reproductive and Obstetric Outcomes *945*; Oocyte Banking *946*; Oocyte Sharing *947*; Oocyte Donor Programs for Stem Cell Research *947*; Remuneration *947*; Disclosure and Counseling *948*; Ethical Concerns Regarding Oocyte Donation *948*; Offenses and their Implications *948*; Sperm Donation *949*; Three-parent Assisted Reproductive Technology *950*

70. **Surrogacy in Assisted Reproductive Technology** 954

Nayana H Patel, Yuvraj D Jadeja, Harsha K Bhadarka, Niket H Patel, Molina N Patel, Harmi Thakkar

What is Surrogacy? *954*; History *954*; Types of Surrogacy *954*; Who Needs Surrogacy? the Indications *954*; Steps Involved in the Surrogacy Process *955*; Risks Associated with Surrogacy *958*; Various Aspects and Concerns Involved in Surrogacy *958*; Surrogacy Legislation: The International Scenario *958*; Surrogacy in India and Guidelines for Surrogacy *959*

71. **Assisted Reproductive Technology Guidelines** 962

(Brig.) RK Sharma

ART Clinic and Bank: Minimal Physical Requirements *963*; ART: Clinics and Banks Classifications as per the Assisted Reproductive Technology (Regulation) Bill, 2021 *964*; ART Team: Essential Qualifications as per the Assisted Reproductive Technology (Regulation) Bill, 2021 *964*; Artificial Insemination with Donor Semen *965*; Oocyte Donation or Embryo Donation *966*; Key Highlights of the Assisted Reproductive Technology (Regulation) Bill, 2021 *966*; Other Duties of Assisted Reproductive Technology Clinic *967*; Need for Assisted Reproductive Technology (Regulation) Bill, 2021 *967*; Concern for Assisted Reproductive Technology (Regulation) Bill, 2021 *967*; Evolution in Surrogacy Law—Legal Insights *968*; Types of Surrogacy *968*; Eligibility Criteria for Couples Intending Surrogacy *969*; Eligibility Criteria for a Surrogate Mother *969*; Abortion During Surrogate Pregnancy *969*; Offenses and Penalties Related to Surrogacy in India *969*; Circumstances for Opting Surrogacy *969*; Analysis of Key Points of Surrogacy (Regulation) Rules, 2022 *969*; Infertility—a Taboo *970*; Assisted Reproductive Technology Bank *971*

72. **Adoption** 973

Himanshu Singhal, Anubhuti Patel

Definition *973*; Types of Adoption *974*; Rules and Regulations of Adoption in India *975*; Pediatrician's Role *977*; Postadoption Family Concerns *977*

73. **LGBTQ and Fertility** 980

Utpala Sen, Gautam Khastgir

Transgender People *981*; Lesbians *982*; Gay Couples *982*; Scenario in India *983*; Support Groups *983*

74. **Transgender Population and Fertility** 986

HK Nagaraj, Arjun N

Gender Affirmation Surgery *986*; Complications of Gender Affirmation Surgery *989*; Fertility Preservation *991*

SECTION 11: OUTCOME FOLLOWING ASSISTED REPRODUCTIVE TECHNIQUE

75. **Maternal and Fetal Outcomes Following Assisted Reproductive Technique** 995

Navya V, Amit J Upadhyay, Kamini A Rao

Possible Causes of Adverse Outcomes at Various Levels *995*; Adverse Obstetric and Perinatal Outcome in Couples with Delay in Time to Pregnancy but without any Treatment *995*; Multiple Pregnancy and Adverse Obstetrical and Perinatal Outcomes *996*; Preterm Delivery *996*; Low Birth Weight *997*; Perinatal Mortality *997*; Other Obstetrical Outcomes *997*; Congenital Anomalies *998*; Chromosomal Disorders *998*; Imprinting Disorders *998*; Preimplantation Genetic Screening *998*; Blastocyst Culture *998*; Fresh Versus Frozen *999*;

Vitrification Versus Slow Freezing *999*; Assisted Hatching *999*; In Vitro Maturation *999*; Long-term Consequences in Assisted Reproductive Technique Born Children *999*; Other Maternal Factors Which Influence the Outcome *999*; Intracytoplasmic Sperm Injection with Ejaculated Versus Nonejaculated Sperm *1000*

76. Early Pregnancy Scan **1004**
Srividhya GK
Normal Sonoembryology *1004*; First-trimester Ultrasound: Normal Landmarks *1005*; Multiple Pregnancy *1010*; First-trimester Complications *1011*; Ectopic Pregnancy *1013*; Heterotopic Pregnancy *1015*; Molar Pregnancy *1015*; Risk Factors for Early Pregnancy Failure *1015*

77. Recurrent Pregnancy Loss: From Diagnostic Dilemmas to Clinical Decisions **1019**
Smitha AP, Sushma Baxi, Sushma Madhuprakash
Defining Pregnancy Loss and Recurrent Pregnancy Loss *1019*; Tip of the Iceberg *1019*; Immunological Milieu in Recurrent Pregnancy Loss *1020*; Natural Killer Cells: Friend or Foe? *1020*; Plasticity of Regulatory T and T Helper 17 Cells *1021*; Interventions in Recurrent Pregnancy Loss *1022*; Tumor Necrosis Factor-alpha Antagonists *1023*; Recent Advances *1024*; Strong Practice Recommendations in Recurrent Pregnancy Loss *1024*

SECTION 12: RECENT ADVANCES

78. Bioengineered Human Endometrium In Vitro **1027**
Satish Patki, Ujjwala Patki, Shweta Patki
Indications of the Culture of Endometrium *1027*; Contraindications *1028*; Three-dimensional Culture System *1028*; Complications *1030*; Study of Window of Implantation on Bioengineered Endometrium *1030*; Limitations of the Present Study and Future Research *1031*

79. Recent Trends in Assisted Reproductive Technique **1033**
Arya Rajendran, Baiju Pookilath
Assisted Reproductive Technique During COVID-19 Pandemic *1033*; Assisted Reproductive Technique and COVID-19 Vaccination *1035*; Newer Diagnostic Modalities in Assisted Reproductive Technique *1035*; Recent Trends in Medical Management in Assisted Reproductive Technique *1038*; Newer Trends in Controlled Ovarian Stimulation *1047*; Advances in Embryology Laboratory Techniques *1048*

80. Uterine Transplantation: Research, Techniques, and Results **1055**
Mats Brännström, Jana EJ Pittman
Animal Research in Uterus Transplantation *1055*; Surgical Techniques in Human Uterus Transplantation *1057*; Results of the only Completed Human Uterus Transplantation Trial *1059*; Results of Uncompleted Studies and Single Cases of Uterus Transplantation *1060*; Live Births after Uterus Transplantation *1062*

81. Ovarian Transplant **1065**
Pravin Mhatre, Jyoti Mhatre
History of Ovarian Transplant *1065*; Animal Experiments *1067*; Human Experiments *1068*; Indications for Ovarian Transplant *1068*; Problems Associated with Ovarian Transplant *1068*; Ovarian Vasculature *1069*; Site of Ovarian Transplantation *1069*; The Solutions *1071*; Journey to the First Transplant *1073*; Government Permission *1073*

82. Novel Ways of Creating Vagina **1075**
Pravin Mhatre, Jyoti Mhatre
Development of Müllerian Duct *1075*; Clinical Presentation *1075*; Use of Peritoneum in Neovaginal Lining *1076*; Procedure *1076*; Research Hypothesis *1078*; Immunohistochemistry *1081*; Role of Stemness Markers and Translational Genes in Creating Neovagina *1089*

83. Genitoplasty **1093**
Prashant Puranik
Embryonal Basis *1093*; Etiology of Vaginal Agenesis and Clinical Presentation *1093*; Differential Diagnosis *1094*; Diagnostic Methods *1095*; Psychological Aspects of Müllerian Aplasia *1096*; Management *1096*; Nonsurgical Creation of a Neovagina *1097*; Surgical Creation of a Neovagina *1097*; Functional Outcomes *1102*; Management of Infertility *1103*; Future Scope *1103*

84. **Endometrial Rejuvenation** 1106
Satish Patki, Shweta Patki, Surhud S Patki, Aditi M Kunte
Role of Endometrium in the Process of Implantation *1106*; Causes and Pathophysiology of Thin Endometrium *1107*; Principles of Endometrial Rejuvenation *1107*; Methods of Endometrial Rejuvenation *1107*

85. **Ovarian Rejuvenation** 1116
Manjunath C Swamy
What are Stem Cells? *1116*; Classification *1116*; Stem Cells "Niche" *1118*; Stem Cell-based Therapy for Female Infertility *1118*; Stem Cell Therapy for Endometrial Regeneration *1120*; Derivatives of Stem Cells: Explored for Regenerating Endometrium *1121*; In Vitro Activation of Ovary *1122*

SECTION 13: MISCELLANEOUS

86. **Batch In Vitro Fertilization** 1127
Sandhya Krishnan
Different Settings where Batch In Vitro Fertilization is Done *1127*; Preparation for a Batch In Vitro Fertilization *1128*; Preparation for a Batch In Vitro Fertilization: Laboratory Aspects *1132*

87. **Frozen Embryo Transfer** 1135
Hrishikesh Pai, Nandita Palshetkar, Rishma Dhillon Pai, Kinjal Shah, Rohan Palshetkar, Arnav Pai
Indications for a Frozen Embryo Transfer *1136*; Different Methods for Endometrial Preparation for Frozen Embryo Transfer *1136*; Ideal Duration of Progesterone Supplementation Before Embryo Transfer *1138*; To Briefly Understand the Technique of Cryopreservation *1139*; Fresh versus Frozen Embryo Transfer *1141*

88. **Evidence-based Practice in Reproductive Medicine** 1145
Parimala Chinta, Mohan S Kamath, Korula George
Controversial Areas in Practice *1145*

89. **Ethical, Legal, and Social Issues of Modern Assisted Reproductive Technology Practice** 1154
Petra De Sutter, Pankaj Talwar
Assisted Reproductive Technology (Regulation) Rules, 2022 *1154*; Surrogacy (Regulation) Rules, 2022 *1157*; Timeline of Assisted Reproductive Technology and Surrogacy Rules (2021–2022) *1157*; Ethical, Legal, and Social Issues *1159*

90. **Quality Management in Assisted Reproductive Techniques Laboratory** 1161
Surbhi Gupta, Divyashree PS
References for Quality Guidelines *1161*; Models for Quality Management *1162*; Components of Quality Control Program *1162*; Emergency Plan in In Vitro Fertilization Laboratory *1175*; Checklist in In Vitro Fertilization Laboratory *1177*; Benefits and Drawbacks of Quality Management System *1177*

91. **Auditing of Clinical Outcomes** 1180
Arati R Rao
Benefits of Audit *1180*; The Audit Cycle *1181*; Sections to be Audited *1181*; Setting Standards *1181*; Selecting Topics for Audit *1182*; In Vitro Fertilization Program Performance Indicators *1182*; Setting Objectives *1183*; Data Collection *1183*; Data Analysis *1183*; Writing an Audit Report *1183*; Recommendations for Change *1184*; Scope of the Audit *1184*; Audit Report *1184*

92. **Periconceptional Challenges and Modifiable Risk Factors: Evidence to Practice** 1185
Revathi S Rajan
Background *1185*; Oxidative Stress *1185*; Immune Regulation in Pregnancy *1185*; Micronutrients and Metabolic Factors *1188*; Post-IVF Pregnancies: Surveillance Patterns and Rationale *1189*; Role of Art/Third-party Reproduction and Preimplantation Genetic Testing for Aneuploidy in Cases with Recurrent Pregnancy Loss *1191*

93. **Emergencies in Infertility** 1193
Arunima Halder
Ovarian Hyperstimulation Syndrome *1193*; Adnexal Torsion *1196*; Emergencies During Oocyte Retrieval *1200*; Emergency after Embryo Transfer *1201*

94. Fetal Reduction 1207
Revathi S Rajan
Background *1207*; Medicolegal Issues and Psychological Impact *1207*; Procedure *1208*; Methods *1208*; Prerequisites *1208*; Technique *1209*; Other Methods *1209*; Failed Reduction *1210*; Selective Reduction *1210*; Studies on Fetal Reduction *1210*

95. COVID-19 and Pregnancy 1212
Varsha Patil, Chandana C
Etiology *1212*; Pathophysiology *1212*; Coronavirus Disease 2019 and Pregnancy *1212*; Clinical Presentation of Coronavirus Disease in Pregnancy *1213*; Effects of Coronavirus Disease on Pregnancy *1213*; Symptoms and Classification of Severity of Coronavirus Disease 2019 *1213*; Preventive Measures to be Taken by Pregnant Women to Avoid Coronavirus Disease 2019 *1213*; Indications for Coronavirus Disease 2019 Testing During Pregnancy *1213*; Computed Tomography Scan Findings of Coronavirus Disease 2019 *1214*; Antenatal Care *1214*; Triaging *1215*; Management of Mild or Asymptomatic Coronavirus Disease 2019 Infection During Pregnancy *1216*; Indications for Inpatient Management *1216*; Treatment of Moderate to Severe Coronavirus Disease 2019 Infection in Pregnancy *1216*; Management of Critically Ill and Severe Hypoxic Coronavirus Disease 2019 Pregnant Patients *1217*; Management of Coronavirus Disease 2019 Pregnant Women in Labor *1217*; Postnatal Care of Coronavirus Disease 2019 Patient *1217*; Use of Personal Protection Equipment in the Management of Suspected/Confirmed Patient of Coronavirus 19 Disease *1219*; How to use Personal Protective Equipment *1219*; Coronavirus Disease 2019 Vaccination in Pregnant Women and Lactating Women *1219*

96. Essentials of Statistics: A Clinician's Perspective 1221
Gautham T Pranesh
Data and its Types *1221*; Summarizing Data *1222*; Normal Distribution and its Properties *1222*; Statistical Tests and Their Application *1223*; Study Designs and Statistical Measures *1224*; Other Applications of Statistics in a Clinical Setting *1228*

VOLUME 2: LABORATORY ASPECTS OF IVF AND ANDROLOGY

SECTION 14: ANDROLOGY

97. Semen Analysis in 21st Century Medicine: A Paradigm Shift 1235
Fahim L Rajwate, Ashish S Reddy, Vasan SS
Semen Analysis *1235*; The American Urological Association Best Practice Policy and the American Society for Reproductive Medicine Practice Committee Report *1236*; The Probabilistic Nature of Human Fertility *1236*; Morphology of Spermatozoa *1237*

98. Sperm Function Tests 1242
Anupama Deenadayal Mettler, Roopini Sathiasai Kumar
Fructose Estimation *1242*; Indices for Abnormal Morphology Calculation *1243*; Tests for Reactive Oxygen Species *1243*; Leukocyte Detection Test *1244*; Sperm Vitality Tests *1244*; Sperm–Mucus Interaction Tests *1245*; Mitochondrial Activity Index Test *1246*; Test for Capacitation *1246*; Tests for Acrosome Reaction *1247*; Hyaluronan Binding Assay *1247*; Competitive Binding Assay *1248*; Sperm Penetration Assay *1248*; Nuclear Chromatin Decondensation Test *1248*; Sperm DNA Fragmentation Index *1248*; Biochemical Assay *1248*; Sperm Selection Using Artificial Intelligence *1250*

99. Selection of Sperm 1253
Muthukumar K
Sperm Selection for Intrauterine Insemination *1253*; Sperm Selection for Intracytoplasmic Sperm Injection *1254*

100. Sperm Chromatin Assessment 1261
Priya Kannan
Clinical Significance *1261*; Causes of Sperm DNA Damage *1262*; Assays for Detection of Sperm DNA Integrity *1262*; Drawback of Sperm DNA Testing *1264*; Clinical Guideline for Use of Sperm DNA Fragmentation *1264*

101. Advanced Sperm Preparation Techniques in Assisted Reproductive Technology 1267

Natchandra Chimote, Bindu Chimote

Simple Wash Method 1268; Migration-Based Techniques 1268; Tips to Maximize the Sperm Yield 1271; Magnetic-Activated Cell Sorting 1272; Glass Wool Filtration 1273; Glass Beads 1274; Sephadex Columns 1274; Transmembrane Migration 1274; Reduction of Semen Viscosity 1274; When to Use a Particular Sperm Preparation Technique 1275; Limitations of Conventional Sperm Preparation Techniques 1275; Advanced Strategies of Sperm Selection 1276; Zeta Potential 1278; Molecular Binding 1278; Hyaluronic Acid Binding 1280; PICSI Dish 1280; Hyaluronan-containing Medium 1280; Microfluidic Isolation of Motile Spermatozoa 1281; Sperm Selection Based on Guidance Mechanisms 1283; Future Development of Sperm Preparation Techniques 1284

102. Semen Banking 1291

Guruprasad Kalthur, Sandhya Kumari, Satish Kumar Adiga

History of Semen Banking 1291; Protocols 1291; Future Direction 1295

SECTION 15: EMBRYOLOGY

103. History of In Vitro Fertilization 1299

Neelima Gupta

History of In Vitro Fertilization 1300; Latest Developments in In Vitro Fertilization Technologies after 2009 1312; The Future 1313

104. In Vitro Fertilization and Embryo Transfer 1319

Alex C Varghese, Shrey Balani, Kannamannadiar Jayaprakasan

Importance of Total Quality 1319; In Vitro Fertilization Laboratory and Culture Systems 1319; Oocyte Abnormalities and Pregnancy Outcomes 1322; Effect of Ovarian Stimulation on Oocyte Quality 1323; Individualized or Patient-Tailored Stimulation Strategies 1323; Oocyte Retrieval 1325; In Vitro Fertilization versus Intracytoplasmic Sperm Injection Insemination 1326; Freeze All Strategy 1328; Embryo Transfer 1328; Training in OPU and ET by Simulators 1329; Artificial Intelligence and Automation 1330

105. Intracytoplasmic Sperm Injection 1334

Alex C Varghese, Kenichiro Hiraoka

Indications for Intracytoplasmic Sperm Injection 1334; Indications for Intracytoplasmic Sperm Injection with Surgically Retrieved Spermatozoa 1335; Location of Intracytoplasmic Sperm Injection Setup 1335; Intracytoplasmic Sperm Injection 1335; Conventional Insemination Versus Intracytoplasmic Sperm Injection 1343; Automation of Intracytoplasmic Sperm Injection 1344

106. Analysis of Fertilization 1351

Shailaja Gada Saxena, Ritu Gada, Dhiraj Gada

Morphological Evaluation of Gametes And Embryos 1351; Time-Lapse Imaging 1354; Metabolomics 1355; Preimplantation Genetic Diagnosis/Screening 1355

107. Morphological Assessment of Oocyte and Embryo 1358

Vijay Mangoli, Ranjana Mangoli

Oocyte 1358; Zygote 1363; Early Cleavage 1364; Cleavage Stage Embryos 1364; Morphological Assessment Using Morphokinetics 1367

108. Blastocyst Culture and Transfer 1370

Rajvi H Mehta, Mohammed Ashraf C, Mir Jaffar

Why Culture Embryos to the Blastocyst Stage In Vitro? 1370; Morphological Evaluation of Blastocysts 1371; Morphology of Poor-Quality Blastocysts 1372; Evaluation of Zygotes and Embryos and Their Potential to Develop Into Blastocysts 1373; Factors Influencing Blastocyst Development 1374; Hatching Phenomenon in a Blastocyst 1374; Cryopreservation of Blastocysts 1374; Advantages and Applications of Blastocyst Culture 1375; Limitations of Blastocyst Transfer 1375

109. Cryopreservation of Oocytes 1380

Goral Gandhi

Indications for Oocyte Freezing 1380; Hurdles Associated with Oocyte Cryopreservation 1380; Factors Affecting Oocyte Survival 1381; Vitrification 1381; Dynamics of Meiotic Spindles of Frozen-Thawed Oocytes 1383;

Time Schedule for Vitrification of Oocytes and Fertilization *1383*; Safety of Vitrification *1383*; Our Results with Oocyte Vitrification *1384*; Our Experience with Oocyte Vitrification *1384*; Immature Oocytes *1384*; Poor Morphology Oocytes *1385*

110. Embryo Cryopreservation 1387
Nitin Laxmikant Lad, Mir Jaffar
Cryoprotective Agents *1387*; Freezing or Slow Freezing *1389*; Vitrification *1389*; "Freeze-All" Strategy *1391*; Safety of Reproductive Cryopreservation *1391*

111. Viral Contamination Risk to Gametes and Embryos in Cryostorage during COVID-19 1393
Prathima Tholeti, Satish Kumar Adiga
SARS-CoV-2 and its Impact on Reproductive Cells *1393*; Fertility Preservation *1394*; Cross-contamination of Viruses in Liquid Nitrogen Cryotanks *1394*; Risk Mitigation Strategies and Safety During Cryostorage *1395*; Cryosystems and Carrier Devices *1395*; Liquid Nitrogen Sterilization *1395*; Washing Procedures to Eliminate Pathogens *1395*; Safety issues *1396*

SECTION 16: ADVANCES IN ASSISTED REPRODUCTIVE TECHNOLOGIES

112. Assisted Hatching in Assisted Reproductive Technology 1401
Gaurav Majumdar
Causes for Impaired Hatching *1401*; Assisted Hatching: Plausible Mechanisms *1401*; Pitfalls of Assisted Hatching *1404*; Patient Selection for Assisted Hatching *1405*; Medical Management *1405*

113. Preimplantation Genetic Screening and Diagnosis: Laboratory Aspects 1407
Krishna Chaitanya M, Durga G Rao, Sushma Baxi, Abhishek Shah
Terminology *1407*; Setting up a State of Assisted Reproductive Technology Laboratory And an Efficient Program for Preimplantation Genetic Screening/Preimplantation Genetic Diagnosis *1408*; Patient Management *1408*; History, Counseling, Consenting, and Documentation *1409*; In Vitro Fertilization Stimulation Protocols *1409*; Choice of Assisted Reproductive Technology for Preimplantation Genetic Screening/Preimplantation Genetic Diagnosis *1409*; Ideal Stage for Embryo Biopsy *1409*; Polar Body Biopsy *1409*; Cleavage Stage Biopsy—Blastomere Biopsy *1410*; Protocol for Embryo Biopsy and Tubing *1410*; Protocol—Blastomere Biopsy *1410*; Advantages of Cleavage Stage Biopsy *1411*; Limitations of Cleavage Stage Biopsy *1411*; Morula Stage Biopsy *1411*; Blastocyst Stage Biopsy *1411*; Protocol For Trophectoderm Biopsy *1411*; Tubing Protocol: Array and Single-Gene Disorders (Blastomere or Trophectoderm) *1412*; Advantages of Trophectoderm Biopsy *1413*; Limitations of Trophectoderm Biopsy *1413*; Noninvasive Methods for Embryo Biopsy *1413*; Cryopreservation of Embryos *1414*; Ideal Platform for Genetic Screening *1414*; Fluorescence In Situ Hybridization *1414*; Errors with Preimplantation Genetic Screening Techniques *1415*; Embryo Transfer *1416*; Follow-up of Pregnancies *1416*; Quality Control and Quality Assurance: Outcome Measures *1416*; Effectiveness and Efficacy of Preimplantation Genetic Screening in the Field of Assisted Reproductive Technology *1417*

114. In Vitro Maturation of Oocytes: A Practical Approach 1420
Varsha Samson Roy
Oocyte Maturation In Vivo *1420*; Advantages and Indications for In Vitro Maturation *1421*; Clinical Aspects of In Vitro Maturation *1421*; In Vitro Maturation Aspiration *1422*; Oocyte Identification *1423*; In Vitro Maturation Culture *1423*; Assessment of Oocyte Maturity *1424*; Fertilization of In Vitro Maturation Oocytes *1424*; Embryo Development *1424*; Protein Synthesis *1424*; Pregnancy Rates with In Vitro Maturation *1425*; Safety of In Vitro Maturation *1425*

115. Ovarian Tissue Cryopreservation and its Eventual Transplantation: Is it Proficient Fertility Preservation Program? 1429
Pankaj Talwar, Pooja Awasthi

116. Polarization Microscopy and its Clinical Applications 1432
Taswin Kaur, Mir Jaffar
Principle *1432*; Device *1433*; Functions of Polarizing Microscope *1434*; Application of Polarizing Microscope *1434*

117. OMICS in Assisted Reproductive Technology 1440
Syed Waseem Andrabi, Nivita Gugnani
Genomic Analysis *1441*; Transcriptomics *1442*; Proteomics *1443*; Metabolomics *1443*

118. **Intracytoplasmic Morphologically Selected Sperm Injection, Physiological Intracytoplasmic Sperm Injection, and its Clinical Significance** 1447

Mohammed Ashraf C

Intracytoplasmic Morphologically Selected Sperm Injection *1448*; Physiological Intracytoplasmic Sperm Injection *1452*; Physiological Intracytoplasmic Morphologically Selected Sperm Injection *1452*

119. **Microfluidics in Assisted Reproductive Technology** 1455

José María de los Santos, Thamara Viloria, Ana Cobo, Josep Lluís Romero, Marcos Meseguer

Manufacturing Microfluidic Devices *1456*; Sperm Isolation *1456*; Oocytes Denudation *1457*; In Vitro Fertilization *1457*; Embryo Culture *1459*; Integrated Platforms *1461*; Microfluidics for Automated Vitrification *1463*

120. **Artificial Intelligence in Assisted Reproductive Technology** 1466

Krishna Chaitanya M, Durga G Rao, Ruchi Narula, Selva Karthick M, Sherin Theresa Mathew

Artificial Intelligence Architecture and Tools Used in Assisted Reproductive Technology *1466*; Why do We Need a Machine Touch? *1467*; Recent Advances of Artificial Intelligence in In Vitro Fertilization and Assisted Reproductive Technology *1468*; Currently Available Tools and Applications *1474*; Lab on a Cloud *1475*; Possible Limitations *1475*; Future Aspects *1476*

SECTION 17: LABORATORY MANAGEMENT

121. **Setting-up an ART Laboratory** 1481

R Suchindra, Anuja Kamath

Layout of an Art Laboratory *1481*; Infrastructure for New Laboratory Set-Up *1482*

122. **Quality Control in IVF Laboratory** 1488

Sanjay Shukla

What is Quality? *1488*; Quality Management *1488*; Quality Control *1489*; Disaster Management *1491*

123. **Embryo Culture Systems** 1494

Goral Gandhi

Culture Media *1494*; Media Systems *1496*; Culture Conditions *1497*; Media Storage and Equilibration *1497*; Incubators *1497*; Air Purification Unit *1498*; Quality Control *1498*; Epigenetic Changes *1498*; Multiple Choice Questions *1499*

124. **Micromanipulators** 1502

Mir Jaffar, Syed Waseem Andrabi, Veena Gangaraju, Mohammed Ashraf C

Micromanipulator *1502*

125. **Troubleshooting in the In Vitro Fertilization Laboratory: Challenging Case Scenarios** 1510

Varsha Samson Roy, Sangita Sharma

Laboratory Quality Management Program *1510*; Equipment *1511*; Air Quality and Culture Conditions *1511*; Disposables and Media *1511*; Operator Skills *1511*; Procedural Aspects *1511*; Patient Factors *1512*; Clinical Aspects *1513*; Challenging Scenarios *1513*

126. **Quality Management in Assisted Reproductive Technology Clinics** 1522

Gautham T Pranesh

Principles of Quality Management *1522*; Developing a Quality Management System in Assisted Reproductive Technology Clinic *1522*; Maintaining Ongoing Compliance to a Quality Management System *1523*; Accreditation, Certification, and Licensing Requirements for Assisted Reproductive Technology Clinics *1524*; Key Elements of a Quality Management System *1524*; Guidelines for Good Practice in In Vitro Fertilization Laboratories *1525*

VOLUME 3: ATLAS OF HUMAN EMBRYOLOGY

127. **Oocyte Cumulus Complex Evaluation** 1533

Kamini A Rao, Divyashree PS

Mature Oocyte Corona Cumulus *1533*; Approximately Mature Oocyte Corona Cumulus *1534*; Immature Oocyte Corona Cumulus *1534*; Postmature Oocyte Corona Cumulus *1535*; Atretic Oocyte Corona Cumulus *1535*

128. Oocyte Nuclear Maturity Evaluation **1537**
Divyashree PS, Kamini A Rao, Anu Kottur
Metaphase II *1538*; Metaphase I *1538*; Germinal Vesicle Oocyte (40×) *1539*; Germinal Vesicle Oocyte (20×) *1539*; Oocytes in Different Stages of Maturation (FIG. 4) *1540*

129. Oocyte Dysmorphisms **1541**
Divyashree PS, Bezar Ghan VV, Kamini A Rao, Mohammed Ashraf C
Granular Cytoplasm *1541*; Vacuoles *1541*; Smooth Endoplasmic Reticulum Cluster *1545*; Refractile Bodies *1545*; Polar Body *1545*; Perivitelline Space *1545*; Zona Pellucida *1552*

130. The Sperm **1557**
Anitha S Kumari K, Dileep Kumar R, Hemanth Kumar MA, Mohammed Ashraf C
Sperm Count and Motility *1557*; Sperm Morphology *1558*; Globozoospermia (Acrosomal Agenesis) *1559*; Sperm Vitality *1560*; Deoxyribonucleic Acid Fragmentation Index *1562*

131. Normal Embryo Development **1564**
Bezar Ghan VV, Divyashree PS, Kamini A Rao
Pronuclear Stage *1565*; Syngamy *1565*; Two-cell Stage *1566*; Four-cell Stage *1566*; Eight-cell Stage *1567*; Compaction *1567*; Early Blastocysts *1568*; Expanded Blastocysts *1568*; Hatching Blastocysts *1569*; Hatched Blastocysts *1569*

132. Embryo Scoring **1570**
Bezar Ghan VV, Divyashree PS, Anitha S Kumari K, Mohammed Ashraf C
Symmetrical Pronuclei *1570*; Nonsymmetrical Pronuclei *1572*; Abnormal Pronuclei *1573*; Two-Cell Grade 1 Embryos *1575*; Two-Cell Grade 2 Embryos *1576*; Four-Cell Grade 1 Embryos *1577*; Four-Cell Grade 2 Embryos *1578*; Four-Cell Grade 3 Embryos *1579*; Eight-Cell Grade 1 Embryos *1580*; Eight-Cell Grade 2 Embryos *1581*; Eight-Cell Grade 3 Embryos *1582*; Grade 1, Day 4 Embryos *1583*; Grade 2, Day 4 Embryos *1584*; Grade 3, Day 4 Embryos *1585*; Early Blastocyst *1586*; Blastocyst *1589*; Expanded Blastocyst *1590*; Hatching Blastocysts *1592*; Hatched Blastocysts *1593*; Morphology of Poor Quality Blastocysts *1594*; Trophoblast Vesicle *1594*; Necrotic Foci *1594*; Vacuoles *1595*; Cytoplasmic Strings *1596*

133. In Vitro Fertilization/Intracytoplasmic Sperm Injection **1597**
Bezar Ghan VV, Divyashree PS
Oocyte Insemination in In Vitro Fertilization *1597*; Intracytoplasmic Sperm Injection *1597*

134. Advanced Techniques **1605**
Anitha S Kumari K, Bezar Ghan VV, Divyashree PS, Dileep Kumar R, Anu Kottur, Kamini A Rao, Mohammed Ashraf C
Physiological Intracytoplasmic Sperm Injection *1605*; Physiological Intracytoplasmic Sperm Injection Dish *1606*; Intracytoplasmic Morphologically Selected Sperm Injection *1608*; Poloscopy *1610*; Principle of Poloscopy *1610*; Time-Lapse Imaging *1613*; 1 Pronuclei *1614*; 3 Pronucleus *1615*; Laser-Assisted Hatching *1618*; Magnetic-Activated Cell Sorting (MACS) of Human Spermatozoa *1621*

135. Cryopreservation **1623**
Bezar Ghan VV, Anitha S Kumari K, Divyashree PS, Mohammed Ashraf C
Cryopreservation of Oocytes *1623*; Cryopreservation of Embryos *1630*; Blastocyst Cryopreservation *1637*; Blastocyst Warming *1640*

136. Assisted Reproductive Technology Laboratory Setting **1645**
Divyashree PS, Hemanth Kumar MA, Dileep Kumar R, Mohammed Ashraf C
Essential Equipment of Assisted Reproductive Technology Laboratory *1645*; Laminar Flow Cabinets *1646*; Heating, Ventilating, and Air-Conditioning *1647*; Incubators *1648*; Microscopes *1649*; Essential Equipment for Clinical Procedures *1654*

137. Embryo Biopsy **1662**
Mohammed Ashraf C, Anuja Kamath
Blastomere Biopsy *1662*; Trophectoderm Biopsy *1663*

Index *1665*

CHAPTER

127 Oocyte Cumulus Complex Evaluation

Kamini A Rao, Divyashree PS

INTRODUCTION

Assessment of oocyte maturity will be difficult immediately after retrieval as it is surrounded by cumulus complex. Although it is not of much importance in intracytoplasmic sperm injection (ICSI), as the oocyte will be evaluated after denudation, evaluation of oocyte cumulus complex (OCC) for the oocyte maturity is important in conventional in vitro fertilization (IVF).

There are conflicting reports regarding correlation of OCC morphology and fertilization and pregnancy rates.[1-4]

Presently we know that evaluation of OCC is not enough to grade oocyte maturity, but we also have to accept that these supporting cells play a vital role in the development of the oocyte. Therefore, in those circumstances where direct evaluation of oocyte is not possible, OCC evaluation is a useful tool in selecting a mature oocyte.

According to Lin and collegues,[3] there are five groups of OCCs based on the morphology of oocyte cytoplasm, cumulus mass, corona cells, and membrane granulosa cells.

Figures 1 to 5 show the oocyte—corona cumulus evaluation.

MATURE OOCYTE CORONA CUMULUS (FIG. 1)

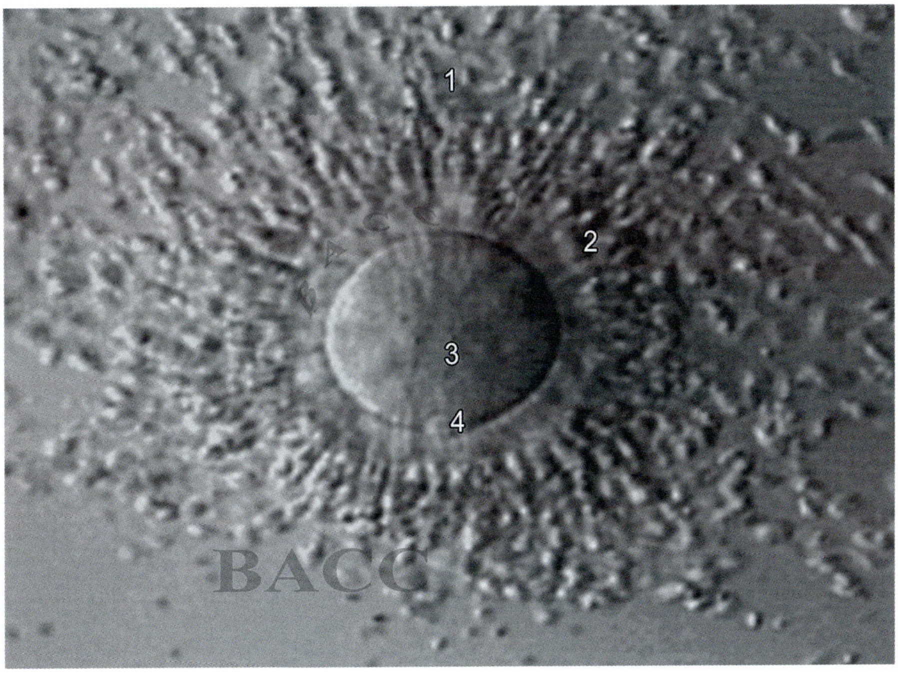

Fig. 1: (1) Expanded cumulus; (2) radiant corona; (3) clear cytoplasm; (4) first polar body.

APPROXIMATELY MATURE OOCYTE CORONA CUMULUS (FIG. 2)

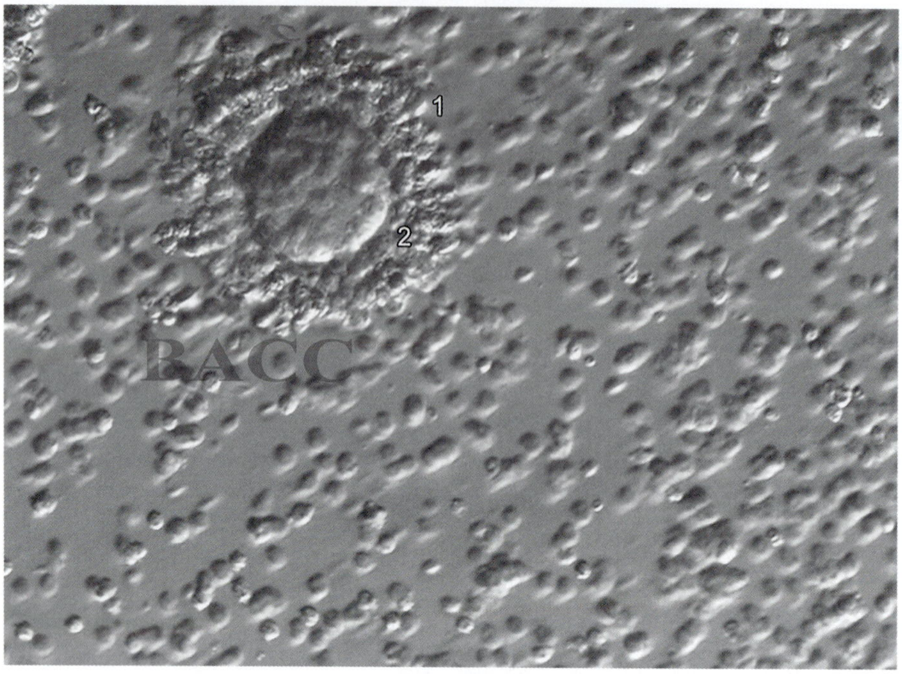

Fig. 2: (1) Expanded cumulus; (2) slightly compact corona.

IMMATURE OOCYTE CORONA CUMULUS (FIG. 3)

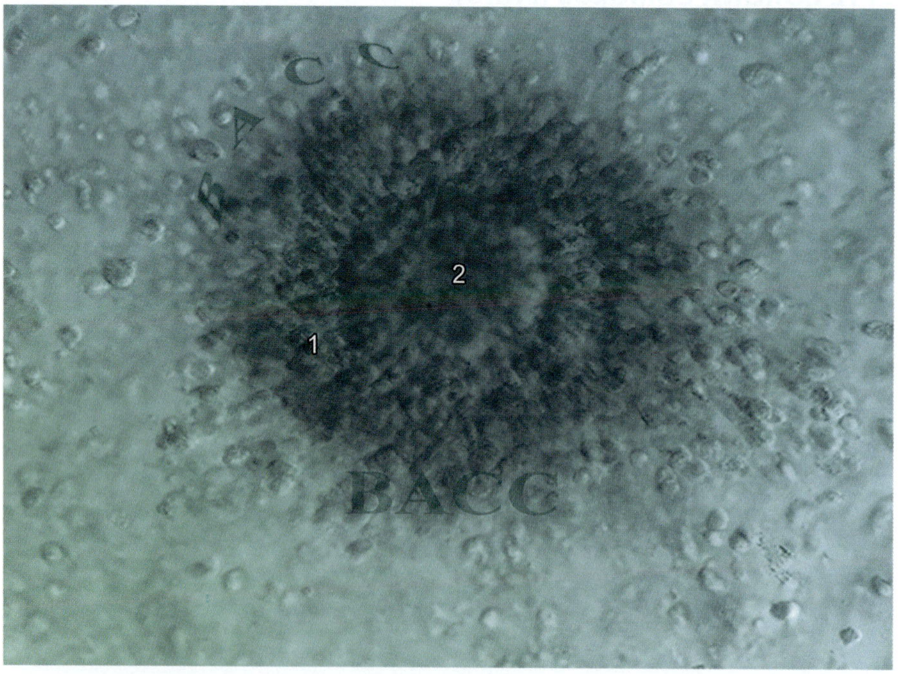

Fig. 3: (1) Adherent compact layer of corona; (2) ooplasm with germinal vesicle (Note: First polar body is not visible).

POSTMATURE OOCYTE CORONA CUMULUS (FIG. 4)

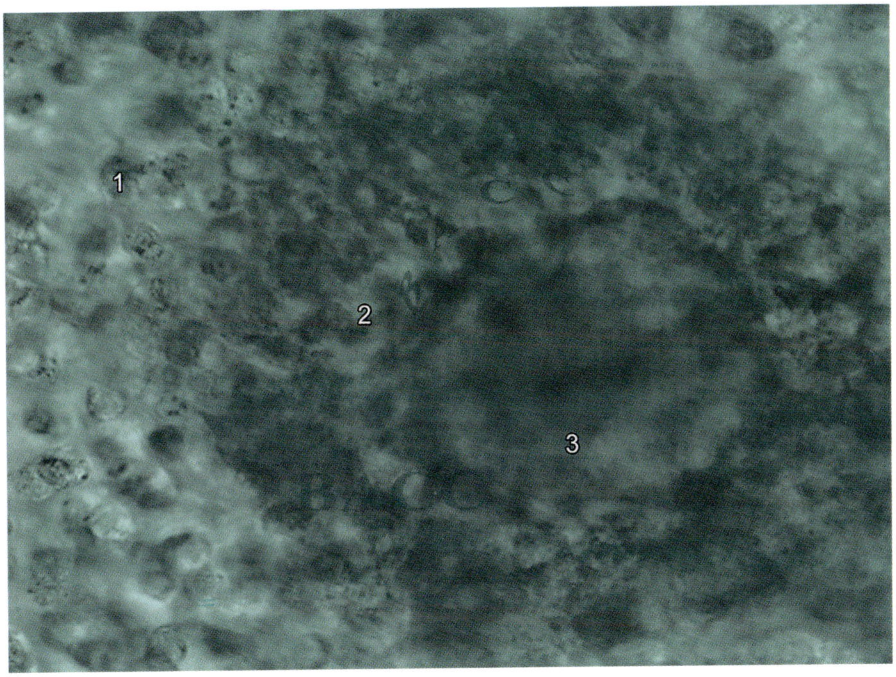

Fig. 4: (1) Expanded cumulus with clumps; (2) irregular, incomplete corona; (3) dark and granular cytoplasm.

ATRETIC OOCYTE CORONA CUMULUS (FIG. 5)

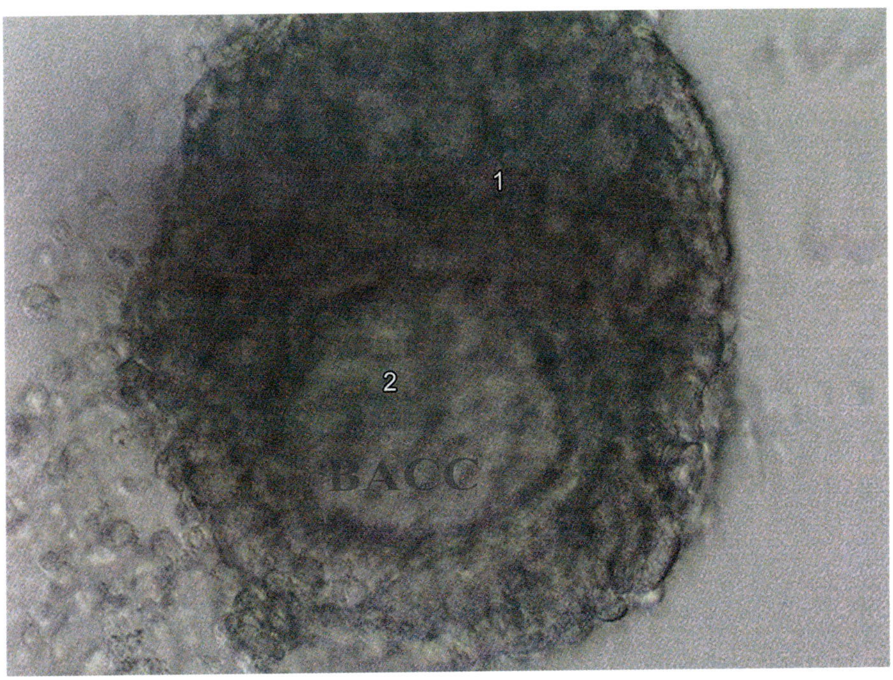

Fig. 5: (1) Clumped and very irregular corona; (2) dark and mishappen cytoplasm.

REFERENCES

1. Rattanachaiyanont M, Leader A, Leveille MC. Lack of correlation between oocyte-corona-cumulus complex morphology and nuclear maturity of oocytes collected in stimulated cycles for intracytoplasmic sperm injection. Fertil Steril. 1999;71:937-40.
2. Ebner T, Moser M, Shebl O, et al. Blood clots in the cumulus-oocyte complex predict poor oocyte quality and post-fertilization development. Reprod Biomed Online. 2008;16:801-7.
3. Ng ST, Chang TH, Wu Tc. Prediction of the rates of fertilization, cleavage, and pregnancy success by cumulus-coronal morphology in an in vitro fertilization program. Fertil Steril. 1999;72:412-7.
4. Lin YC, Chang SY, Lan KC, et al. Human oocyte maturity in vivo determines the outcome of blastocyst development in vitro. J Assist Reprod Genet. 2003;20:506-12.

CHAPTER 128

Oocyte Nuclear Maturity Evaluation

Divyashree PS, Kamini A Rao, Anu Kottur

INTRODUCTION

The goal in assisted reproductive technologies is not only to obtain, but also to identify, the best quality oocyte. This is because the health of embryo, fetuses, neonates and adults is unquestionably rooted in a healthy oocyte. Indeed, we first need to know how to differentiate between the mature and immature oocytes and also to identify different oocyte abnormalities, so that we can reliably produce it.

Denudation is a prerequisite for intracytoplasmic sperm injection (ICSI), as only denuded oocytes can be successfully manipulated by the holding pipette. This ancillary effect of ICSI allows us to focus on oocyte nuclear maturity and also its morphological abnormalities.

Currently, oocyte nuclear maturity is assessed by the presence of an extruded first polar body (IPB) in the perivitelline space (PVS) and by the absence of germinal vesicle (GV).

Germinal vesicle: The chromatin in the meiotically arrested oocytes is encapsulated by a nuclear structure known as the germinal vesicle.

First polar body: As a part of reductional division, oocytes undergo disproportionate cytokinesis and extrusion of half of their genetic material within the IPB.

During controlled ovarian hyperstimulation cycles, approximately 85% of the oocytes are metaphase II (MII), 10% are GV and 5% are metaphase I (MI)[1] **(Figs. 1 to 4)**.

Metaphase II oocyte ***(Fig. 1)****:* Otherwise called mature oocyte or egg should have following characteristics:[2,3]

- Round, clear zona pellucida
- Small PVS containing a single unfragmented IPB
- Cytoplasm that is pale and moderately granular and with no inclusions.

Germinal vesicle oocyte: Germinal vesicle is present in the ooplasm.

Metaphase I oocyte: No visible GV in the ooplasm and no IPB in the PVS.

METAPHASE II (FIG. 1)

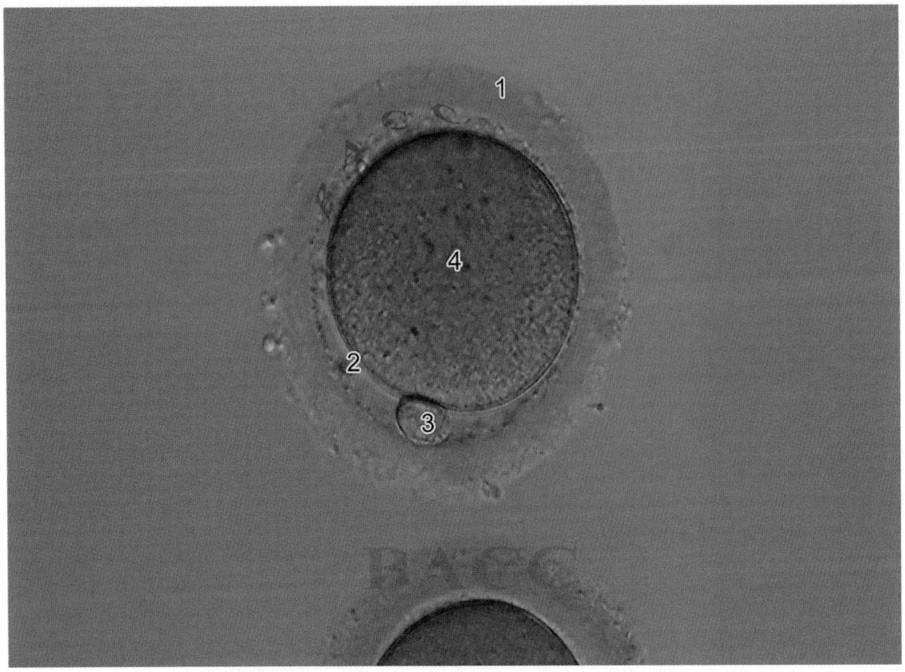

Fig. 1: (1) Round, clear zona pellucida; (2) small perivitelline space; (3) single unfragmented first polar body; (4) pale, moderately granular ooplasm.

METAPHASE I (FIG. 2)

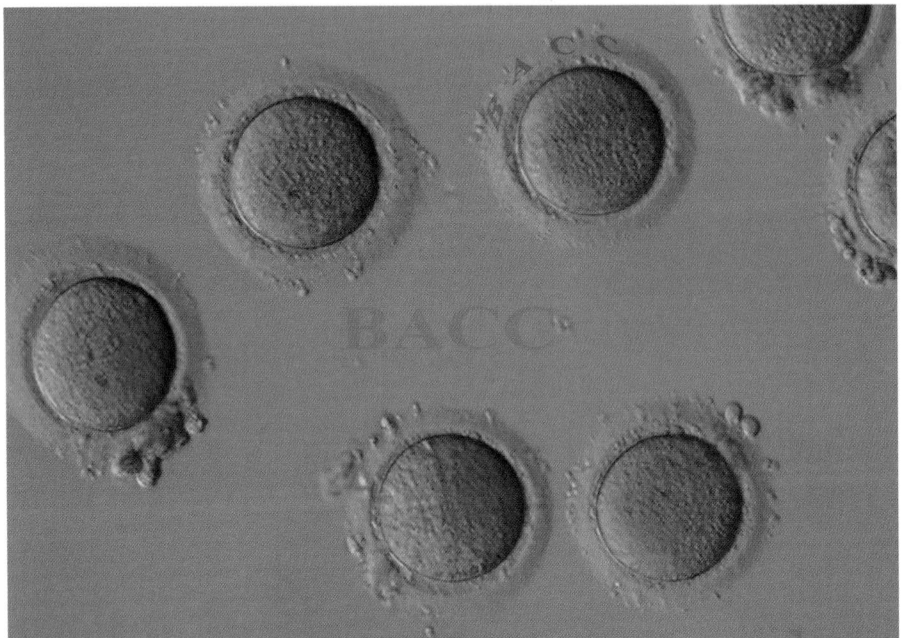

Fig. 2: Metaphase I oocytes. (*Note:* No germinal vesicle in the ooplasm; no visible first polar body).

GERMINAL VESICLE OOCYTE (40×) (FIG. 3A)

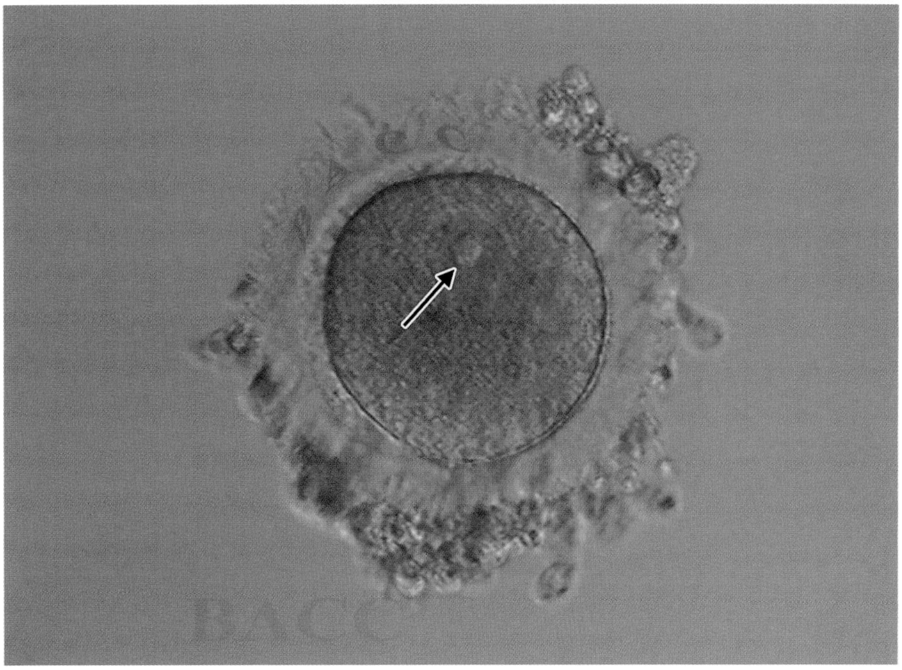

Fig. 3A: Oocyte recovered at the germinal vesicle stage, note the presence of germinal vesicle (arrow).

GERMINAL VESICLE OOCYTE (20×) (FIG. 3B)

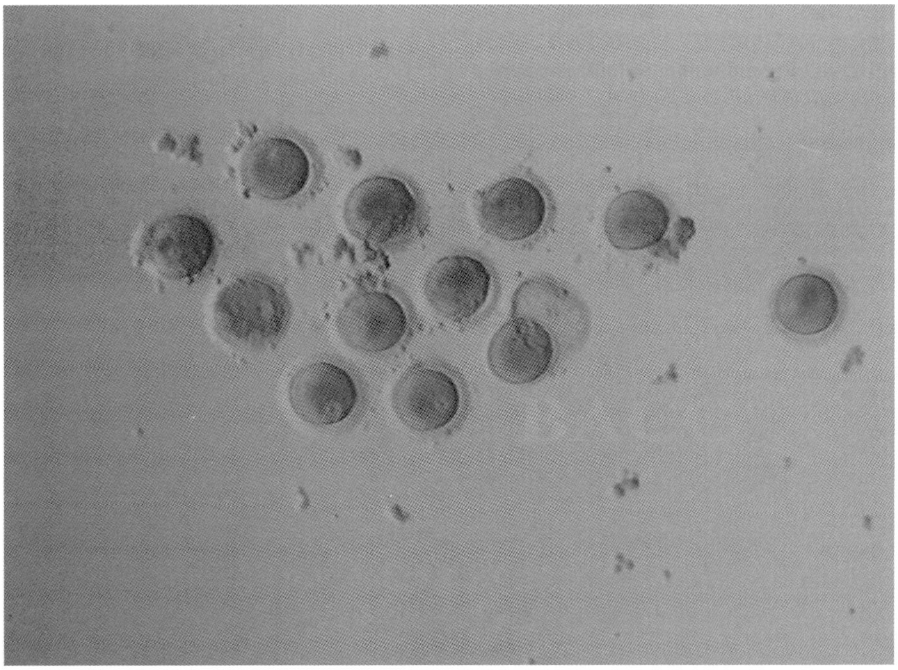

Fig. 3B: All oocytes are at germinal vesicle stage and despite overnight incubation did not proceed to germinal vesicle breakdown.

OOCYTES IN DIFFERENT STAGES OF MATURATION (FIG. 4)

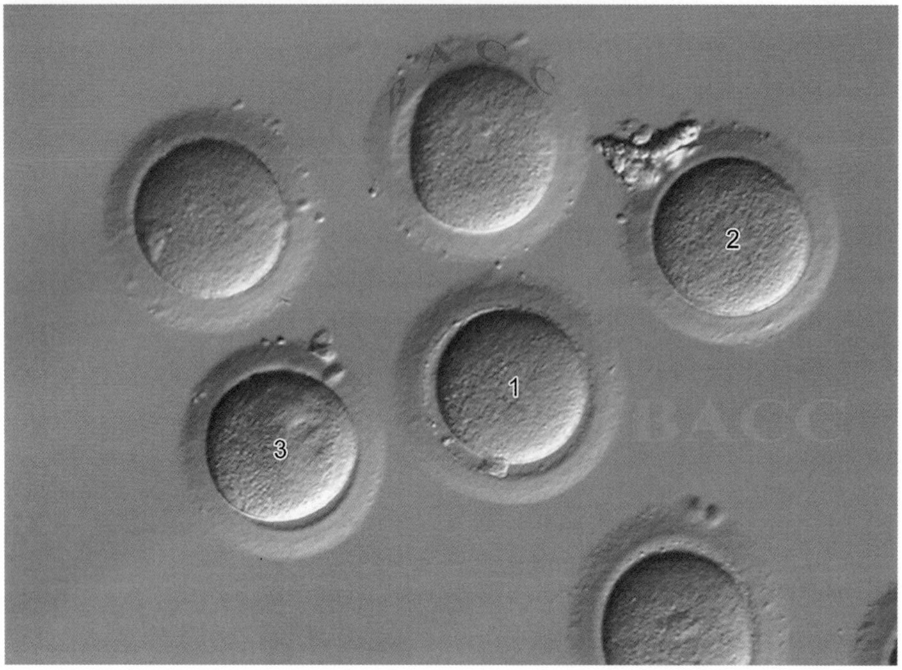

Fig. 4: (1) Metaphase II oocyte with the presence of first polar body; (2) metaphase I oocyte without first polar body and germinal vesicle; (3) GV oocyte with the presence of germinal vesicle.

REFERENCES

1. Ubaldi F, Rienzi L. Micromanipulation techniques in human fertility: PZD, SUZI, ICSI, MESA, PESA, FNA and TESE. In: Revelli A, Tur-Kaspa I, Holte JG, Massobrio M (Eds). Biotechnology of Human Reproduction. Oxford: Parthenon Publishing; 2003. pp. 315-36.
2. Xia P. Intracytoplasmic sperm injection: correlation of oocyte grade based on polar body, perivitelline space and cytoplasmic inclusions with fertilization rate and embryo quality. Hum Reprod. 1997;12:1750-5.
3. Balaban B, Urman B. Effect of oocyte morphology on embryo development and implantation. Reprod Biomed Online. 2006;12:608-15.

CHAPTER 129

Oocyte Dysmorphisms

Divyashree PS, Bezar Ghan VV, Kamini A Rao, Mohammed Ashraf C

INTRODUCTION

In the previous chapter, description regarding an "ideal" oocyte has been given. However, all the ideal characteristics may not be found in all the oocytes retrieved during controlled ovarian hyperstimulation (COH), this is true even in donor in vitro fertilization (IVF) cycles.

Following denudation, specific anomalies or dysmorphisms of the oocytes may be detected by examination with light microscopy. These anomalies or dysmorphisms have been observed in a high proportion (63%) of metaphase II (MII) oocytes obtained after retrieval.[1,2]

Oocyte abnormalities can be broadly categorized as shown in the **Flowchart 1**.

GRANULAR CYTOPLASM

Granularity can be observed within the cytoplasm and it may be either homogeneously or centrally placed **(Figs. 1 and 2)**.

Severity of granularity is based on its depth and diameter (>50%—severe) **(Fig. 3)**.[3]

VACUOLES

Vacuoles are membrane-bound cytoplasmic inclusions filled with fluid virtually identical with perivitelline fluid. Vacuoles vary in size as well as in number **(Figs. 4A to C)**. They can be present in the oocyte on the collection day (day 0) or may be artificially created by intracytoplasmic sperm injection (ICSI) (day 1) or may be seen in embryos

Flowchart 1: Category of oocyte abnormalities.

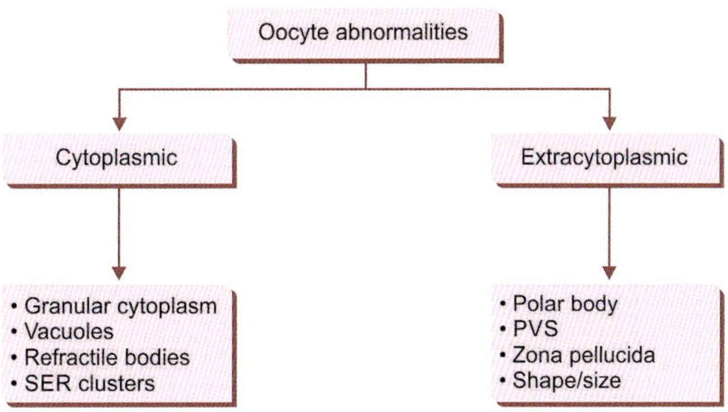

(PVS: perivitelline space; SER: smooth endoplasmic reticulum)

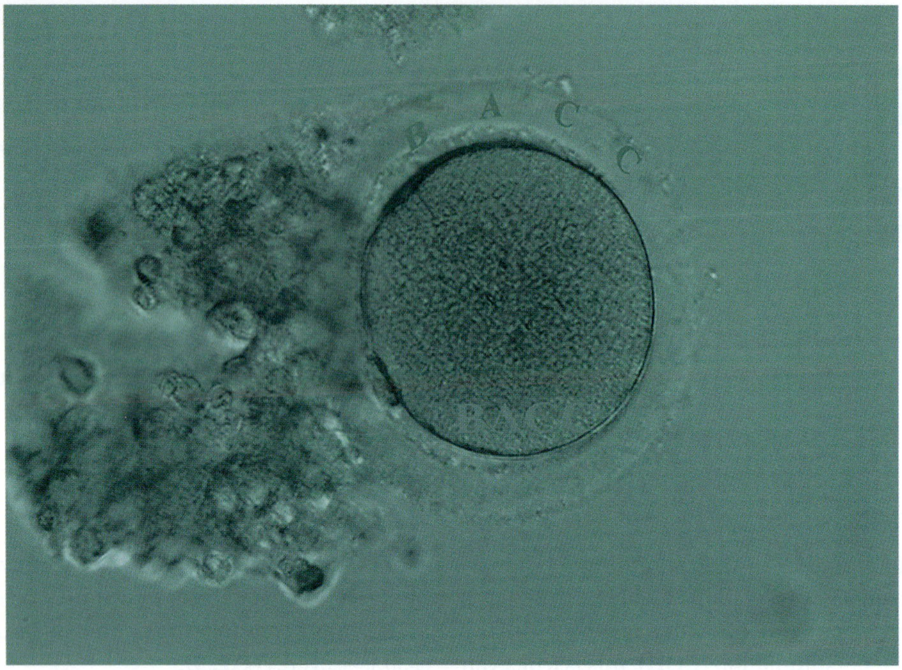

Fig. 1: Oocyte having homogeneous granular cytoplasm.

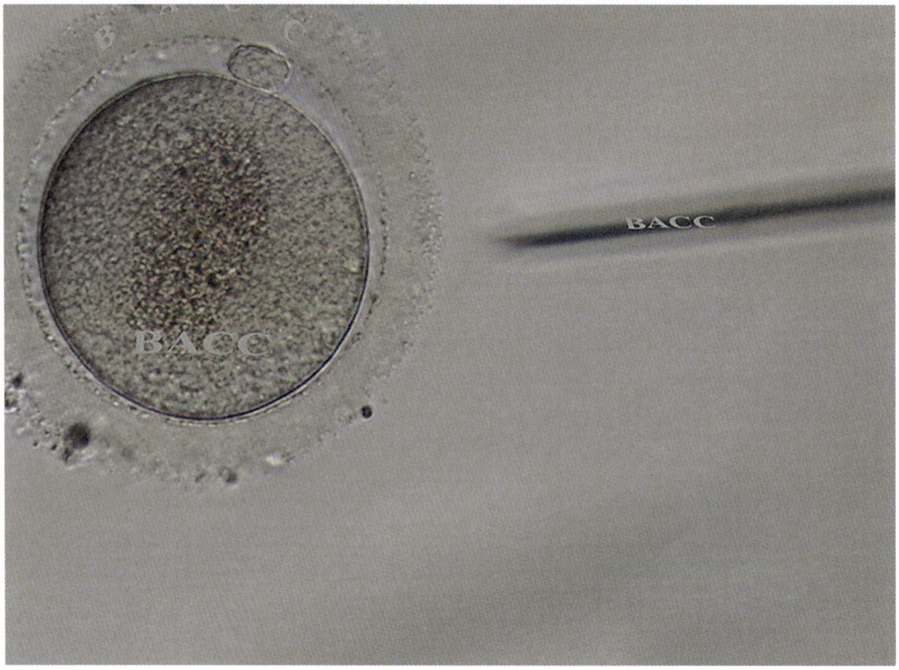

Fig. 2: Oocyte with centrally placed granularity.

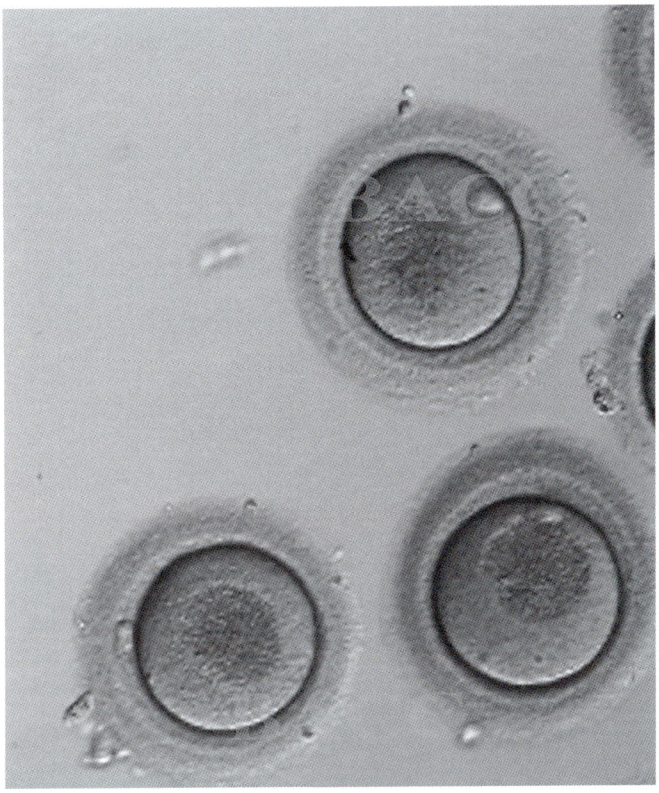

Fig. 3: MII oocytes showing a very large centrally located granular area occupying the majority of the cytoplasm. This granularity is typical of organelle clustering.

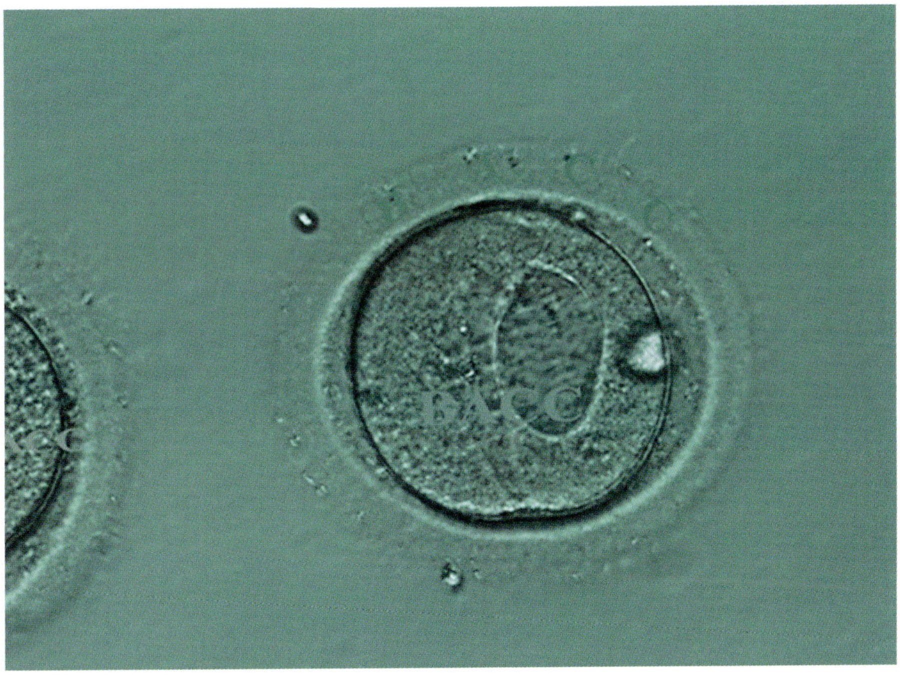

Fig. 4A: Single large vacuole in metaphase II oocyte.

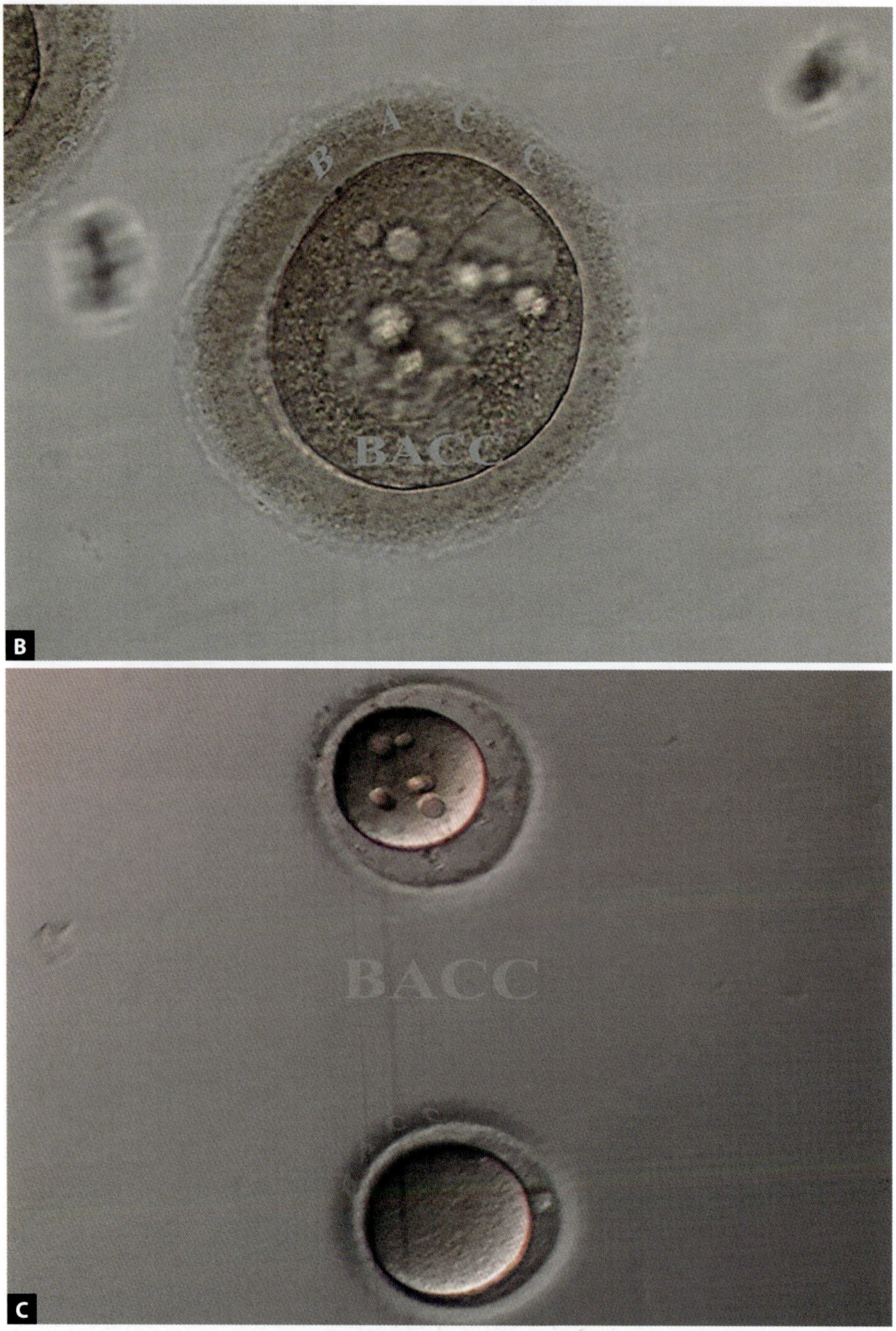

Figs. 4B and C: Multiple vacuoles.

associated with developmental arrest. The later the vacuole arouse, the poorer the oocyte perform on blastocyst formation.[4]

SMOOTH ENDOPLASMIC RETICULUM CLUSTER

Under inverted microscopy, smooth endoplasmic reticulum (SER) clusters can be morphologically distinguished from fluid-filled vacuoles. SER clusters are pronuclear sized, flat clear disk-like structures **(Fig. 5)**. Presence of SER cluster has been associated with poor fertilization and embryo development.[5,6]

REFRACTILE BODIES

The refractile body, so called because of its nature under bright-field microscopy. The evolution of this structure and its relationship to oocyte maturity and viability are not yet fully understood **(Figs. 6A and B)**.

POLAR BODY

First polar body is believed to indicate the postovulatory age of the oocyte. Different authors have found a significant relationship between first polar body (IPB) morphology and blastocyst formation, implantation and ongoing pregnancy **(Figs. 7A to F)**.[7]

According to Ebner et al.[8] categories of IPB have been described:

- *Grade 1:* Round or ovoid, intact (smooth surface)
- *Grade 2:* Round or ovoid, intact (rough surface)
- *Grade 3:* Fragmented
- *Grade 4:* Broken in two
- *Grade 5:* Huge IPB

PERIVITELLINE SPACE

Abnormalities of perivitelline space (PVS) could be enlargement at one or more areas or PVS granularity/fragments **(Figs. 8A to D)**.

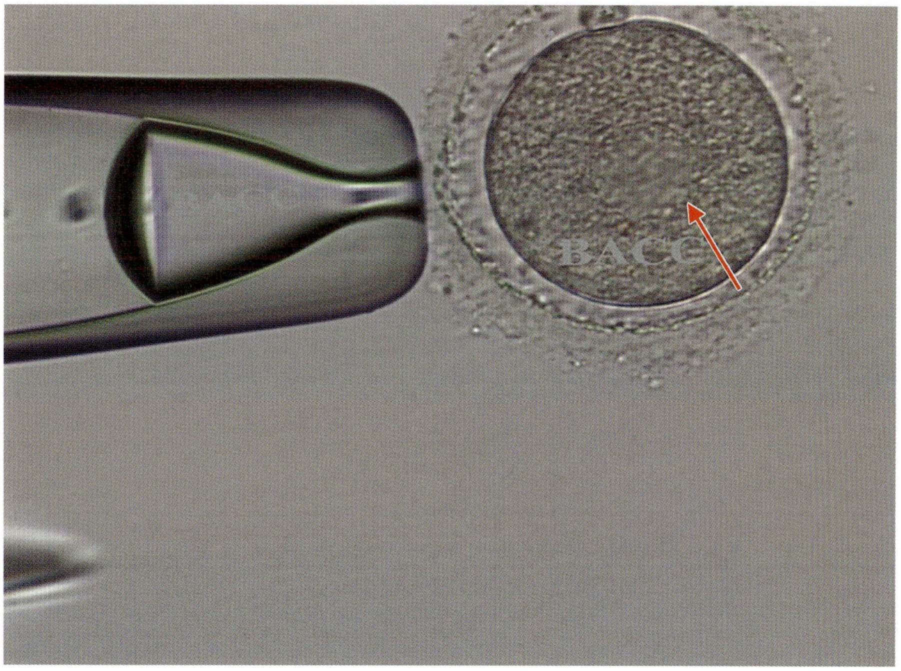

Fig. 5: Oocyte with smooth endoplasmic reticulum (SER) cluster (arrow).

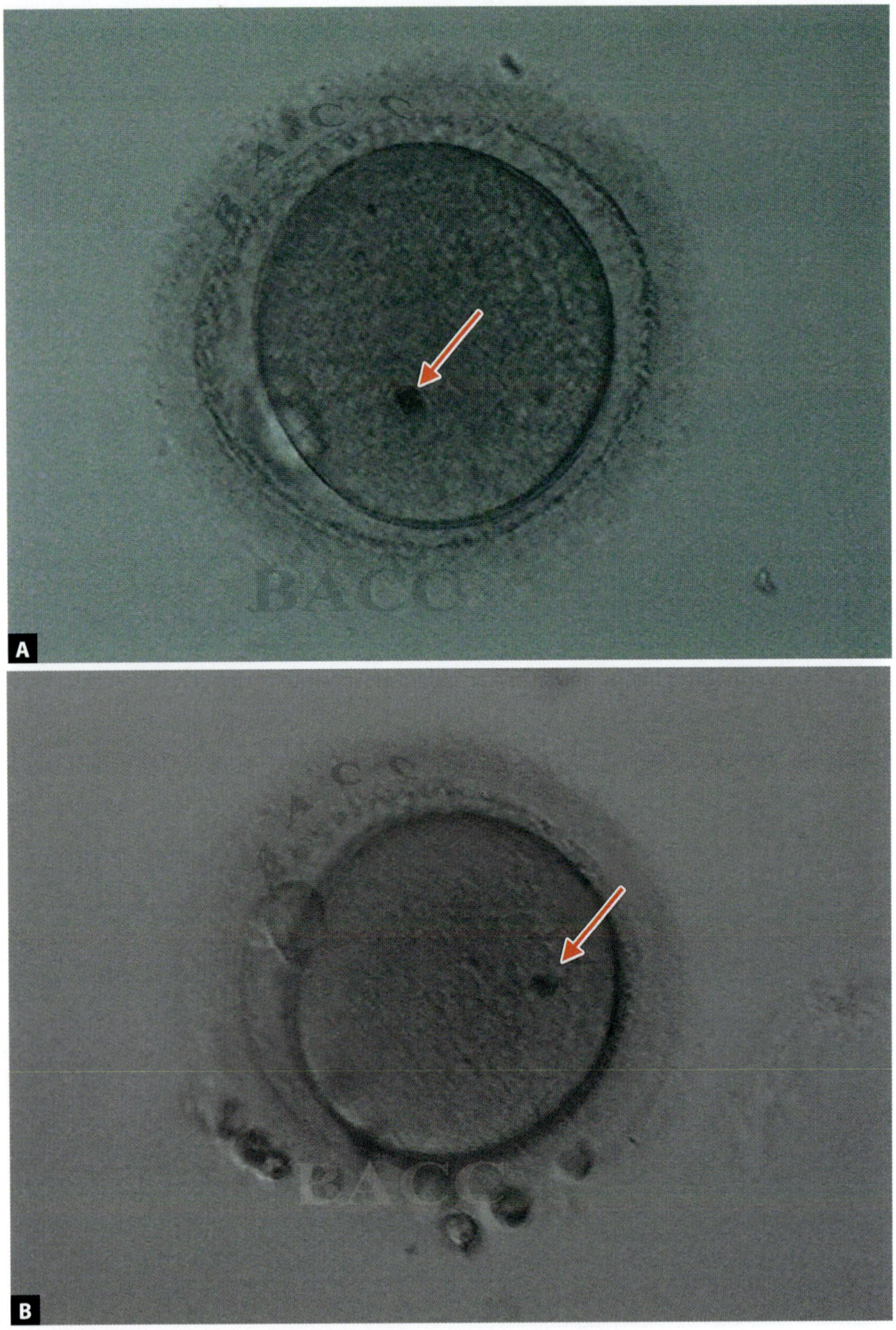

Figs. 6A and B: Refractile body (arrows).

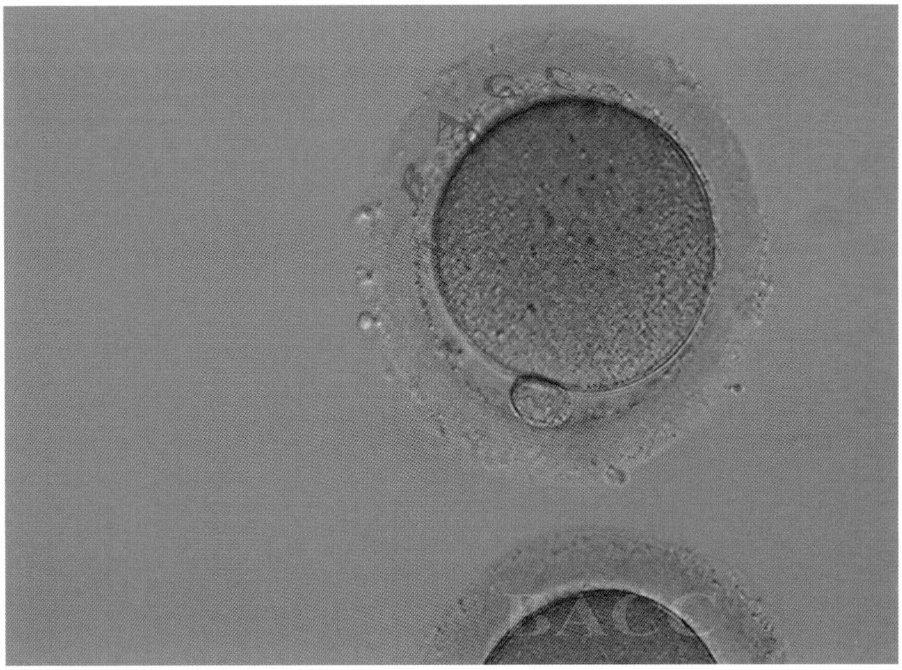

Fig. 7A: Polar body with smooth surface.

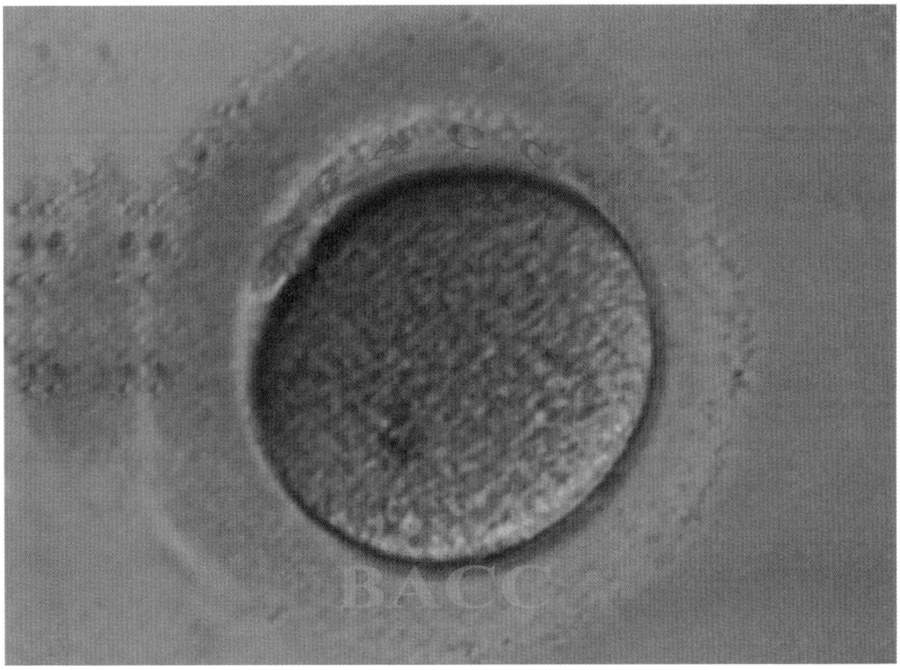

Fig. 7B: Polar body with rough surface.

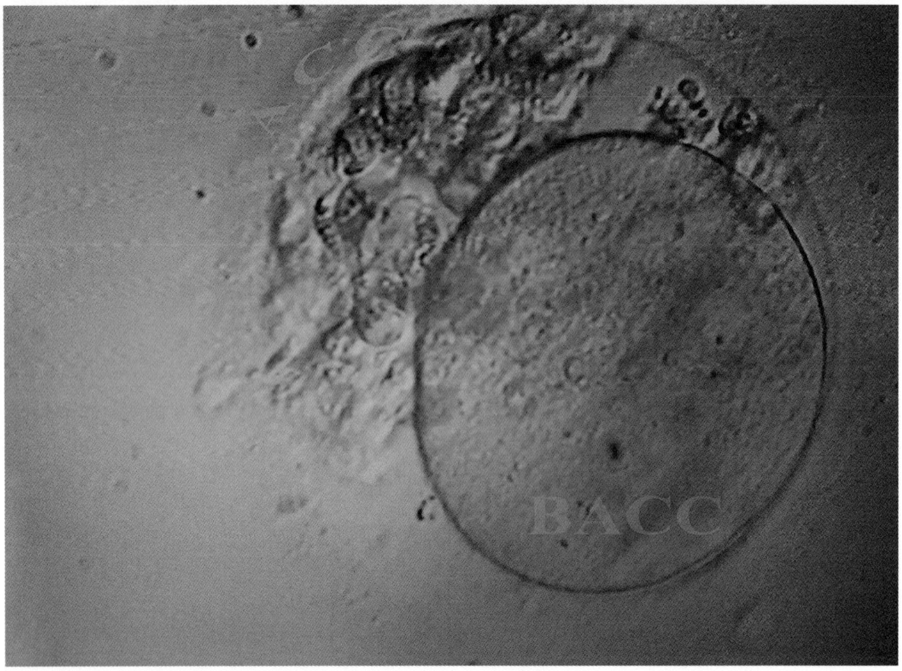

Fig. 7C: Fragmented polar body.

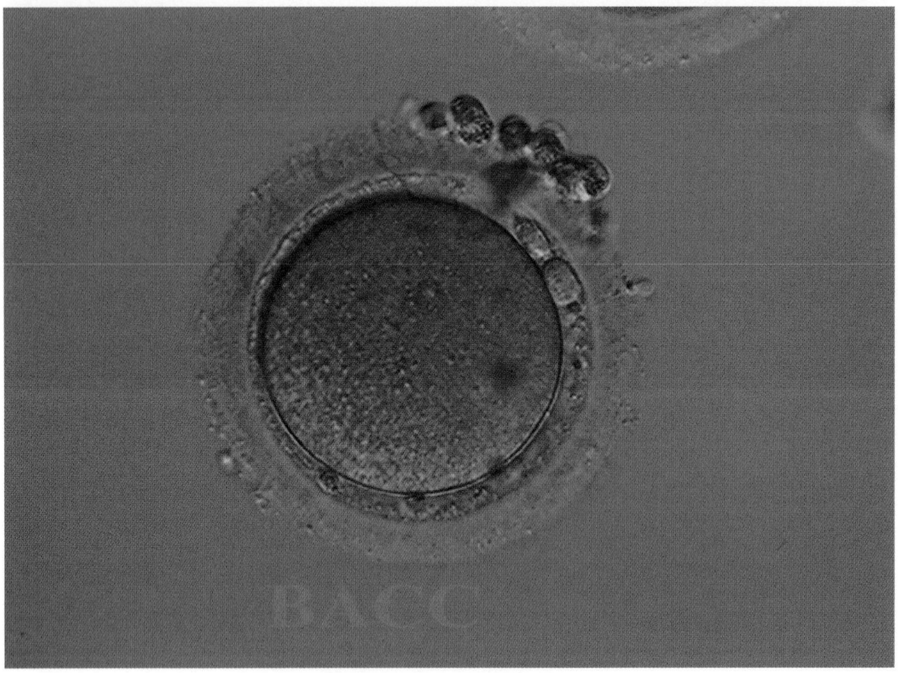

Fig. 7D: Polar body broken into two.

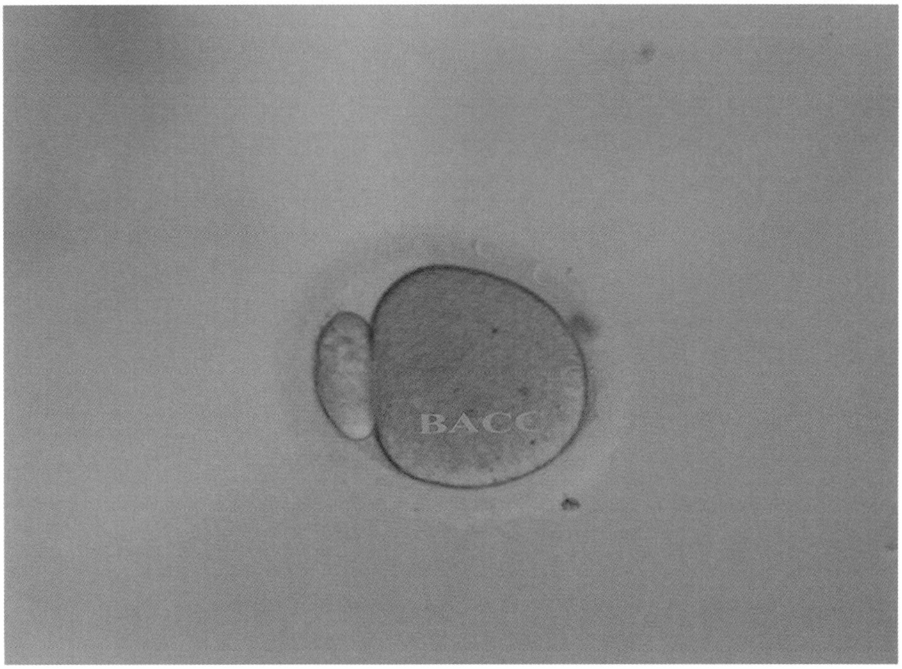

Fig. 7E: Large first polar body.

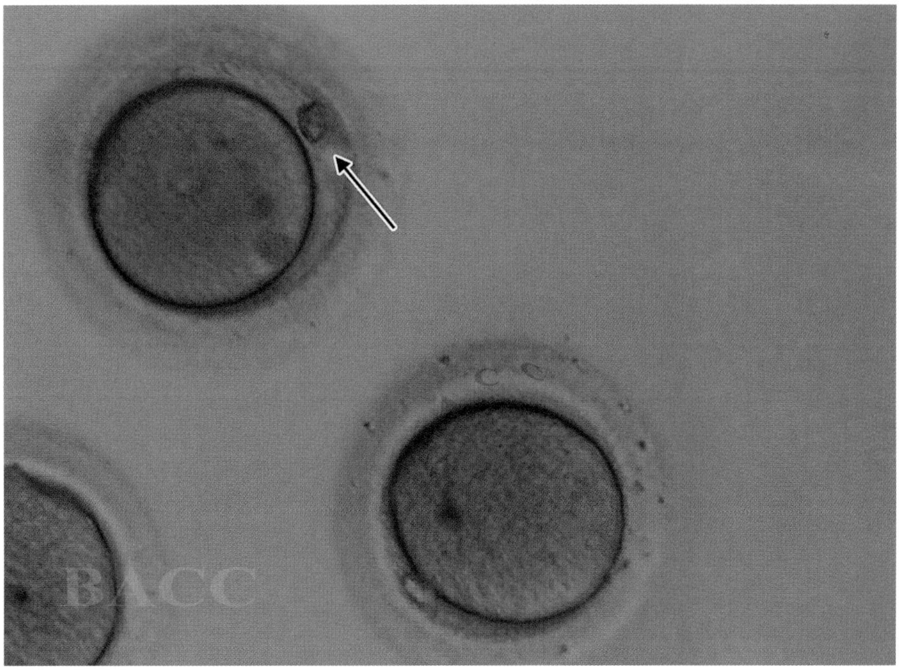

Fig. 7F: First polar body detached from ooplasm (arrow).

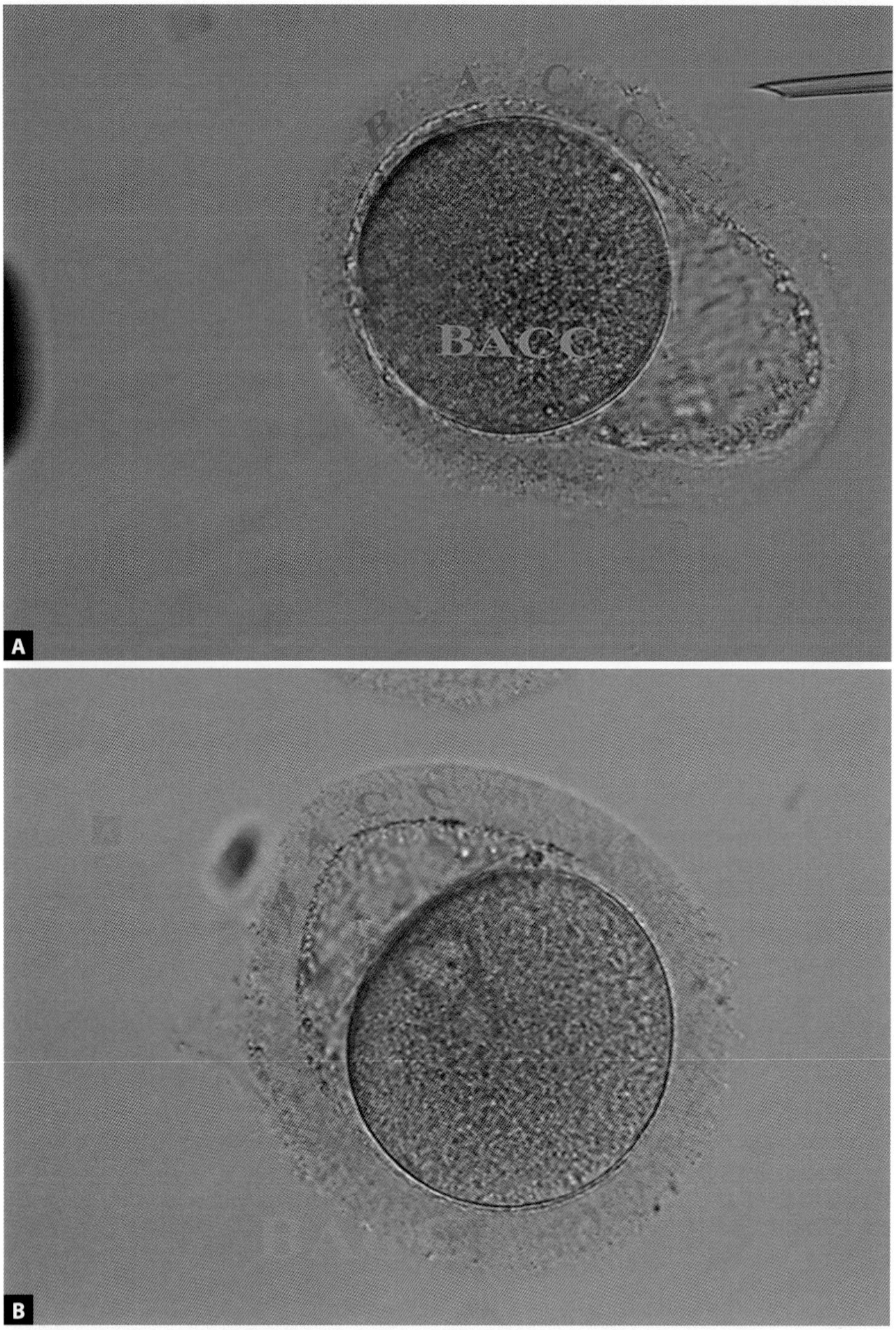

Figs. 8A and B: Increased perivitelline space with septa.

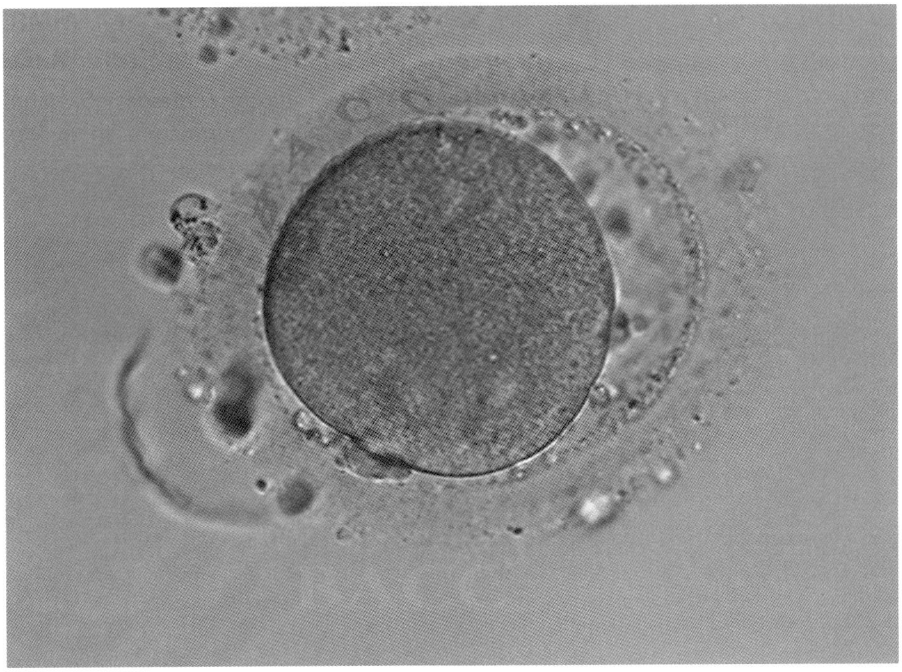

Fig. 8C: Increased perivitelline space with granulations.

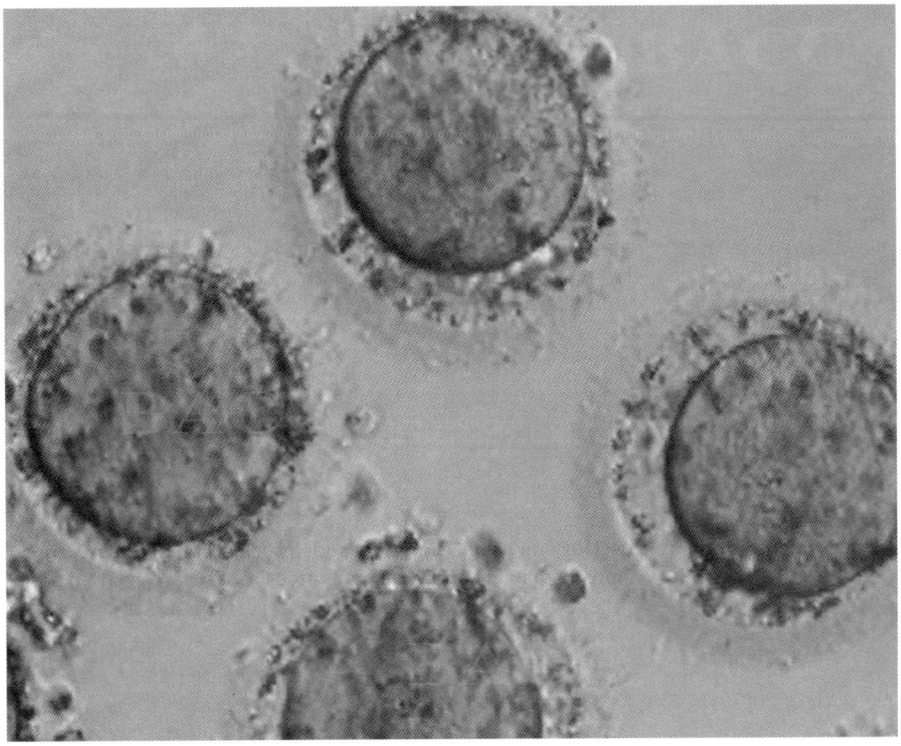

Fig. 8D: Increased perivitelline debris in the perivitelline space (PVS).

ZONA PELLUCIDA

The zona pellucida (ZP) is a transparent, extracellular matrix composed of defined glycoproteins built in a typical fibrogranular structure by noncovalent interactions.[9] Abnormalities of ZP can be in its thickness and sometimes even absent zona **(Figs. 9A to H)**.

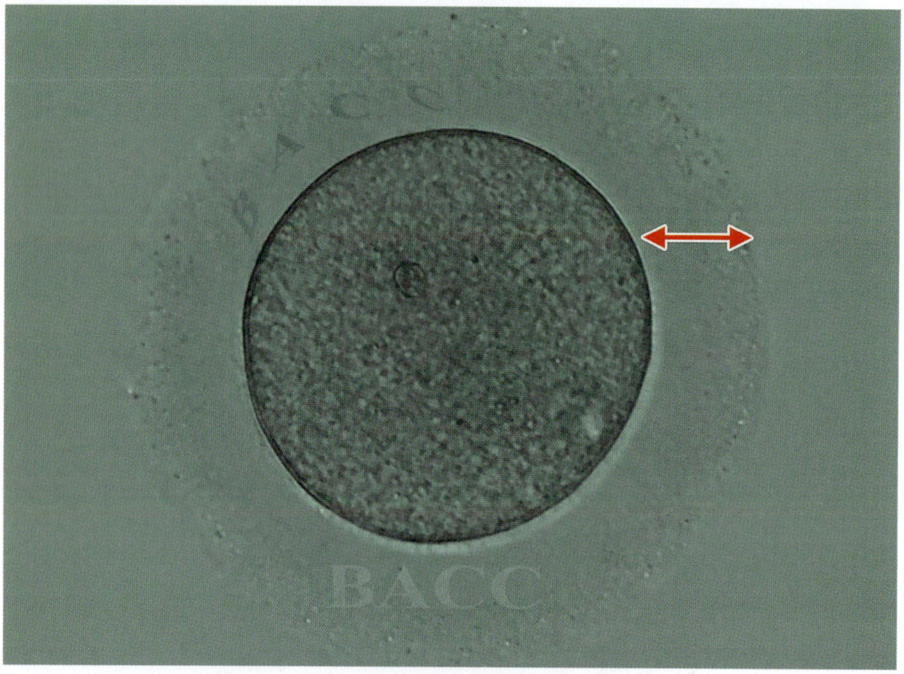

Fig. 9A: Thick zona pellucida surrounding the oocyte.

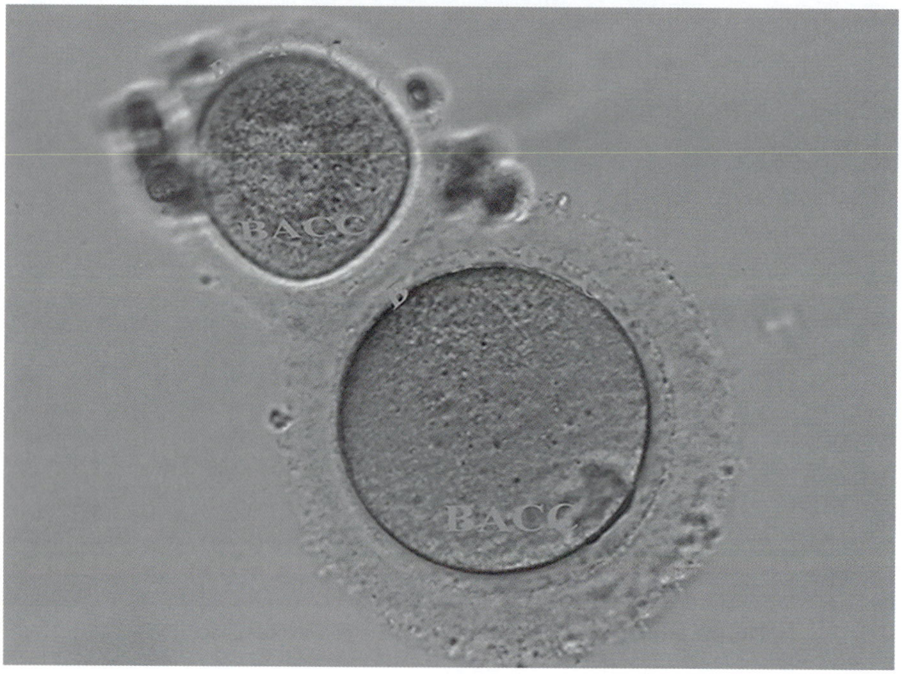

Fig. 9B: Two oocytes were recovered within a single zona pellucida, the smaller oocyte has a germinal vesicle and larger oocyte is metaphase I.

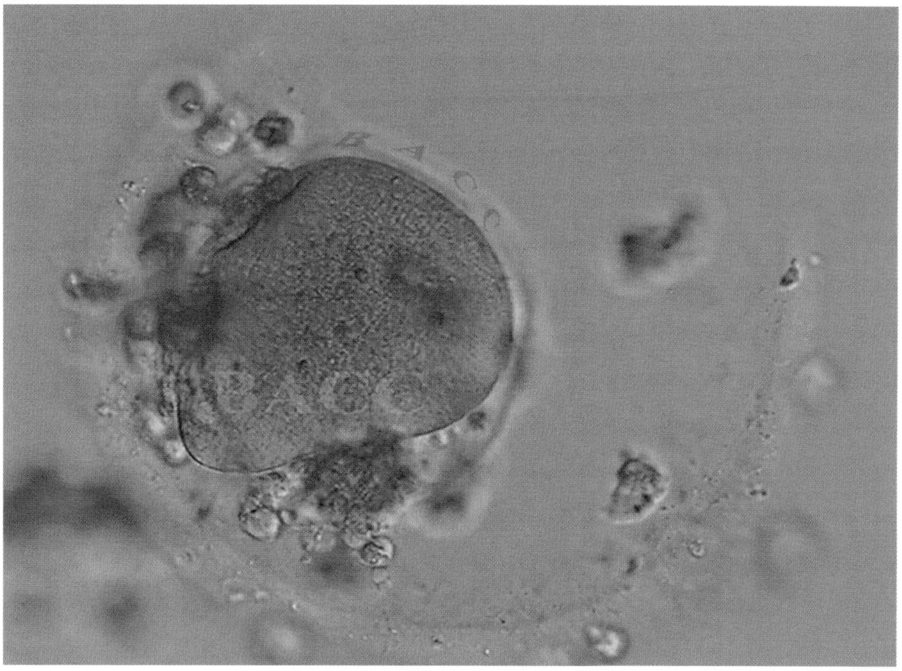

Fig. 9C: Oocyte with double zona.

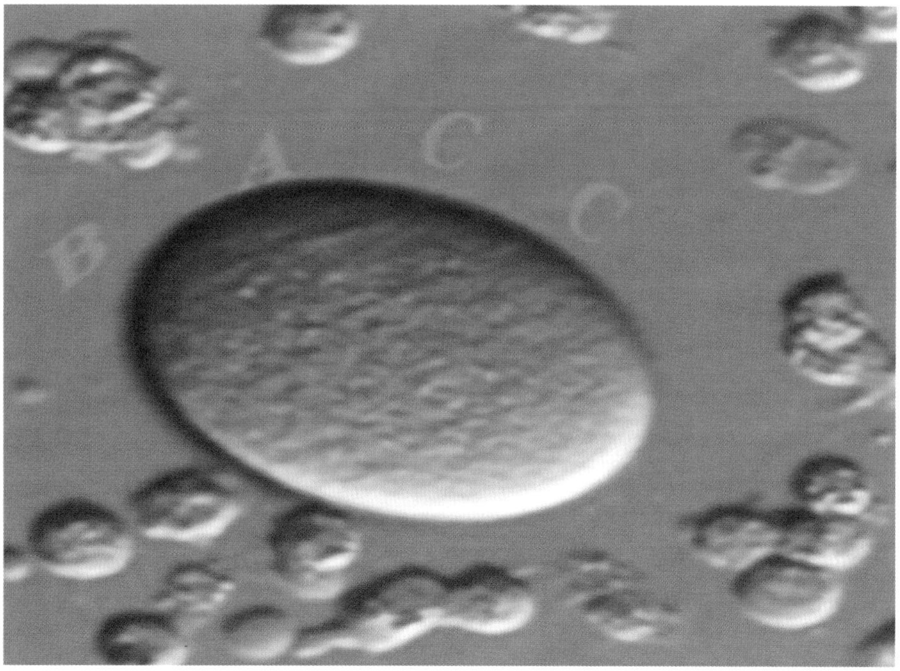

Fig. 9D: Oocyte with absent zona (one of the reason could be high suction pressure due to which zona pellucida can break).

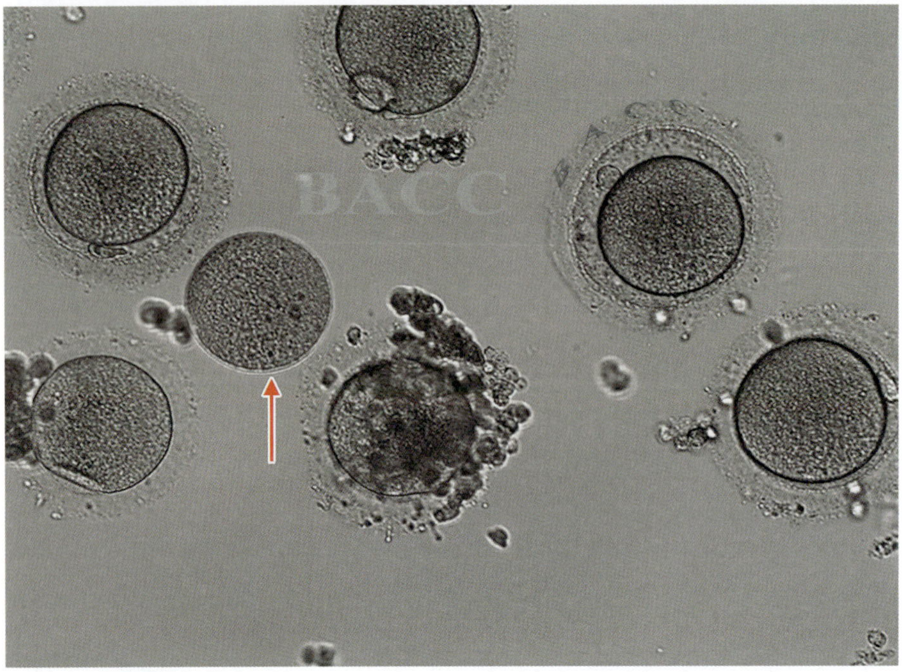

Fig. 9E: Oocyte cohort with one of the oocyte having absent zona (arrow).

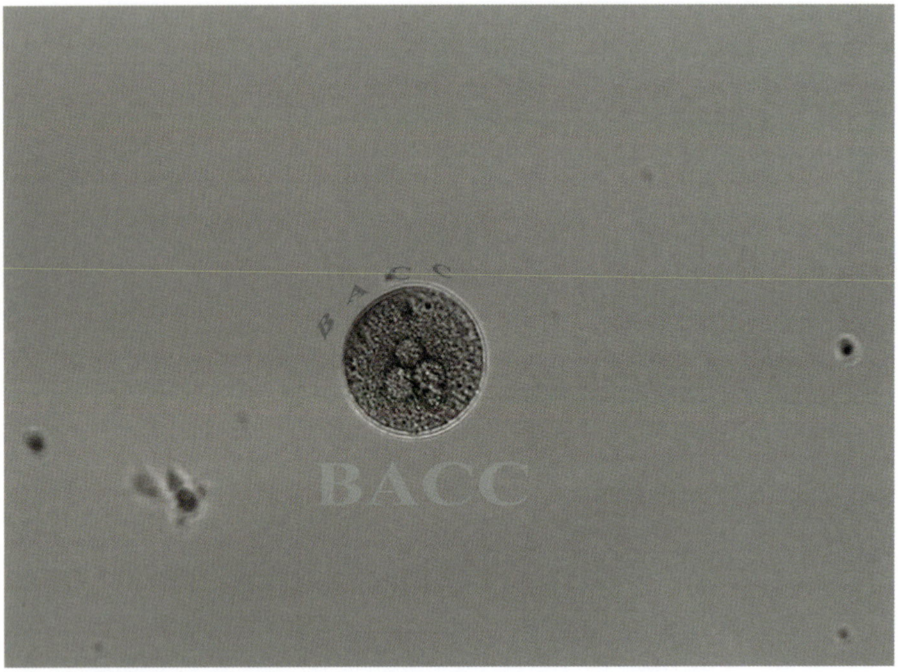

Fig. 9F: The same oocyte at 18 hours postinsemination showing evidence of fertilization, with two pronuclei, and a single vacuole.

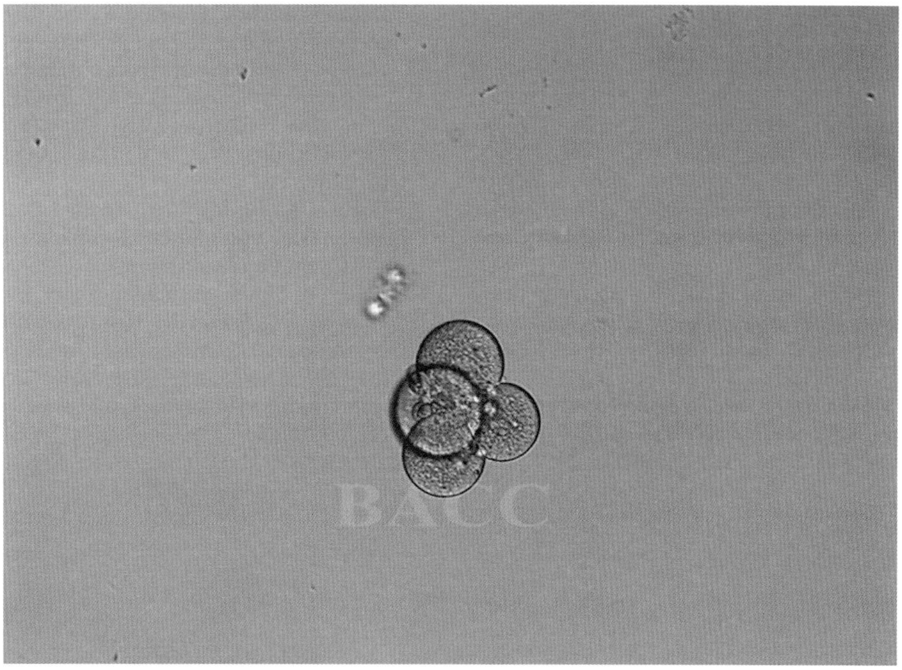

Fig. 9G: Four-cell embryo, with absent zona. (200x magnification). This is the same embryo which was obtained after fertilizing the oocyte with empty zona shown in the previous figures. The embryo got arrested at four-cell stage.

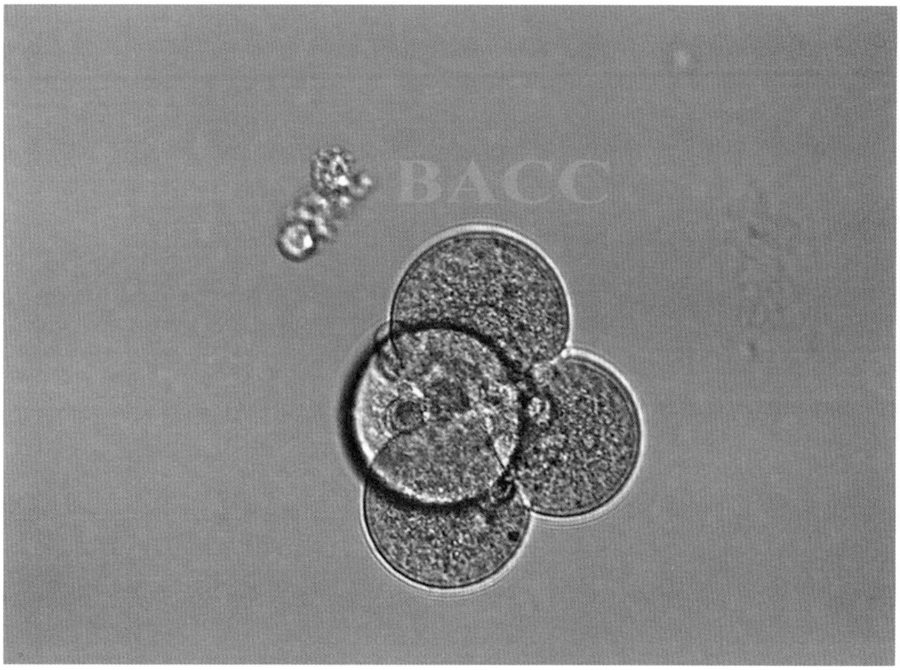

Fig. 9H: Four-cell embryo, with absent zona. (400x magnification)

REFERENCES

1. De Sutter P, Dozortsev D, Qian C, et al. Oocyte morphology does not correlate with fertilization rate and embryo quality after intracytoplasmic sperm injection. Hum Reprod. 1996;11:595-7.
2. Balaban B, Urman B, Sertac A, et al. Oocyte morphology does not affect fertilization rate, embryo quality and implantation rate after intracytoplasmic sperm injection. Hum Reprod. 1998;13:3431-3.
3. Kahraman S, Yakin K, Donmez E, et al. Relationship between granular cytoplasm of oocytes and pregnancy outcome following intracytoplasmic sperm injection. Hum Reprod. 2000;15:2390-3.
4. Ebner T, Moser M, Sommergruber M, et al. Occurrence and developmental consequences of vacuoles throughout preimplantation development. Fertil Steril. 2005;83:1635-40.
5. Otsuki J, Okada A, Morimoto K, et al. The relationship between pregnancy outcome and smooth endoplasmic reticulum clusters in MII human oocytes. Hum Reprod. 2004;19:1591-7.
6. Sá R, Cunha M, Silva J, et al. Ultrastructure of tubular smooth endoplasmic reticulum aggregates in human metaphase II oocytes and clinical implications. Fertil Steril. 2011;96:143-9.e.7.
7. Ebner T, Moser M, Sommergruber C, et al. First polar body morphology and blastocyst formation rate in ICSI patients. Hum Reprod. 2002;17:2415-8.
8. Ebner T, Moser M, Yaman C, et al. Elective transfer of embryos selected on the basis of first polar body morphology is associated with increased rates of implantation and pregnancy. Fertil Steril. 1999;72:599-603.
9. Oehninger S. Biochemical and functional characterization of the human zona pellucida. Reprod Biomed Online. 2003;7(6):641-8.

CHAPTER 130

The Sperm

Anitha S Kumari K, Dileep Kumar R, Hemanth Kumar MA, Mohammed Ashraf C

INTRODUCTION

The sperm cell is a specialized cell and plays a role in transfer of paternal deoxyribonucleic acid (DNA) and activation of the mature egg. It is composed of three parts—head, mid-piece and tail. The head is connected to the mid-piece by a short region, the neck.

During evaluation of male infertility, semen analysis is the cornerstone of laboratory evaluation and helps to define the severity of male factor.

The semen analysis provides information on semen volume as well as sperm concentration, motility and morphology.[1]

Components of sperm evaluation include:

- Sperm count **(Figs. 1A and B)**
- Sperm motility **(Figs. 1A and B)**
- Sperm morphology **(Figs. 2A to C)**
- Globozoospermia **(Figs. 3A and B)**
- Sperm vitality **(Figs. 4A to C and 5A to C)**
- Sperm DNA fragmentation **(Figs. 6A and B)**

SPERM COUNT AND MOTILITY

Makler chamber is designed specifically for assessing the sperm concentration and motility. The advantage of Makler chamber is that no dilution is required to assess the semen sample **(Figs. 1A and B)**.

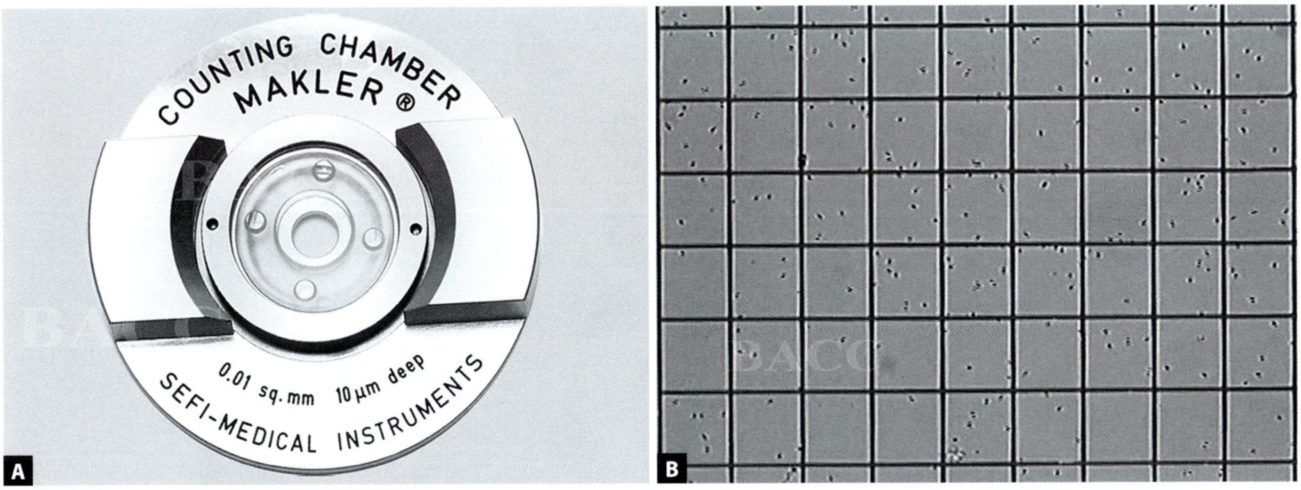

Figs. 1A and B: (A) Makler chamber; (B) Makler chamber charged with sperms at 200x magnification.

SPERM MORPHOLOGY (FIGS. 2A TO C)

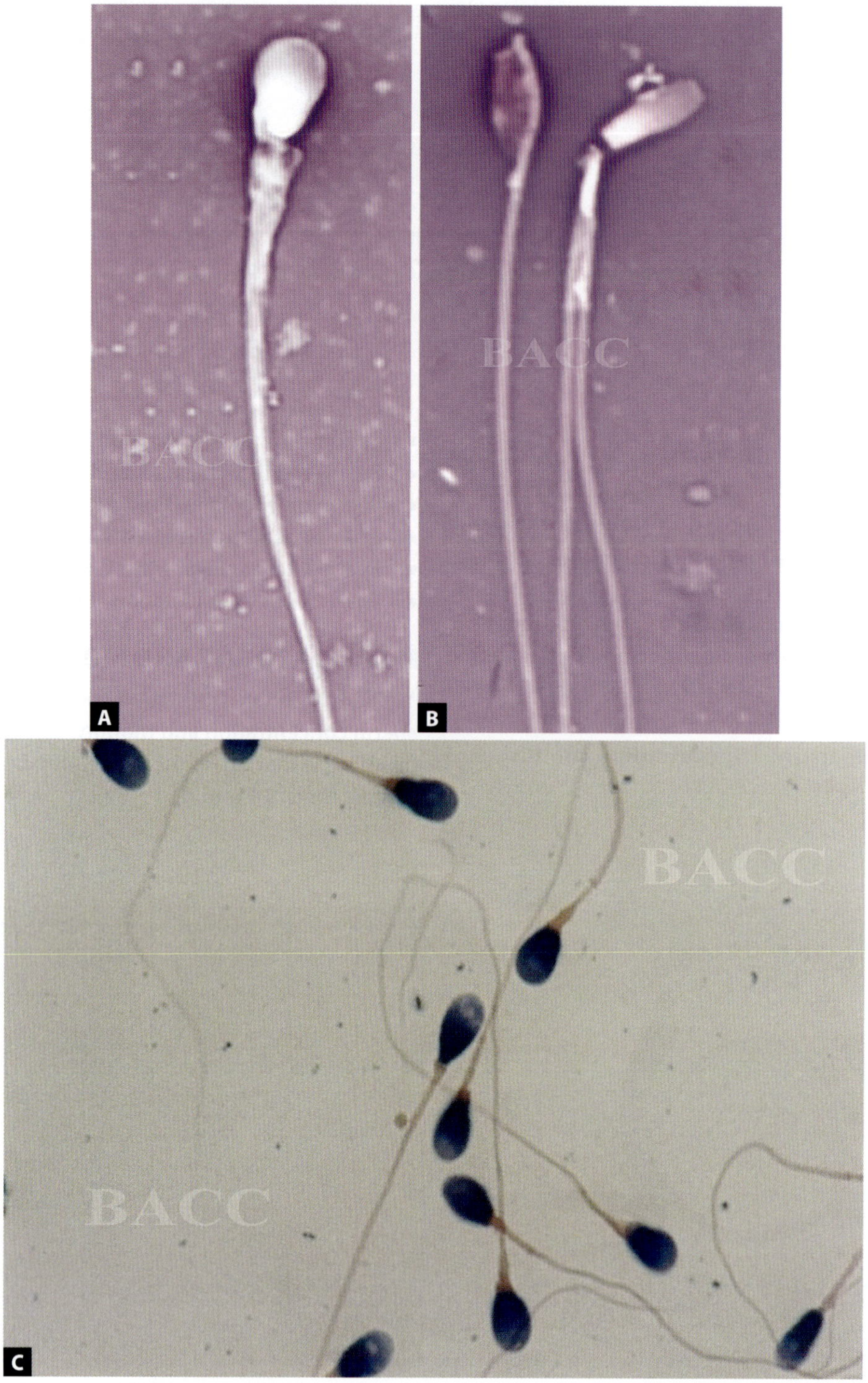

Figs. 2A to C: Sperm morphology. (A) Eosin-Nigrosin stained smear showing sperm with defective mid-piece; (B) Eosin-Nigrosin stained smear showing sperm abnormalities. Sperm on the left showing amorphous head and sperm on the right showing duplication of tail; and (C) Sperm morphology with papanicolaou stain.

GLOBOZOOSPERMIA (ACROSOMAL AGENESIS)

Globozoospermia (round headed sperm syndrome) exhibits a partial or a complete lack of acrosome and acrosomal enzymes which make the sperm completely unable to penetrate the zona pellucida **(Figs. 3A and B)**.

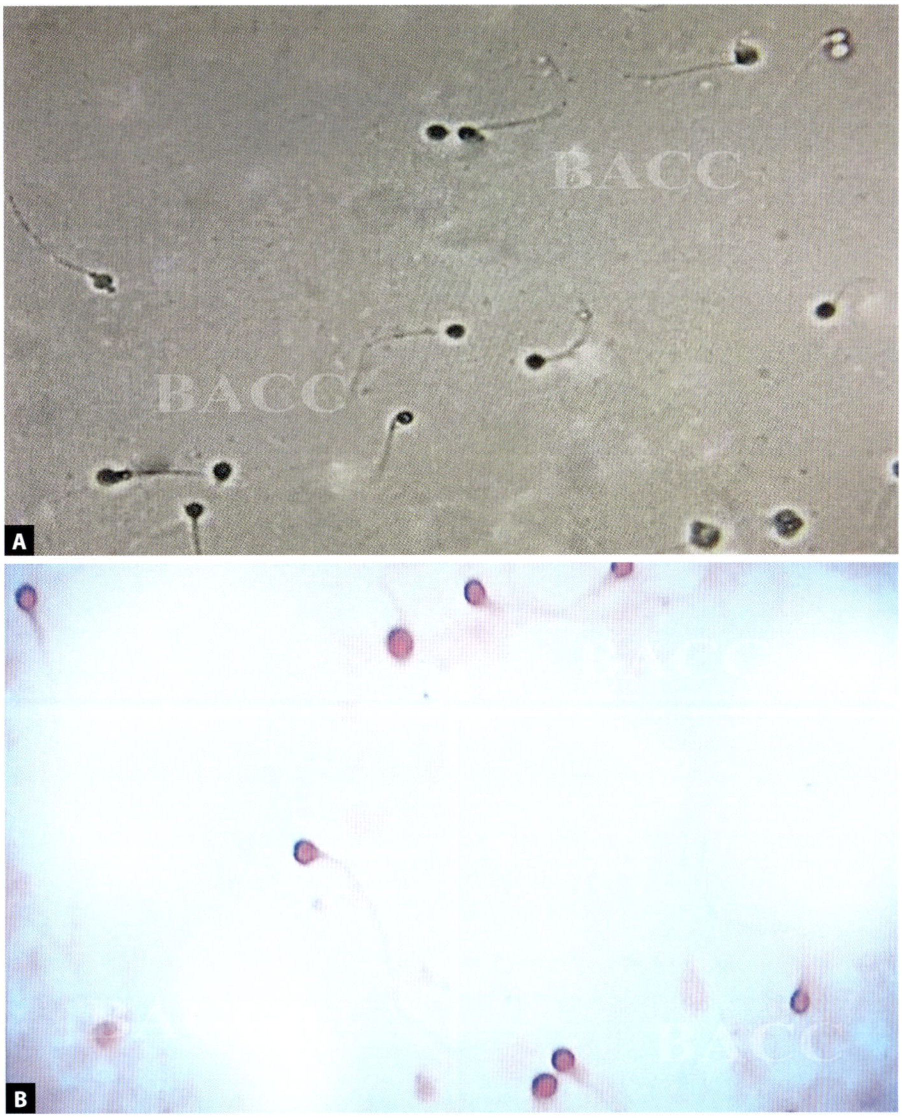

Figs. 3A and B: (A) Depicts globozoospermia in real time; (B) Depicts globozoospermia with eosin-hematoxylin staining technique.

SPERM VITALITY

Sperm vitality is a technique evaluated by assessing the membrane integrity of the cells. The two techniques exclusively used for sperm vitality include dye-exclusion method and hypo-osmotic swelling test.

Sperm Vitality by Hypo-osmotic Swelling Test

Hypo-osmotic swelling (HOS) test is used to determine the viability of the sperm. In the HOS test, viable non-motile sperm will swell and also show the curling of tail when incubated in a hypo-osmotic solution as shown in **Figures 4A to C**.

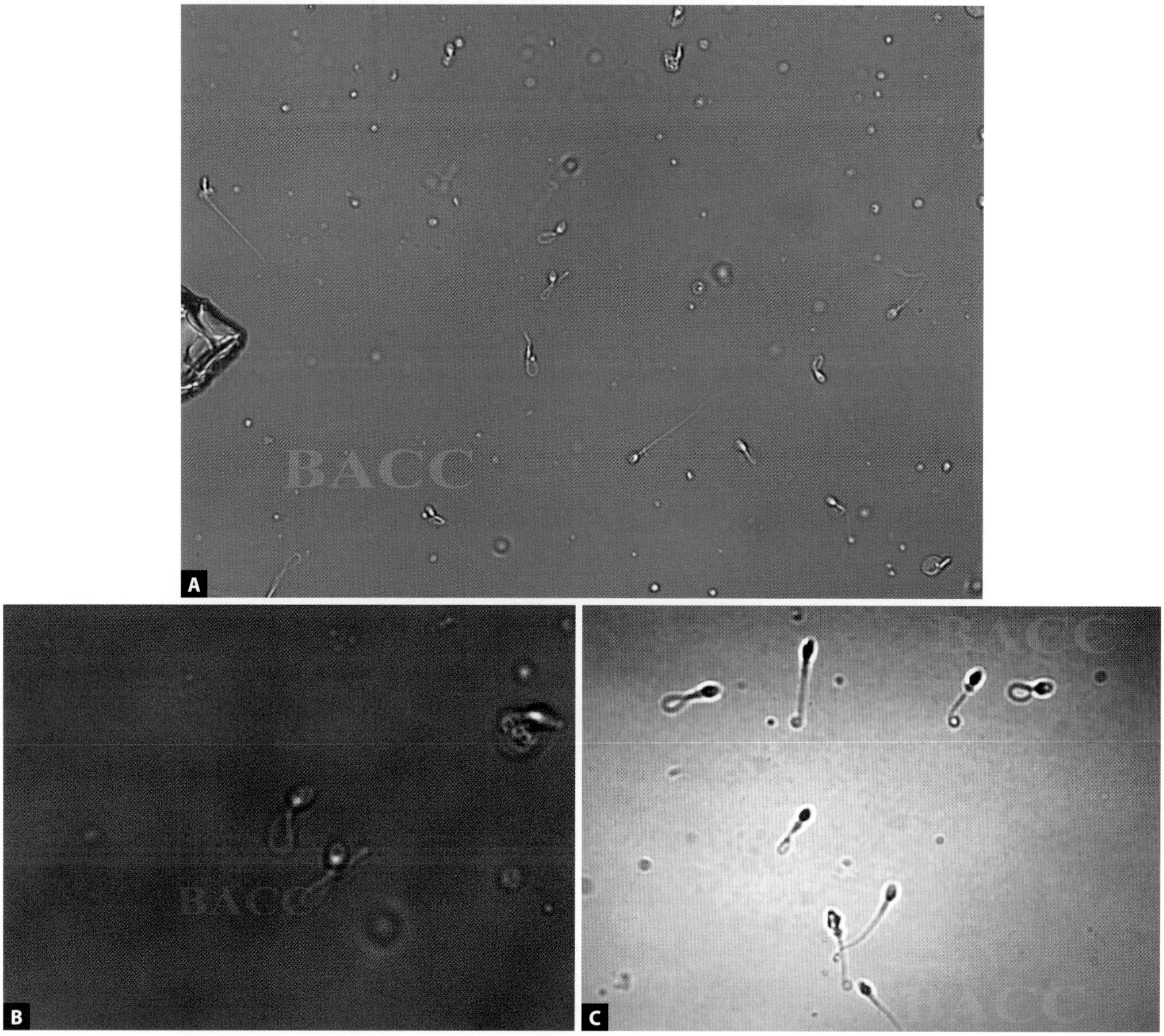

Figs. 4A to C: (A) Hypo-osmotic swelling test (200×); (B and C) Hypo-osmotic swelling test (400×).

Sperm Vitality by Dye Exclusion Method

In this method, the nonvital (dead cells) allows the entry of membrane-impermeant stains where the live one does not allow the diffusion of stain **(Figs. 5A to C)**.

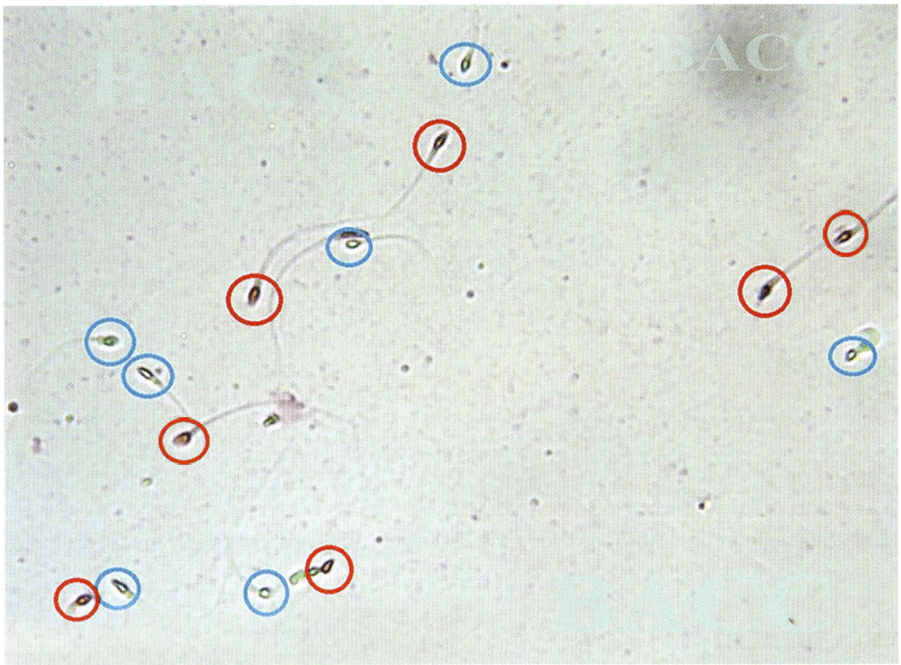

Fig. 5A: Dye-exclusion method with eosin stain. Red circle indicates spermatozoa with red or dark pink heads and are considered dead (membrane damaged). Blue circle indicates spermatozoa with white heads and is considered alive (membrane intact).

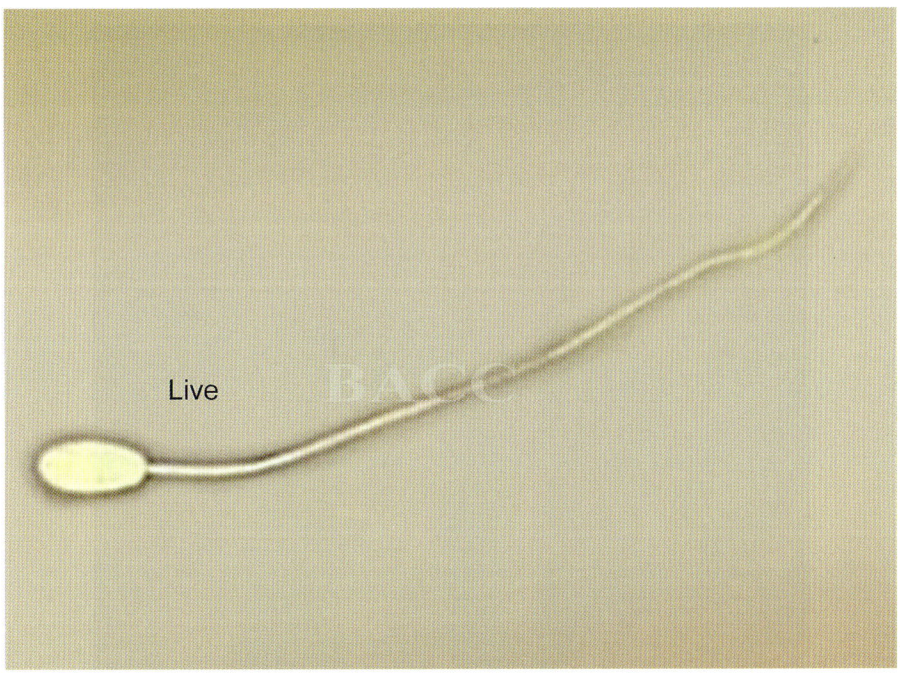

Fig. 5B: Sperm viability by staining. Eosin-Nigrosin stained smear showing, non-uptake of the dye by the sperm, indicating viability.

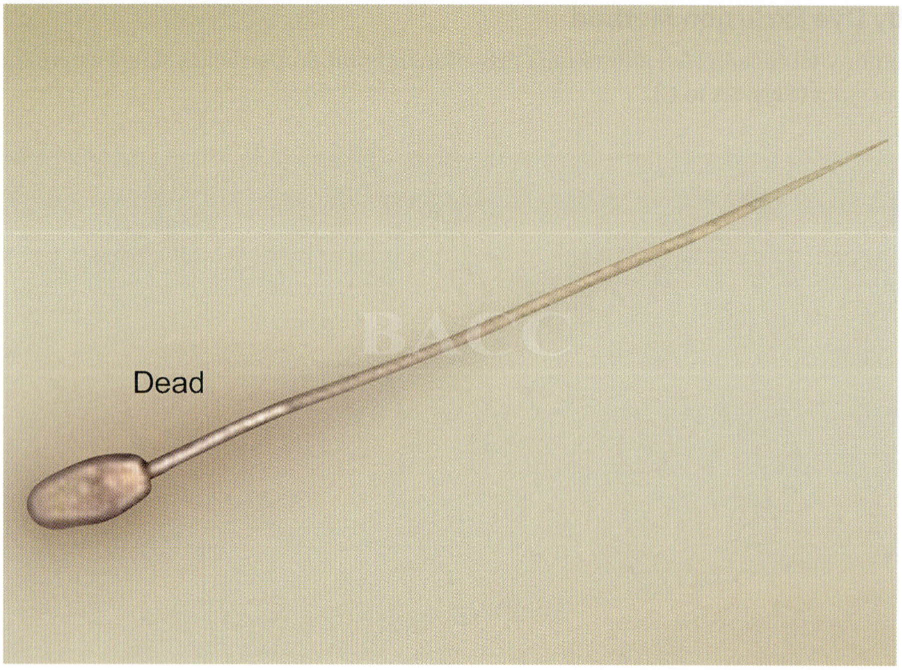

Fig. 5C: Sperm viability by staining. Eosin-Nigrosin stained smear showing, uptake of the dye by the sperm, indicating nonviability.

DEOXYRIBONUCLEIC ACID FRAGMENTATION INDEX

Deoxyribonucleic acid (DNA) integrity is important for normal embryo development. The term "DNA fragmentation" refers to denatured or damaged sperm DNA that cannot be repaired **(Figs. 6A and B)** shows the image of DNA fragmentation index (DFI).

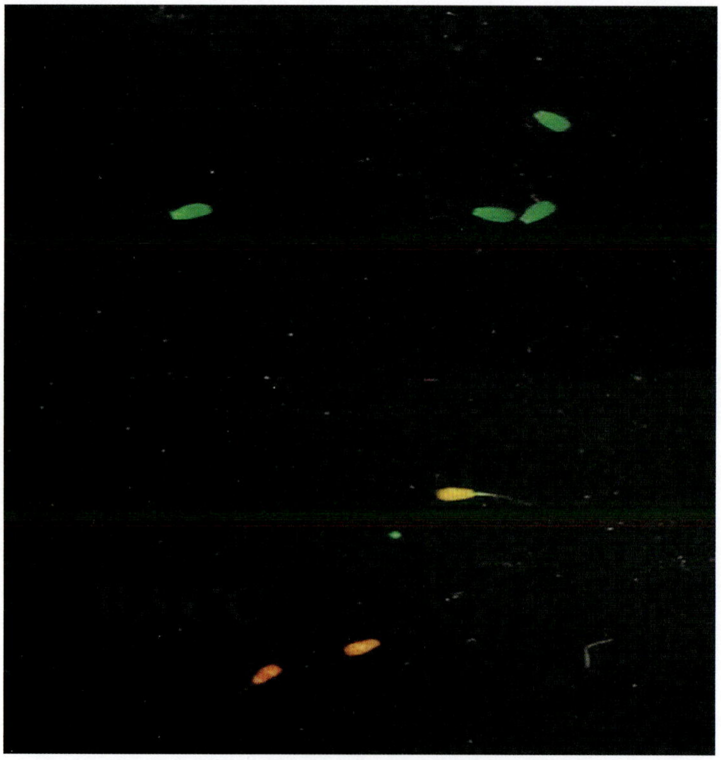

Fig. 6A: Deoxyribonucleic acid fragmentation index.

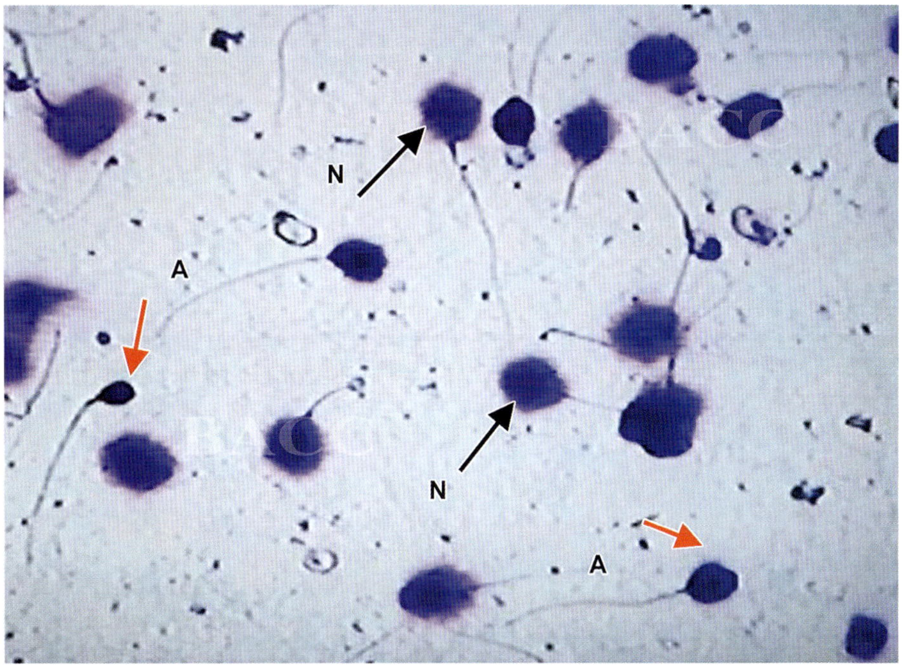

Fig. 6B: Deoxyribonucleic acid fragmentation index (DFI) using halosperm (based on SCD technique) where the normal forms show the halo and the sperms with abnormal DNA does not show halo. "A" represents sperms with fragmented DNA and "N" represents sperm cells with normal DNA.

REFERENCE

1. World Health Organization. WHO laboratory manual for the examination and processing of human semen, 2010.

CHAPTER 131

Normal Embryo Development

Bezar Ghan VV, Divyashree PS, Kamini A Rao

INTRODUCTION

Knowledge of the nature of embryo growth, and the handling and scoring of quality in human embryos are significant aspects for embryologists in in vitro fertilization (IVF) clinics.

Timing and reporting of observation of fertilized oocytes and embryos is very critical. This is because comparison of results between different laboratories becomes much easier and standardized.

According to Istanbul consensus 2011,[1] the expected stage of development at different points of time was standardized which is depicted in **Table 1** and **Figures 1 to 8**. The times given reflect the times at which these events occur in the majority of patients/cases.

TABLE 1: Timing of observation of fertilized oocytes and embryos and expected stage of development at each time point.

Type of observation	*Timing (hour postinsemination)*	*Expected stage of development*
Fertilization check (2 PN)	17 ± 1	Pronuclear stage
Syngamy check	23 ± 1 (post-ICSI) 28 ± 1 (post-IVF)	Expect 50% to be in syngamy (up to 20% may be at the two-cell stage)
Early cleavage	26 ± 1	Post-ICSI two-cell stage
Day-2 embryo assessment	44 ± 1	Four-cell stage
Day-3 embryo assessment	68 ± 1	Eight-cell stage
Day-4 embryo assessment	92 ± 2	Morula
Day-5 embryo assessment	116 ± 2	Blastocyst

(ICSI: intracytoplasmic sperm injection; IVF: in vitro fertilization; PN: pronuclear)

PRONUCLEAR STAGE (FIG. 1)

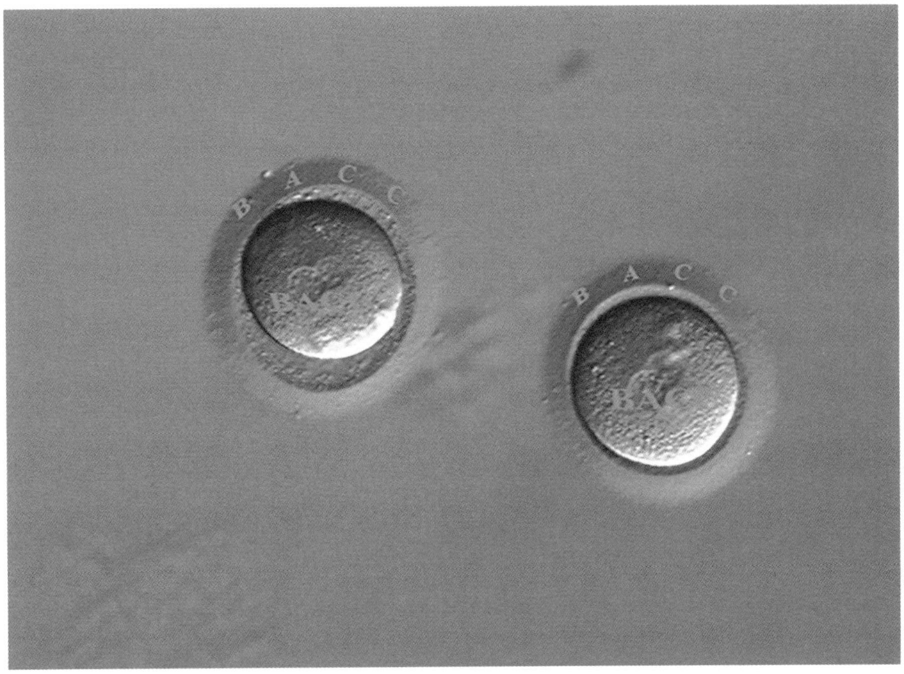

Fig. 1: Normally fertilized human oocytes in pronuclear stage, showing two prominent pronuclei and distinct nuclear precursor bodies.

SYNGAMY (FIG. 2)

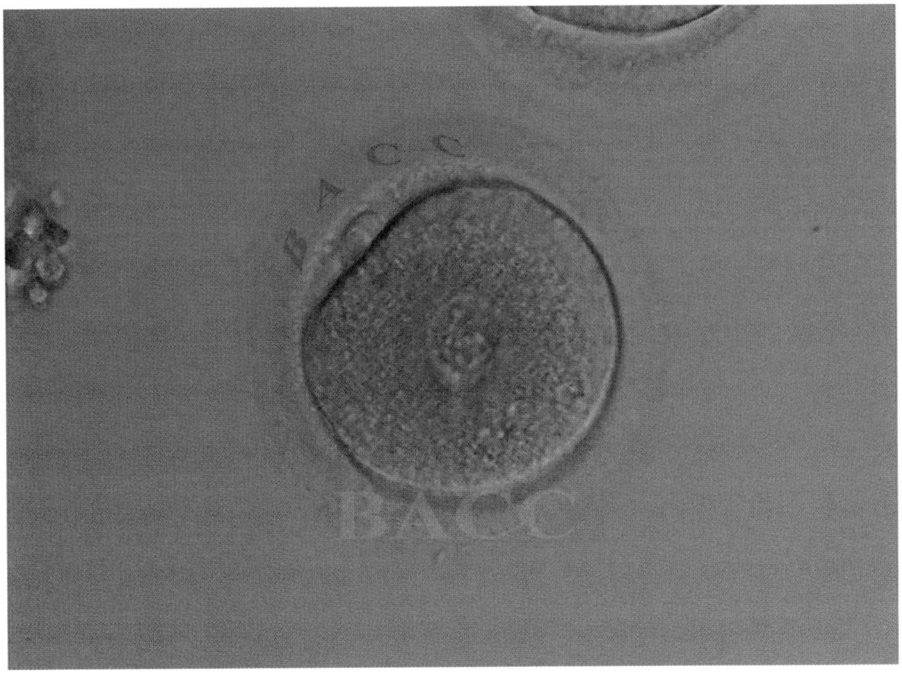

Fig. 2: Normally fertilized oocyte in syngamy. Note the fusion of two pronuclei.

TWO-CELL STAGE (FIG. 3)

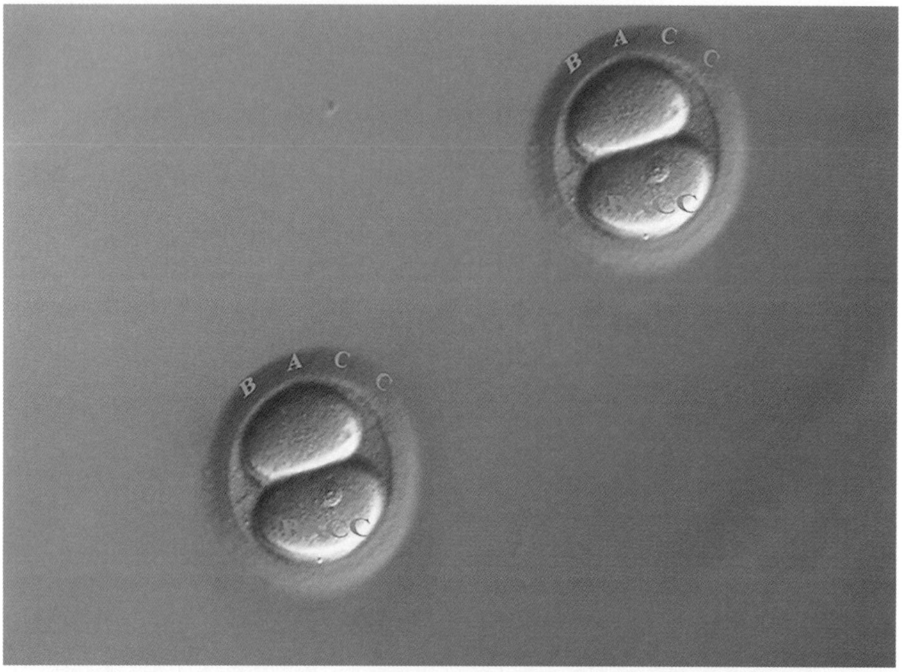

Fig. 3: Two-cell human embryo at 26 hours postinsemination. Nuclei are not visible and the elongated appearance of individual cells depicts further cell division is impending.

FOUR-CELL STAGE (FIG. 4)

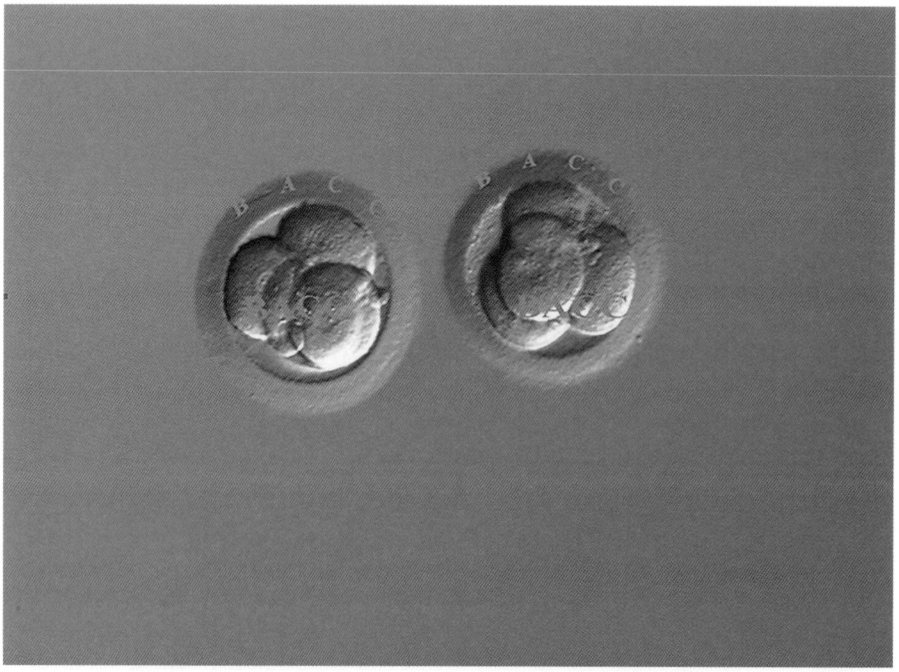

Fig. 4: Four-cell stage human embryo, 44 hours postinsemination.

EIGHT-CELL STAGE (FIG. 5)

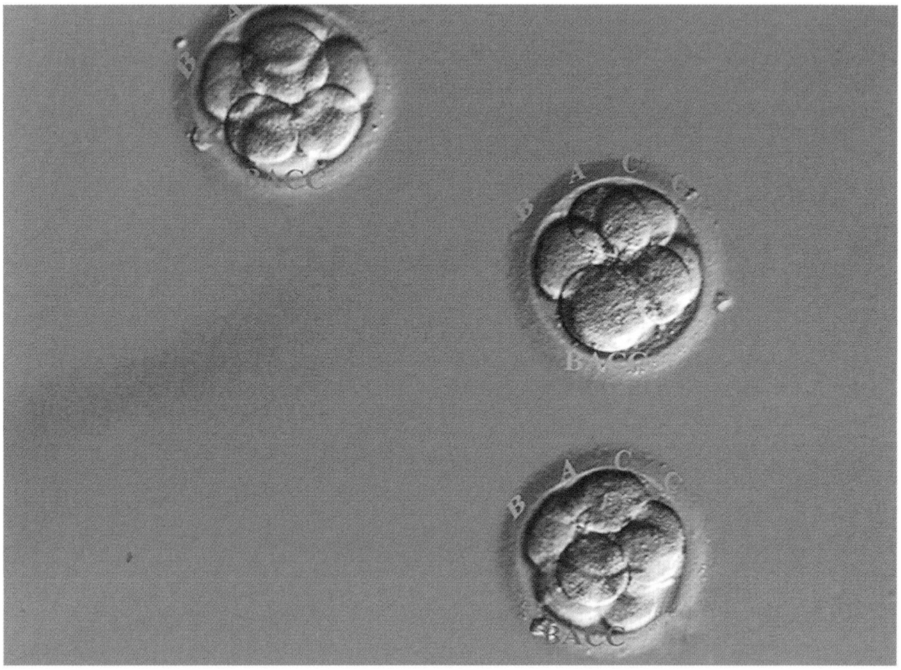

Fig. 5: An eight-cell embryo, 68 hours postinsemination.

COMPACTION (FIG. 6)

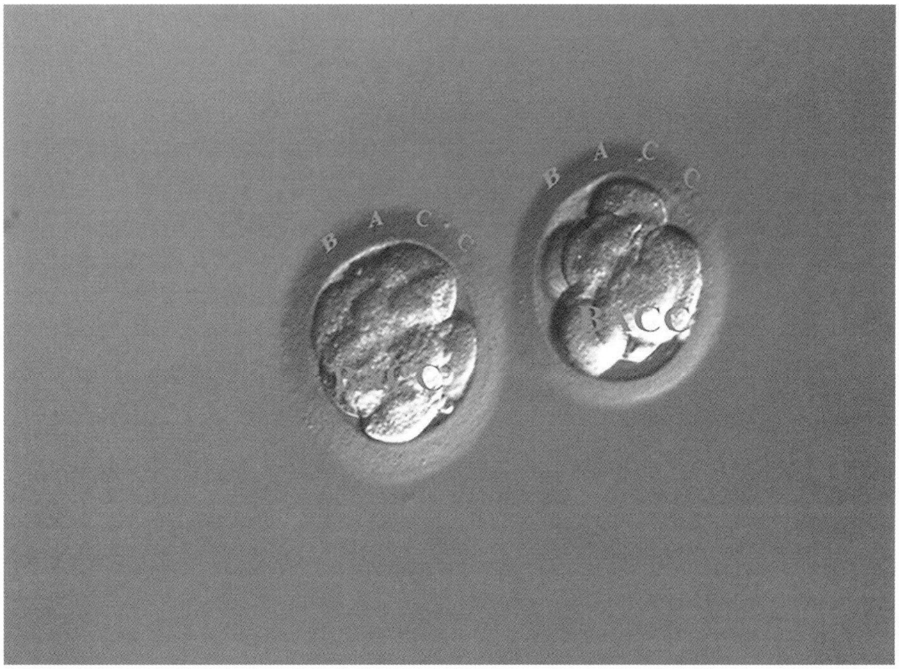

Fig. 6: Human embryo, 92 hours postinsemination. Note compaction, with cell membranes closely applied as tight junctions begin to form.

EARLY BLASTOCYSTS (FIG. 7A)

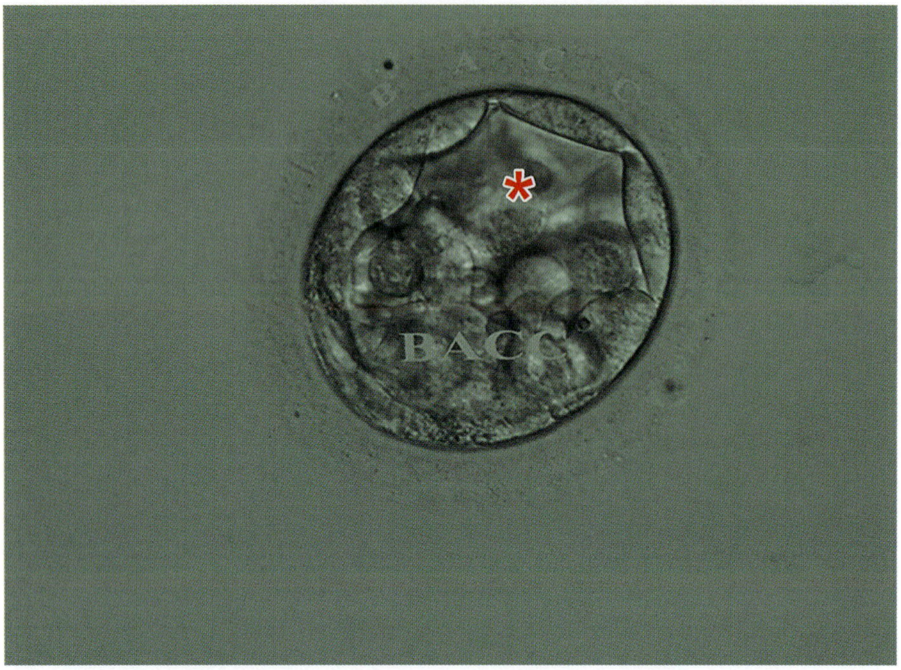

Fig. 7A: Human embryo in early blastocyst stage. Note the appearance of early cavity (asterix).

EXPANDED BLASTOCYSTS (FIG. 7B)

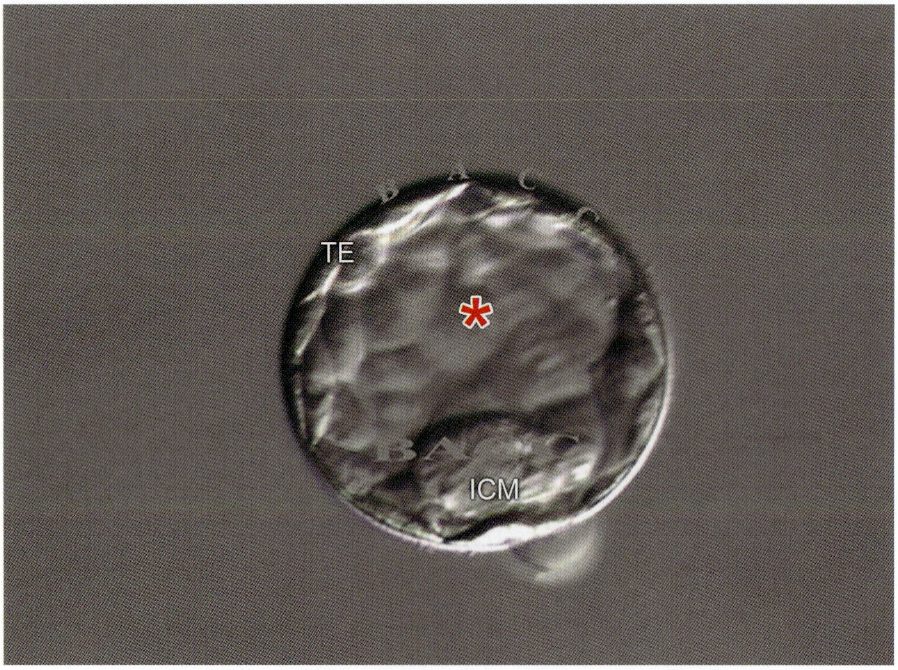

Fig. 7B: Fully expanded blastocyst, showing distinct inner cell mass (ICM), trophectoderm (TE) cells and blastocele cavity (asterix).

HATCHING BLASTOCYSTS (FIG. 7C)

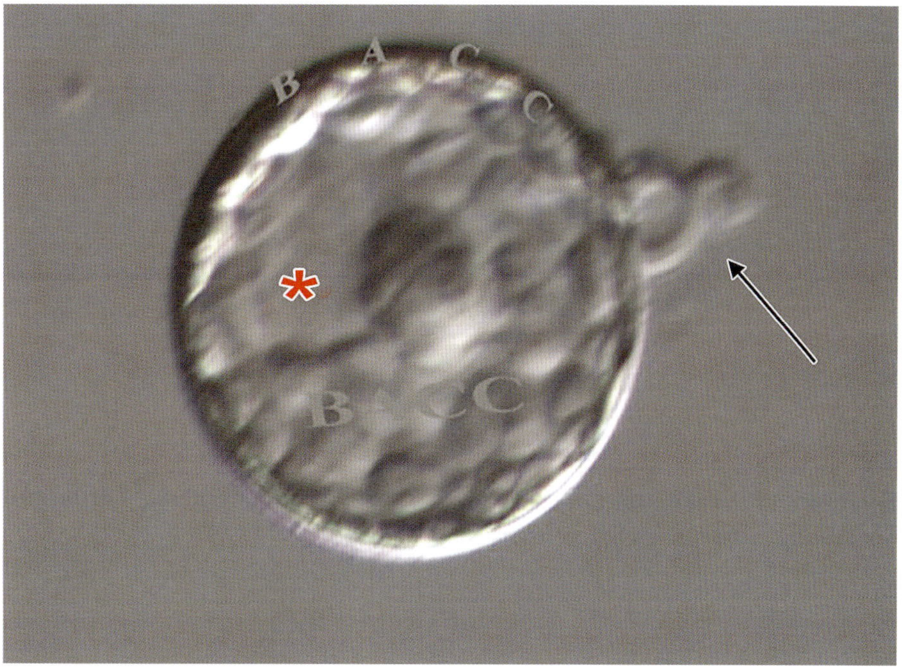

Fig. 7C: Early hatching of the blastocyst. Note the breaching of zona at the point of hatching (arrow) asterix-blastocele cavity.

HATCHED BLASTOCYSTS (FIG. 8)

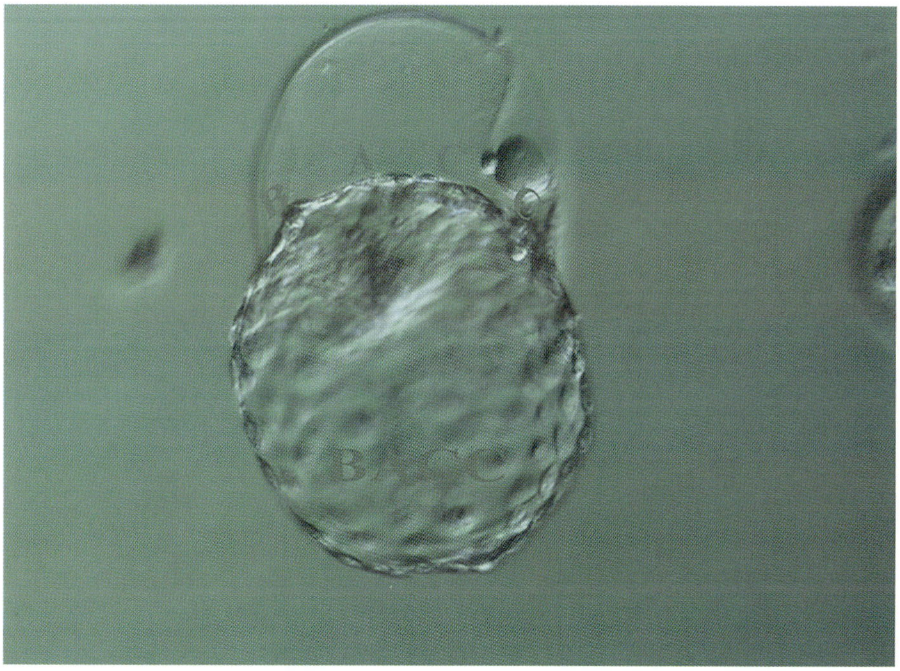

Fig. 8: Fully hatched blastocyst. Note the empty zona after blastocyst hatching.

REFERENCE

1. ALPHA Scientists in Reproductive Medicine and ESHRE Special Interest Group Embryology. Istanbul consensus workshop on embryo assessment: proceedings of an expert meeting. Reprod BioMed Online. 2011;22:632-46.

CHAPTER 132

Embryo Scoring

Bezar Ghan VV, Divyashree PS, Anitha S Kumari K, Mohammed Ashraf C

INTRODUCTION

For standardized reporting and to minimize diversities in reporting of embryo scoring, Istanbul global consensus scoring system for embryo[1] has been used in the present chapter **(Tables 1 to 4)**.

TABLE 1: Consensus scoring system for pronuclei (Figs. 1 to 3).

Category	*Rating*	*Description*
1	Symmetrical	Equivalent to Z1 and Z2
2	Nonsymmetrical	Other arrangements, including peripherally sited pronuclei
3	Abnormal	Pronuclei with 0 or 1 nucleolar precursor bodies (NPBs)

SYMMETRICAL PRONUCLEI (FIGS. 1A TO C)

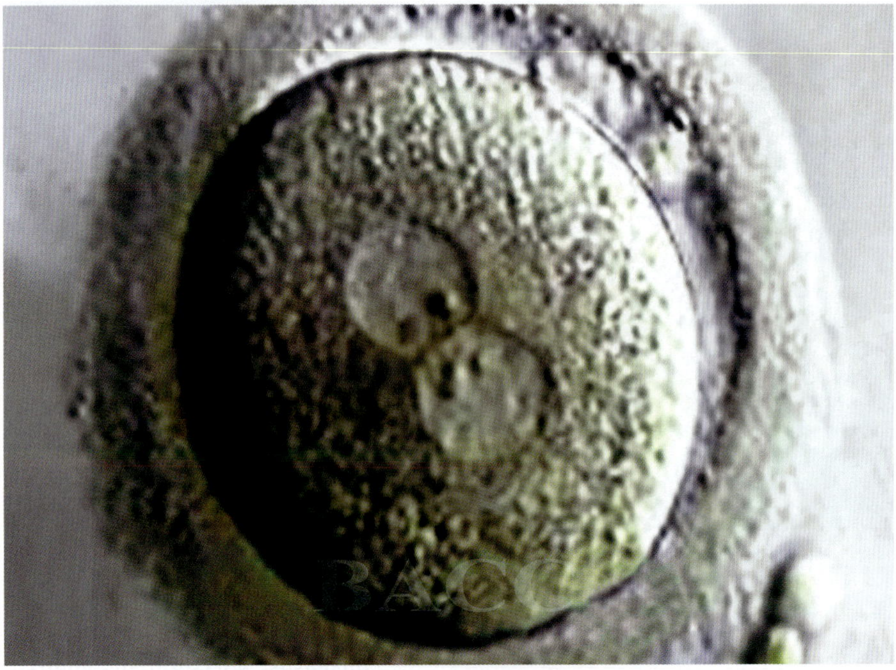

Fig. 1A: Human embryo in the pronuclear stage with two symmetrical pronuclei, equal number of nuclear precursor bodies (NPBs2), in juxtaposition and two polar bodies at 1 o'clock position.

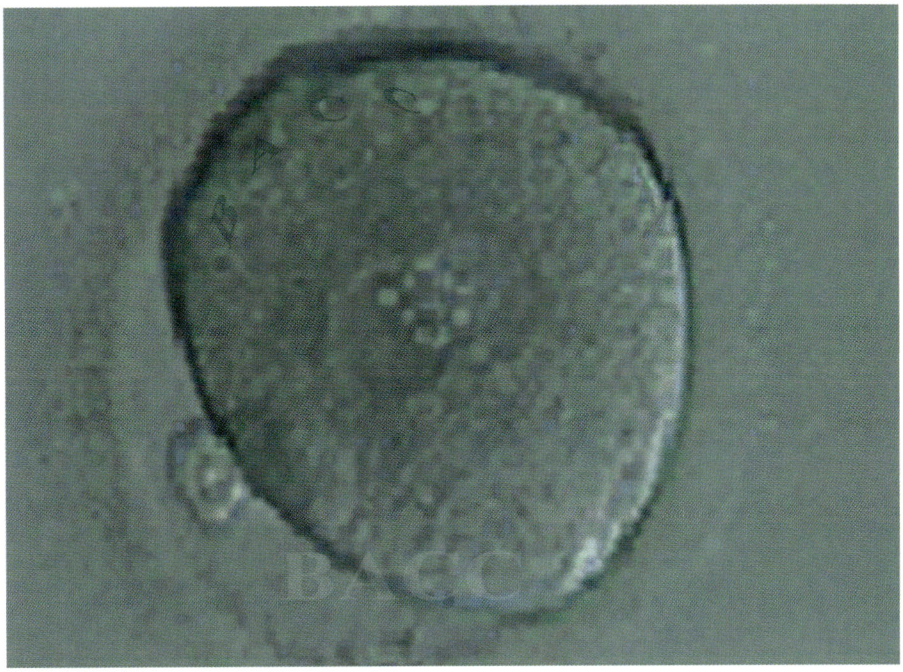

Fig. 1B: Pronuclear stage embryo with centrally located symmetrical pronuclei, juxtaposed and equal nuclear precursor bodies (NPBs3), two interposed polar bodies at 8 o'clock position.

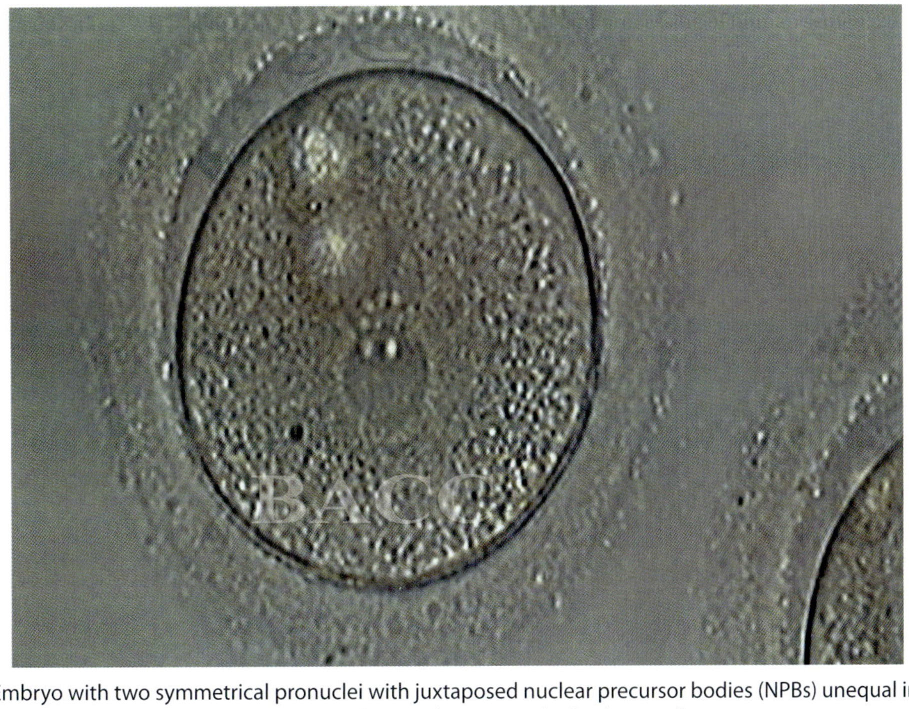

Fig. 1C: Embryo with two symmetrical pronuclei with juxtaposed nuclear precursor bodies (NPBs) unequal in number. Two polar bodies can be seen at the background.

NONSYMMETRICAL PRONUCLEI (FIGS. 2A AND B)

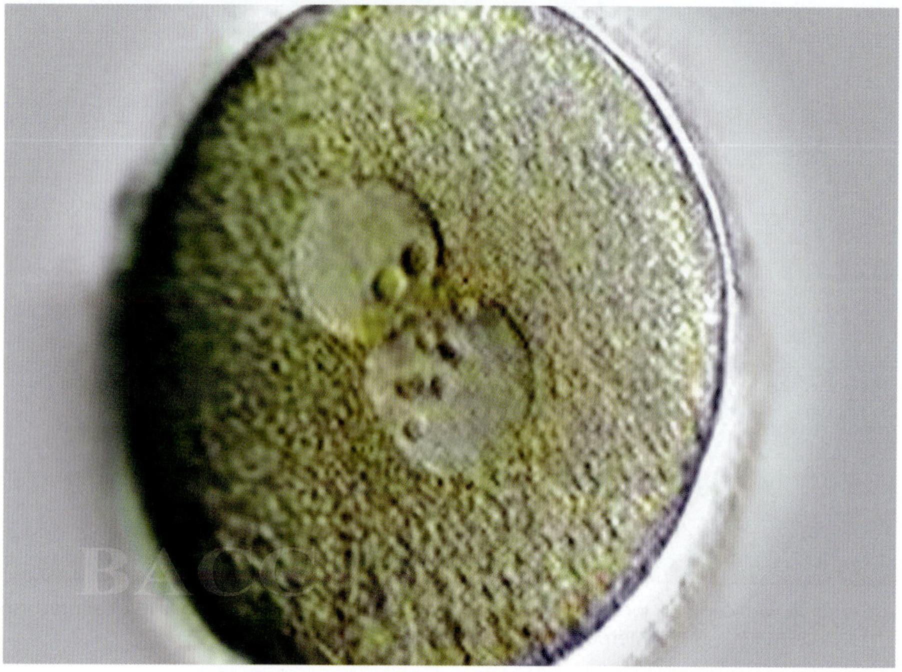

Fig. 2A: Human embryo in pronuclear stage, with two unequal pronuclei, and juxtaposed nuclear precursor bodies (NPBs) unequal in number.

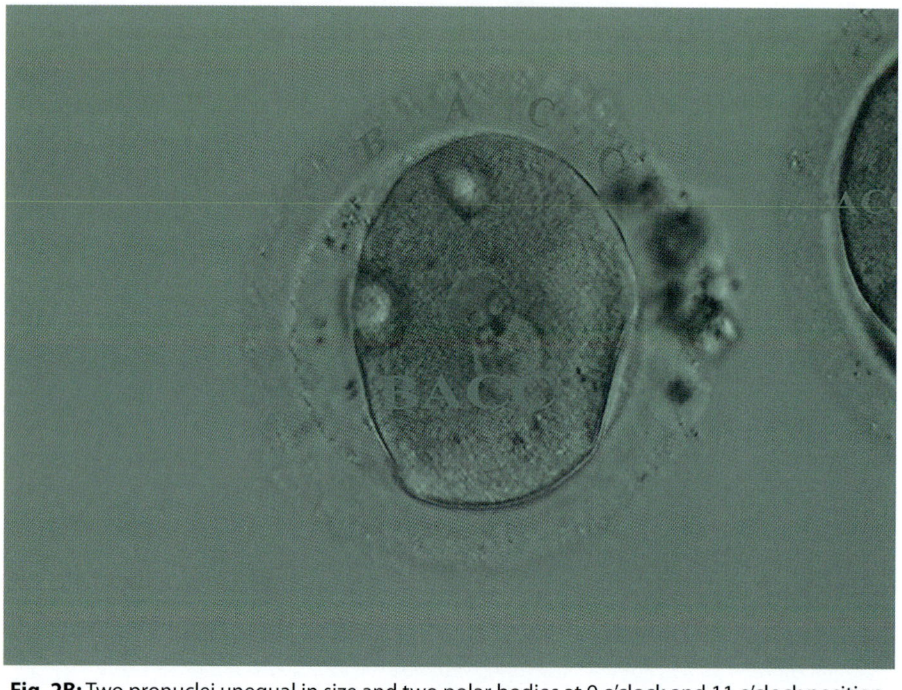

Fig. 2B: Two pronuclei unequal in size and two polar bodies at 9 o'clock and 11 o'clock position.

ABNORMAL PRONUCLEI (FIGS. 3A TO C)

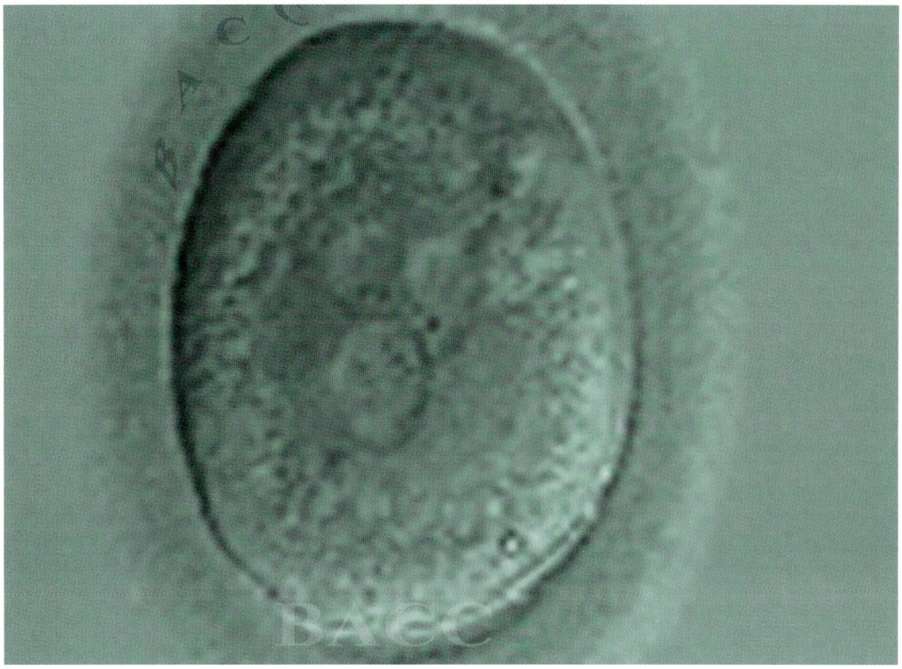

Fig. 3A: Abnormal zygote with three pronuclei.

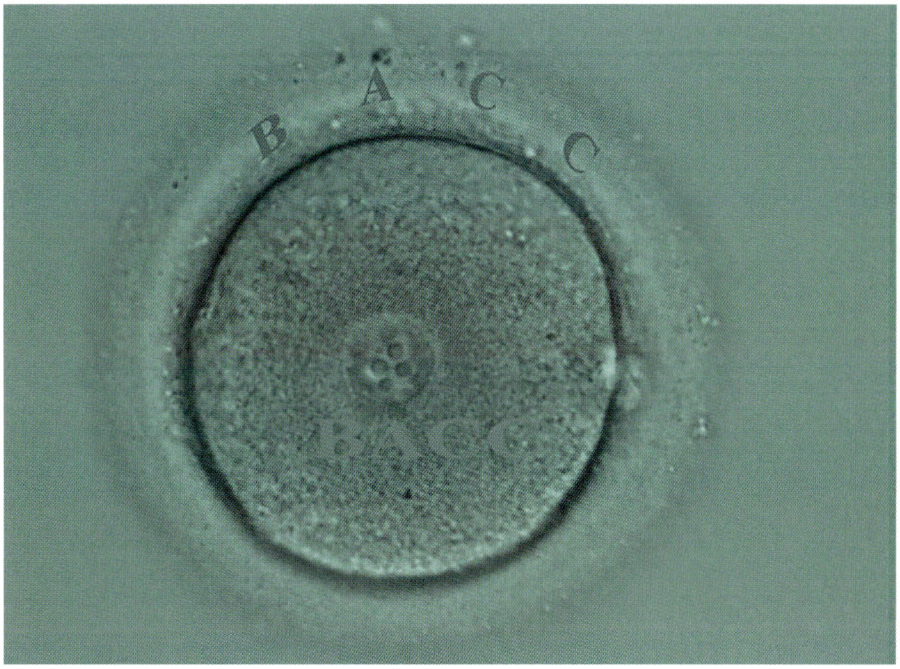

Fig. 3B: An unfertilized, parthenogenetically activated human oocyte showing one prominent pronucleus and one of the two polar bodies.

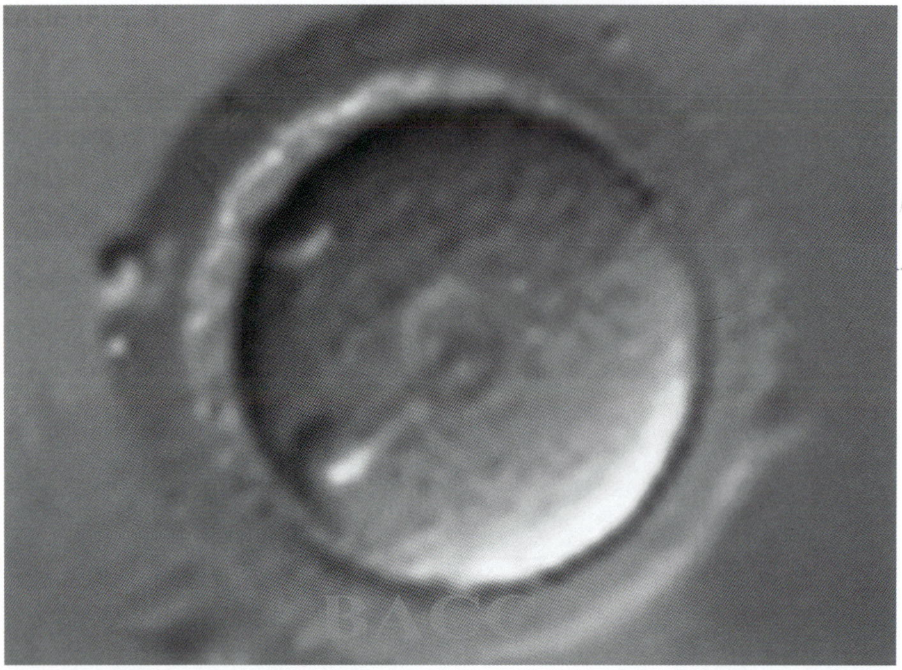

Fig. 3C: Abnormal zygote with single bulls-eye pronucleus (pronucleus with single NPB) and two polar bodies.

TABLE 2: Consensus scoring system for cleavage-stage embryos (in addition to cell number) (Figs. 4 to 6).

Grade	*Rating*	*Description*
1	Good	<10% fragmentation Stage-specific cell size No multinucleation
2	Fair	10–25% fragmentation Stage-specific cell size for majority of cells No evidence of multinucleation
3	Poor	Severe fragmentation (>25%) cell-size not stage-specific Evidence of multinucleation

TABLE 3: Consensus scoring system for day 4 embryos (Figs. 7A to F).

Grade	*Rating*	*Description*
1	Good	Entered into a fourth round of cleavage Evidence of compaction that involves virtually all the embryo volume
2	Fair	Entered into a fourth round of cleavage Compaction involves the majority of the volume of the embryo
3	Poor	Disproportionate compaction involving less than half of the embryo, with two or three cells remaining as discrete blastomeres

TWO-CELL GRADE 1 EMBRYOS (FIGS. 4A AND B)

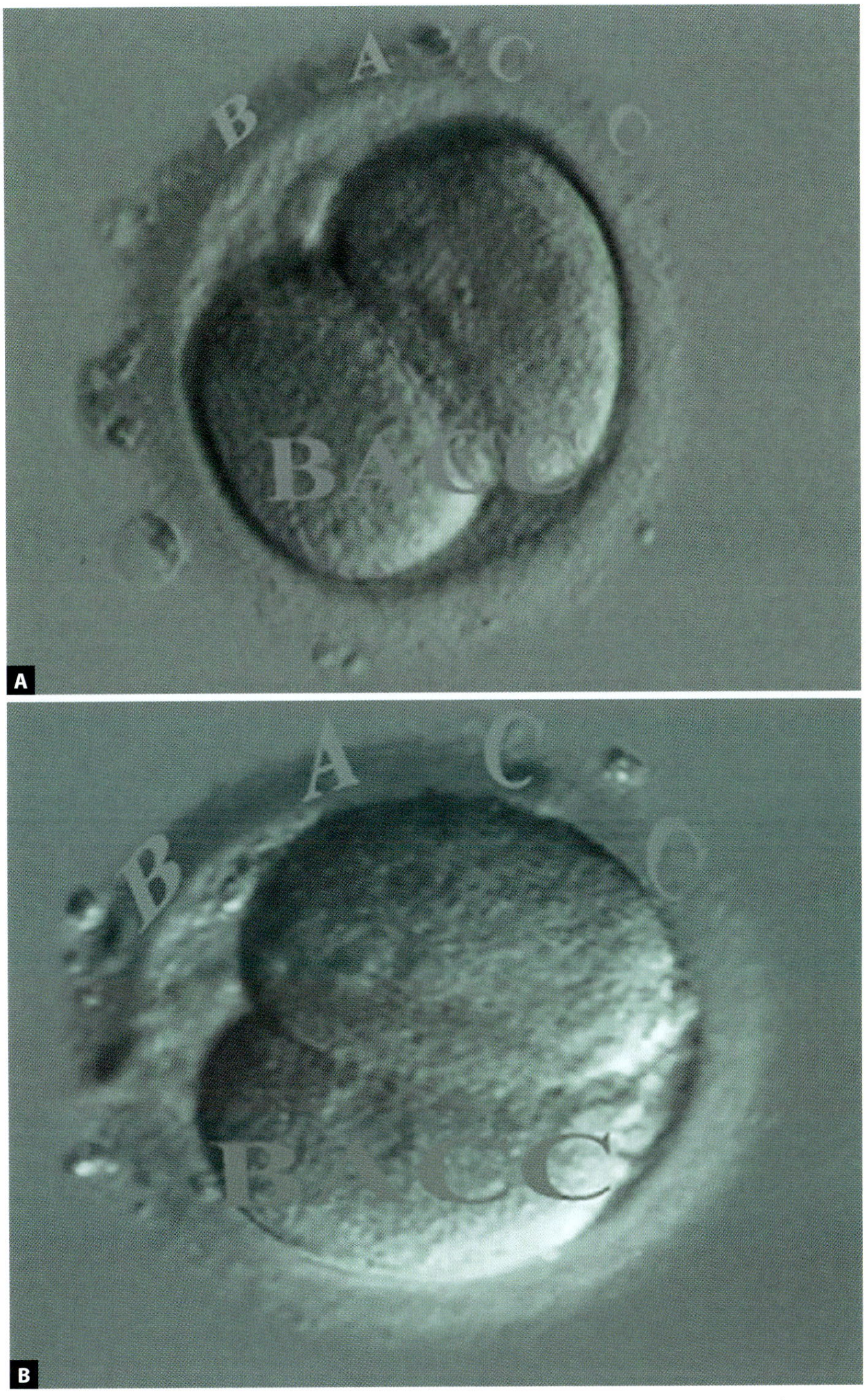

Figs. 4A and B: Two-cell, grade 1 human embryos. Note the stage-specific cell size and less than 10% fragmentation.

TWO-CELL GRADE 2 EMBRYOS (FIGS. 4C AND D)

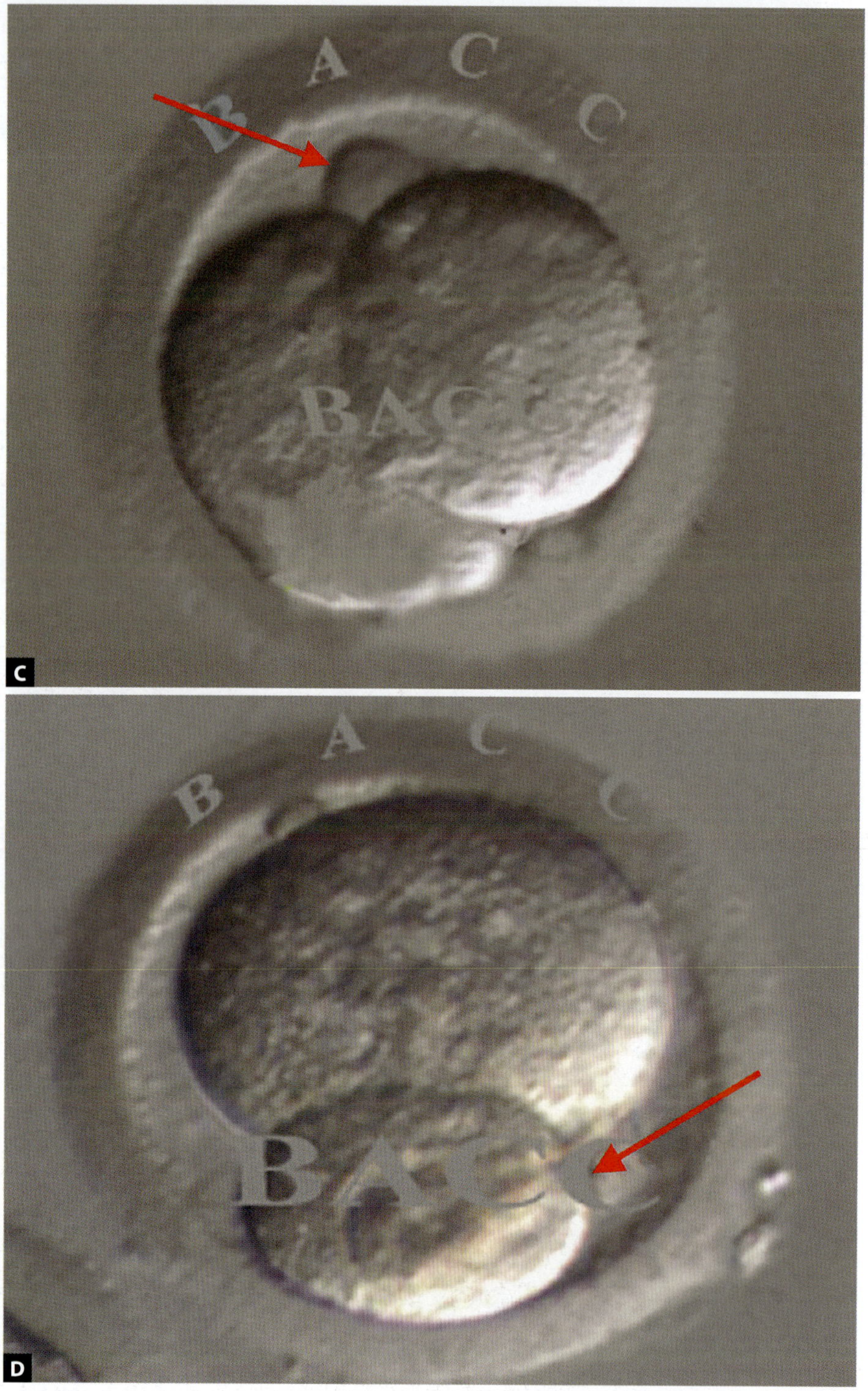

Figs. 4C and D: Two-cell, grade 2 human embryos. Note unequal blastomeres and fragmentation (arrows).

FOUR-CELL GRADE 1 EMBRYOS (FIGS. 5A AND B)

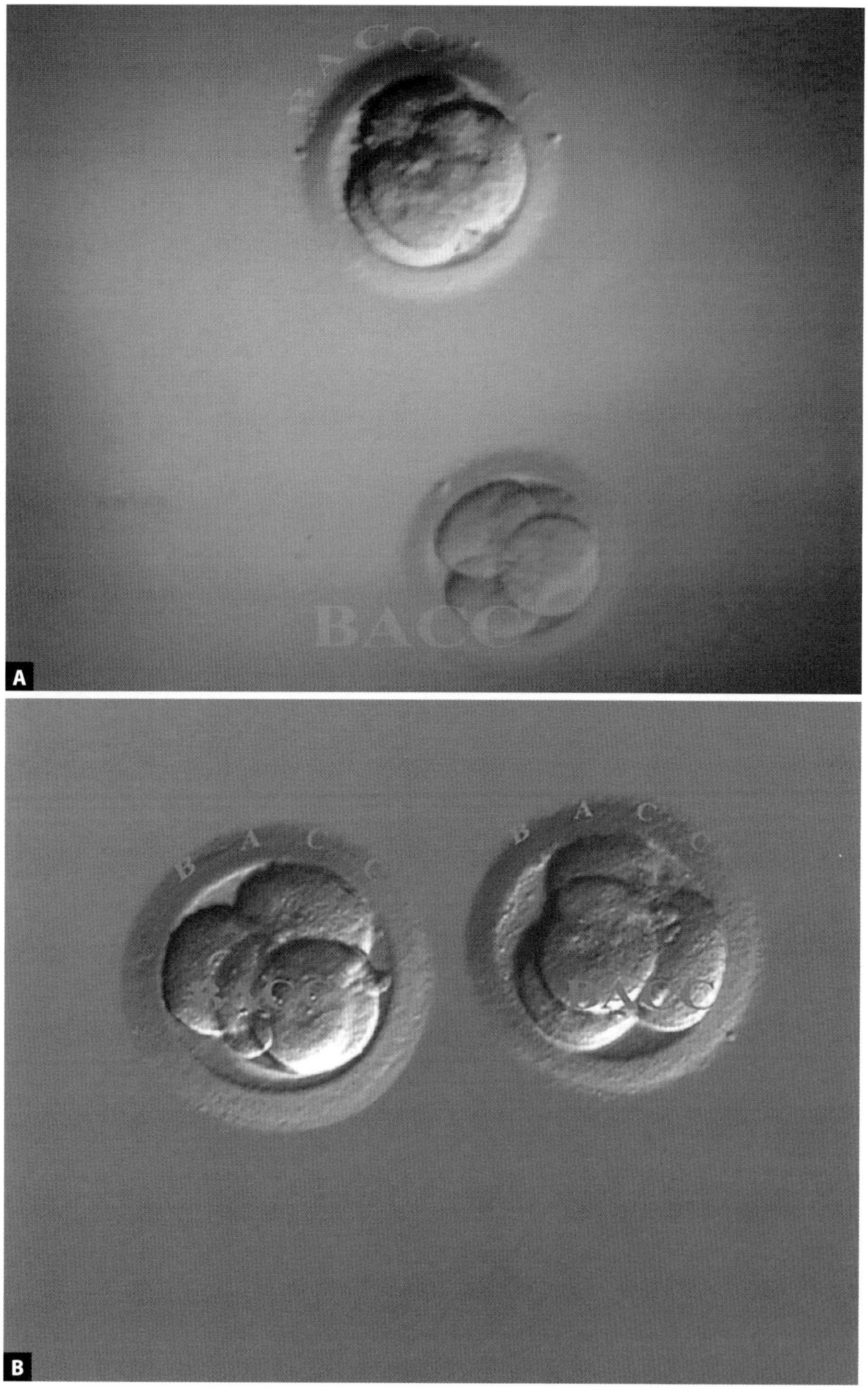

Figs. 5A and B: Four-cell, grade 1 human embryos. Note the stage-specific cell size and no fragmentation.

FOUR-CELL GRADE 2 EMBRYOS (FIGS. 5C AND D)

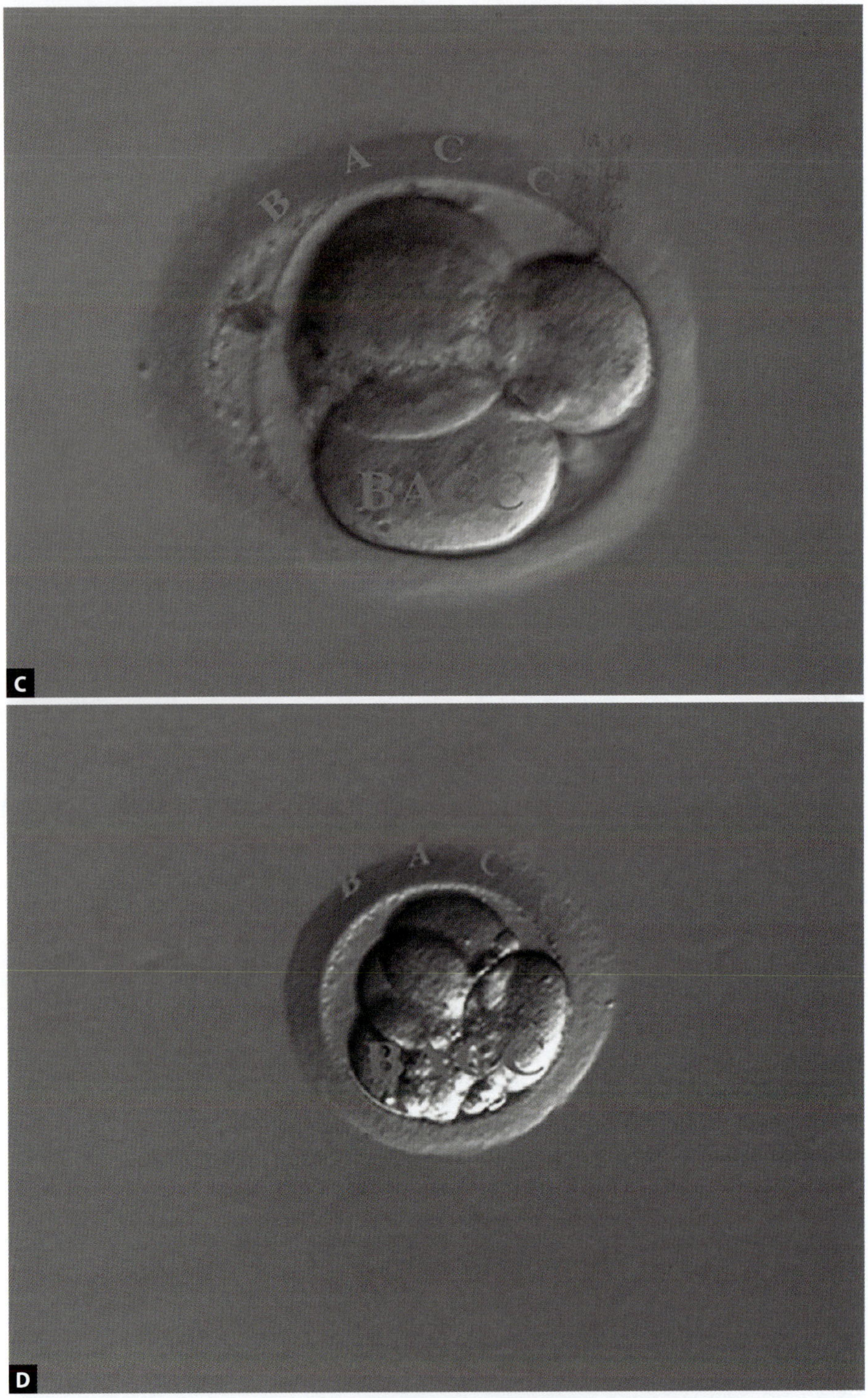

Figs. 5C and D: Four-cell, grade 2 human embryos (Note stage-specific cell size for majority of cells in Figure C and less than 25% fragmentation in Figure D).

FOUR-CELL GRADE 3 EMBRYOS (FIGS. 5E AND F)

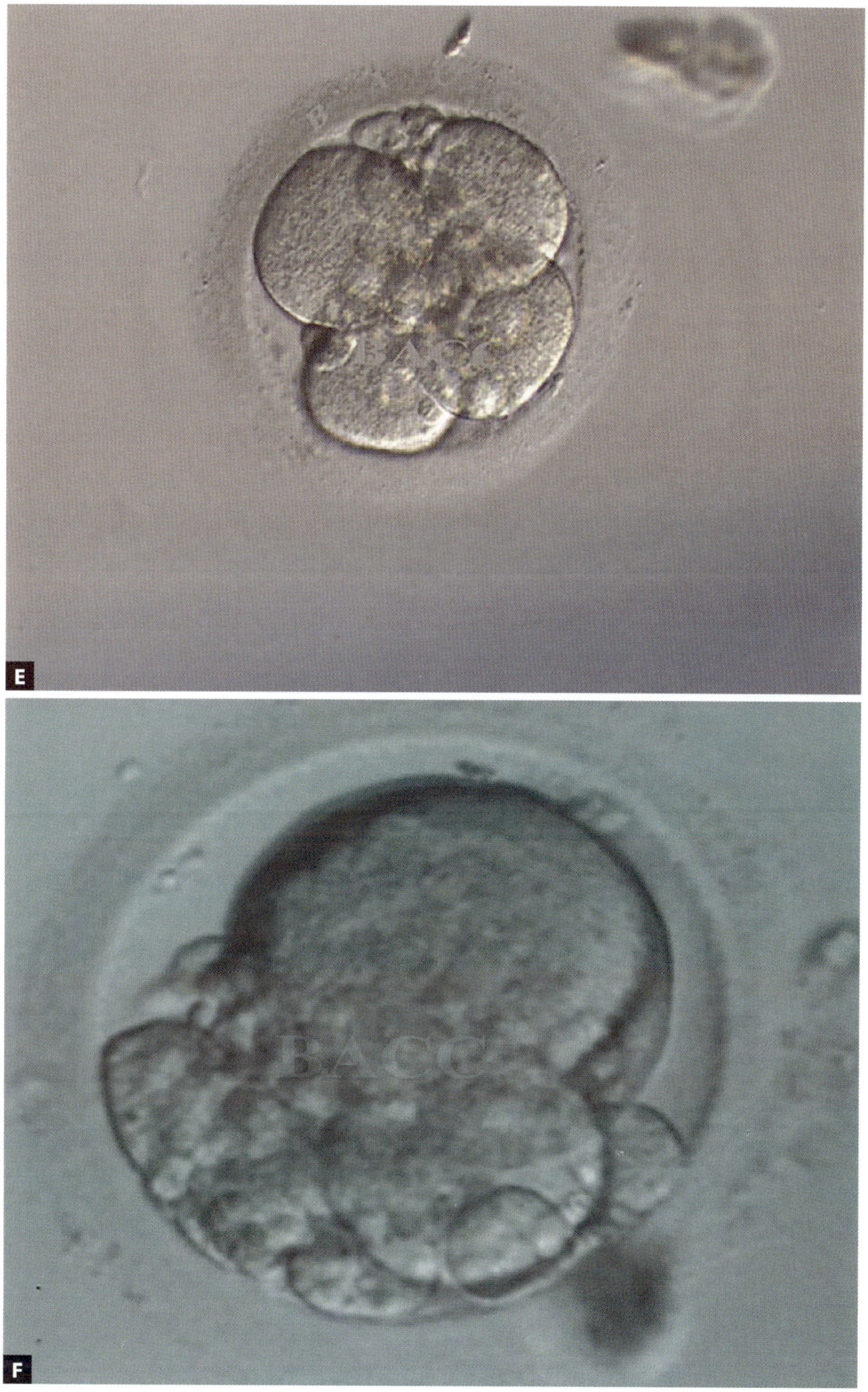

Figs. 5E and F: Four-cell, grade 3 human embryos (Note more than 25% fragmentation in Figure E, unequal blastomeres with fragmentation in Figure F).

EIGHT-CELL GRADE 1 EMBRYOS (FIGS. 6A AND B)

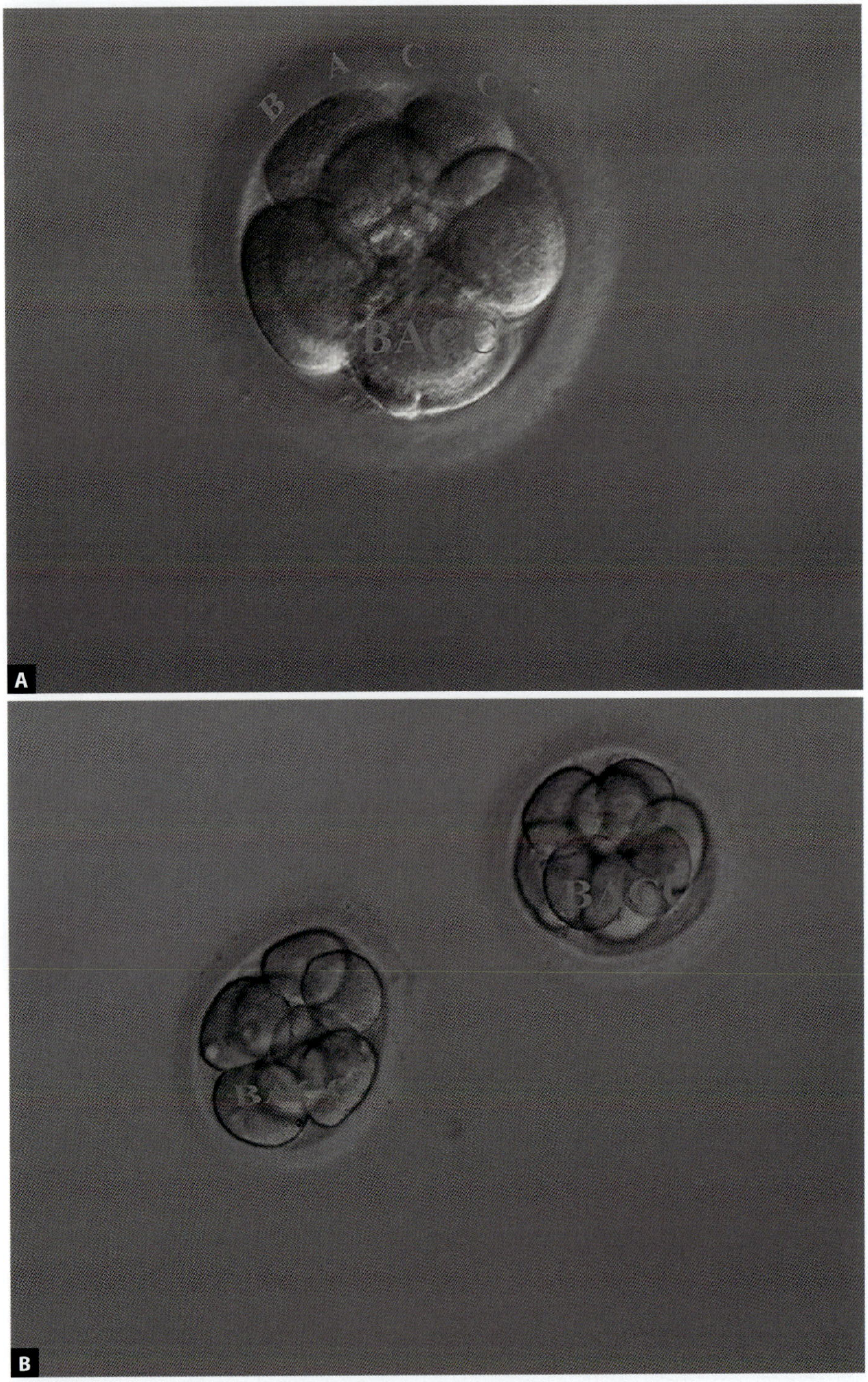

Figs. 6A and B: Eight-cell, grade 1 human embryos. Note the stage-specific cell size and no fragmentation.

EIGHT-CELL GRADE 2 EMBRYOS (FIGS. 6C AND D)

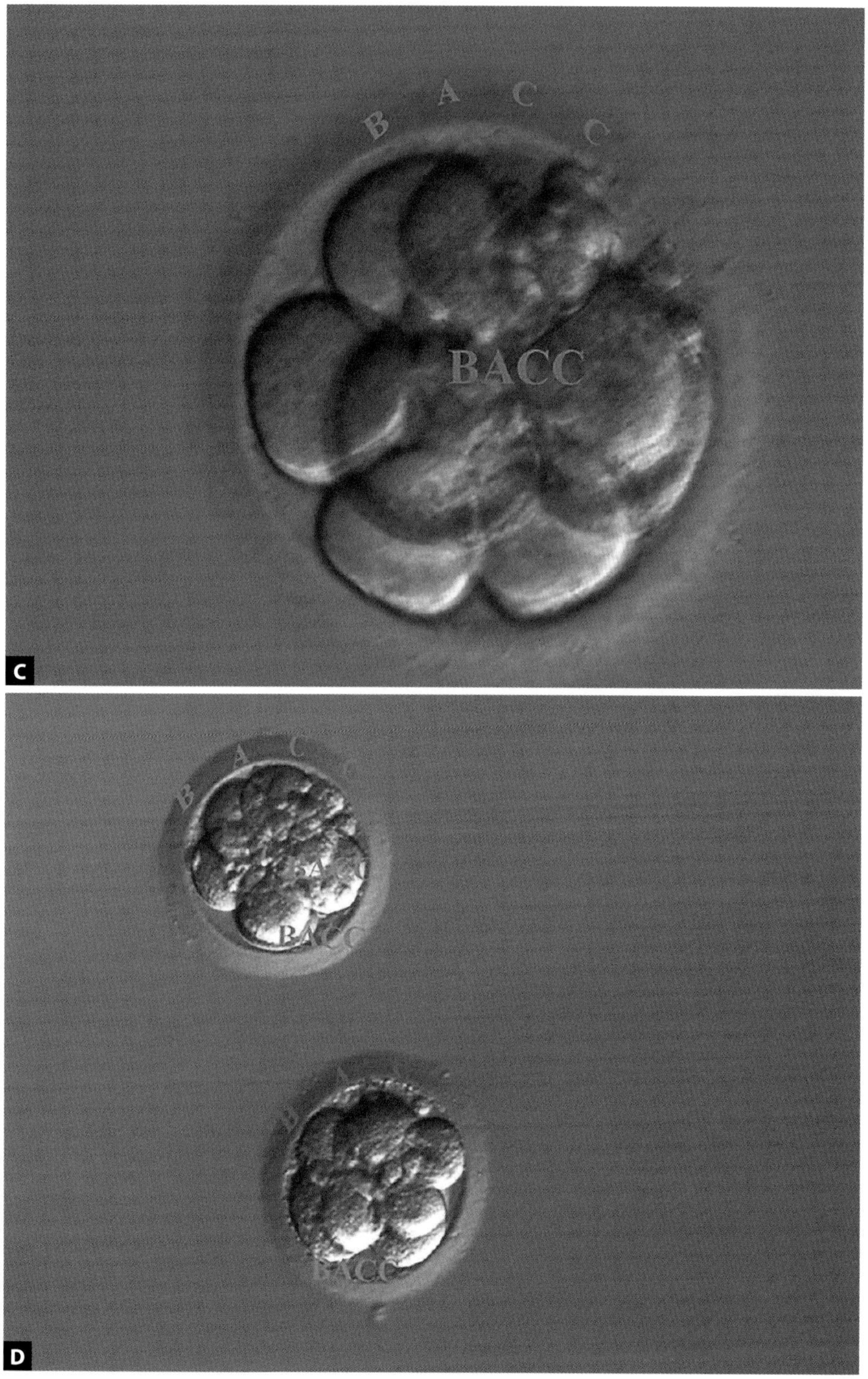

Figs. 6C and D: Eight-cell, grade 2 human embryos. Note less than 25% fragmentation.

EIGHT-CELL GRADE 3 EMBRYOS (FIGS. 6E AND F)

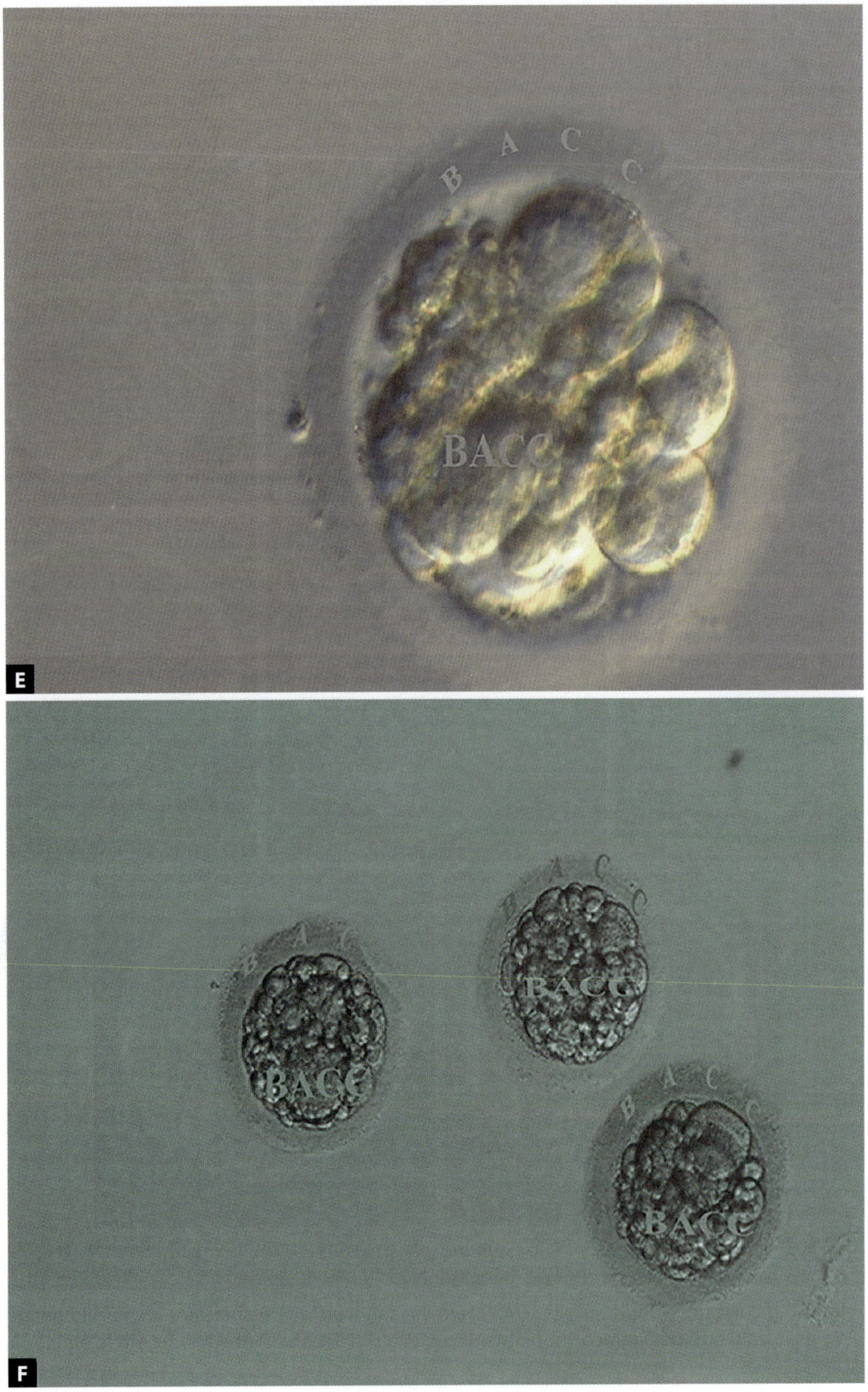

Figs. 6E and F: Eight-cell, grade 3 human embryos. Note more than 25% fragmentation.

GRADE 1, DAY 4 EMBRYOS (FIGS. 7A AND B)

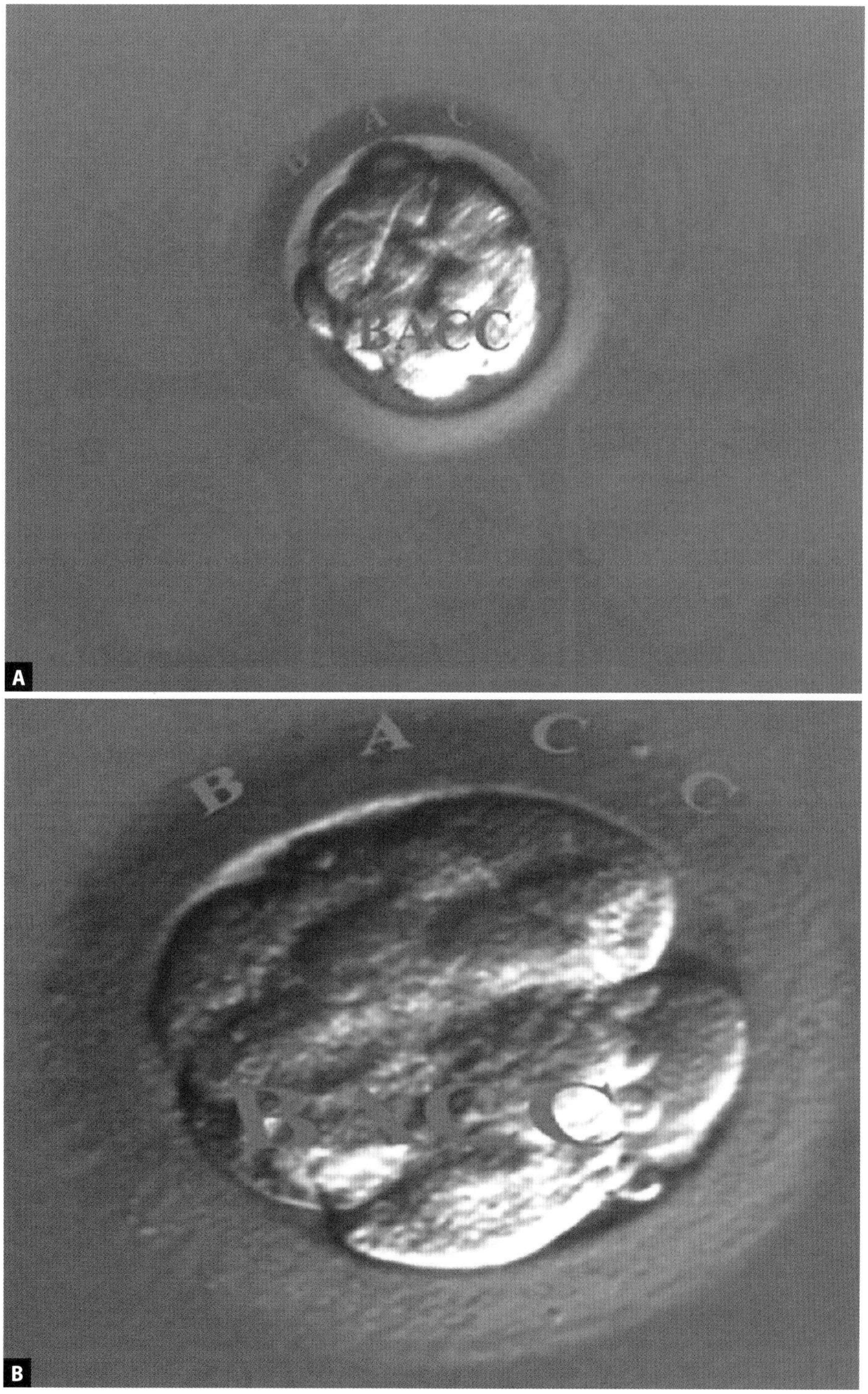

Figs. 7A and B: Grade 1, day 4 embryos with evidence of compaction involving almost all the embryo volume.

GRADE 2, DAY 4 EMBRYOS (FIGS. 7C AND D)

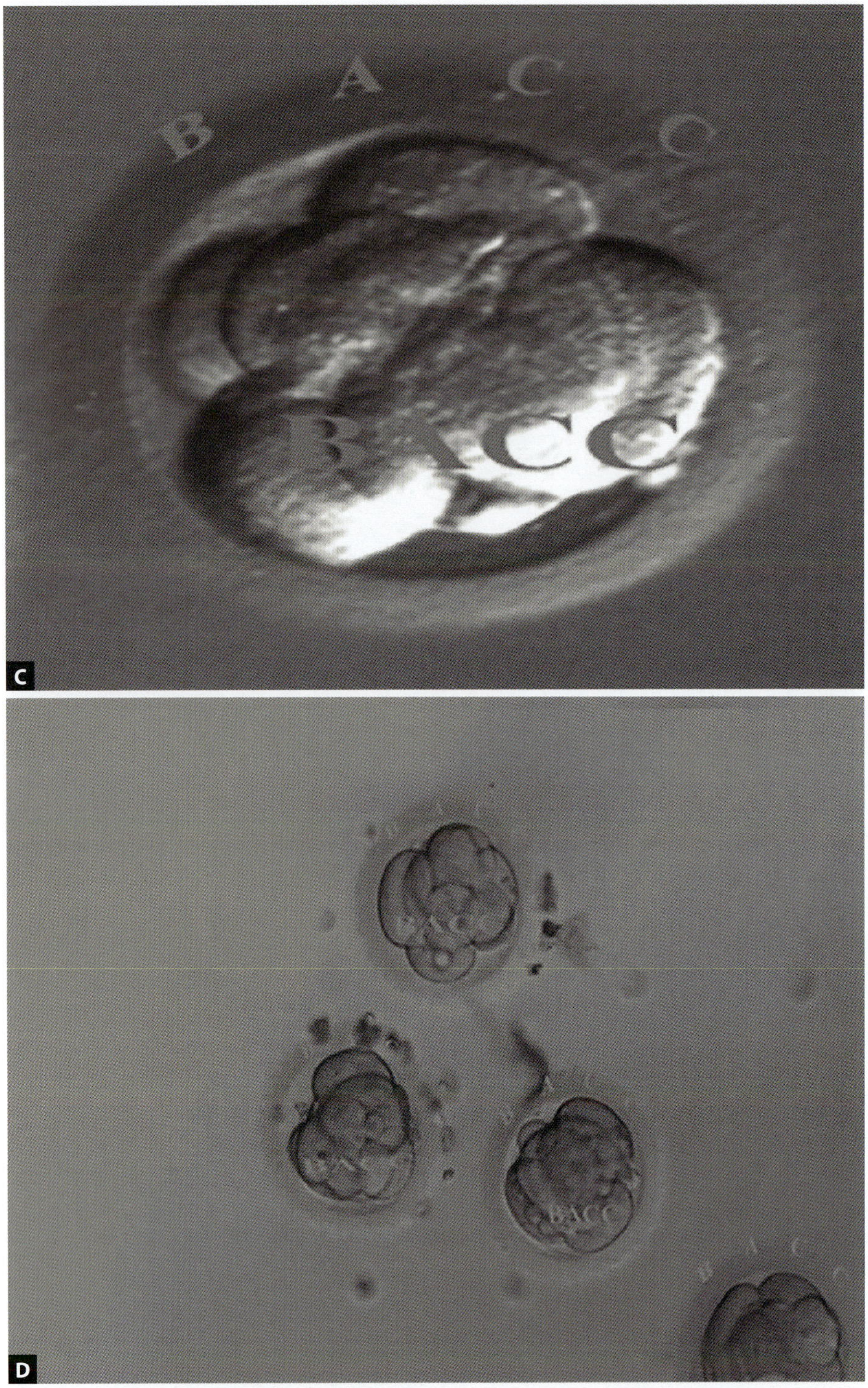

Figs. 7C and D: Grade 2, day 4 embryos with compaction involving majority of the embryo volume.

GRADE 3, DAY 4 EMBRYOS (FIGS. 7E AND F)

The scoring system for blastocysts is a combination of the stage of development and of the grade of the inner cell mass (ICM) and of the trophectoderm (TE). It is a numerical interpretation of the Gardner scale.[2,3] The "*stages of development*" is graded as:

- *Early blastocyst*: Cavity is just beginning to form and cell types not distinguishable.
- *Expanded blastocyst*: Cavity is fully formed, contains 100–125 cells, and is still contained in zona pellucida (ZP).

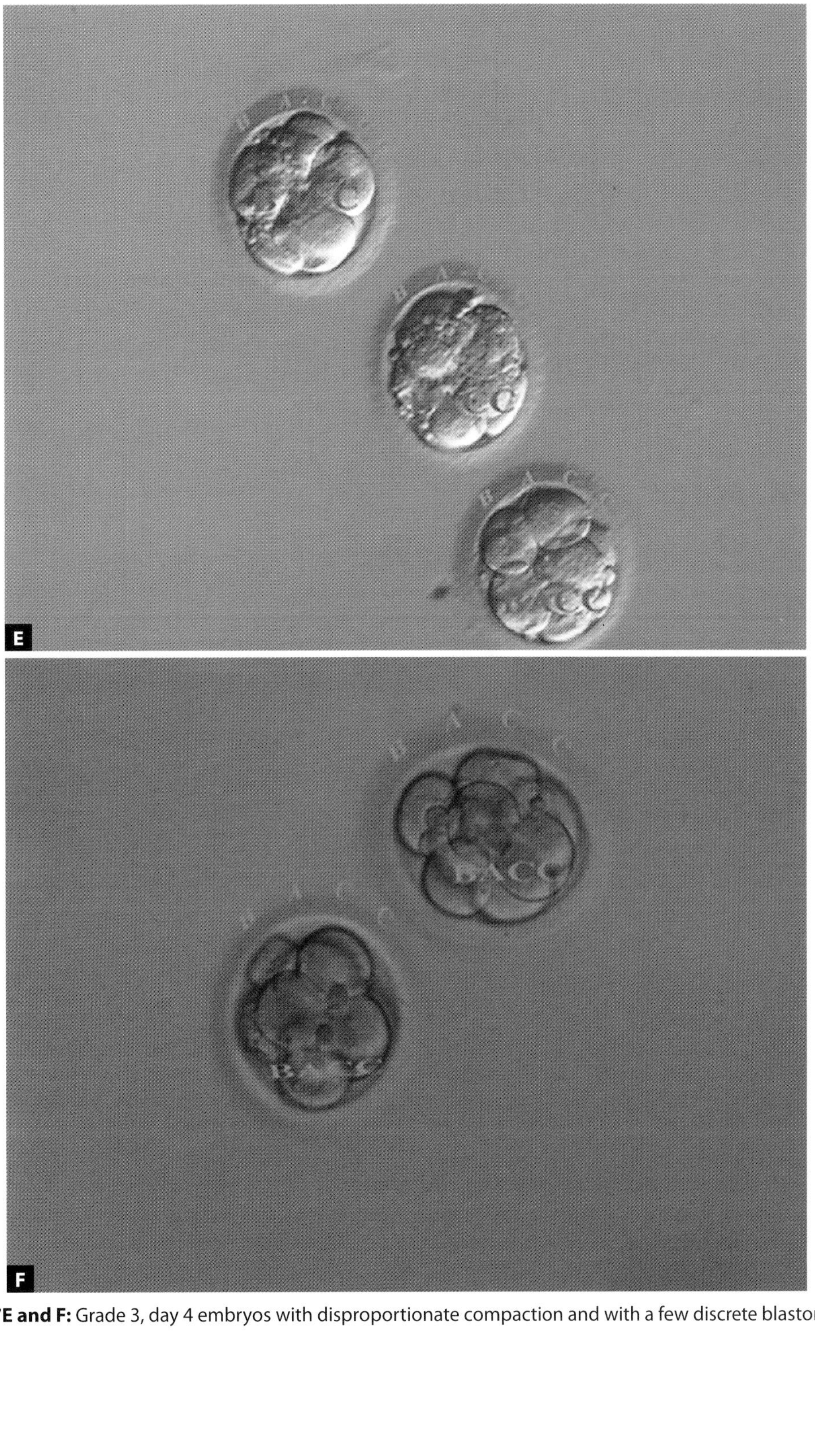

Figs. 7E and F: Grade 3, day 4 embryos with disproportionate compaction and with a few discrete blastomeres.

TABLE 4: Consensus scoring system for blastocysts.

	Grade	Rating	Description
Stage of development	1 2 3 4		Early Blastocyst Expanded Hatched/Hatching
Inner cell mass	1	Good	Prominent, easily discernible, with many cells that are compacted and tightly adhered together
	2	Fair	Easily discernible, with many cells that are loosely grouped together
	3	Poor	Difficult to discern, with few cells
Trophectoderm	1	Good	Many cells forming a cohesive epithelium
	2	Fair	Few cells forming a loose epithelium
	3	Poor	Very few cells

- *Hatched blastocyst*: Embryo is outside the ZP and contains more than 150 cells.

In the **Figures 8 to 12,** different blastocysts in different stages of development and in different grades have been explained. **Figures 8A to E** show early blastocyst in different grades. **Figures 9A and B** show blastocysts in different grades. **Figures 10A to E** show expanded blastocysts. **Figures 11A and B** show hatching blastocyst. **Figures 12A and B** show hatched blastocyst.

EARLY BLASTOCYST (FIGS. 8A TO E)

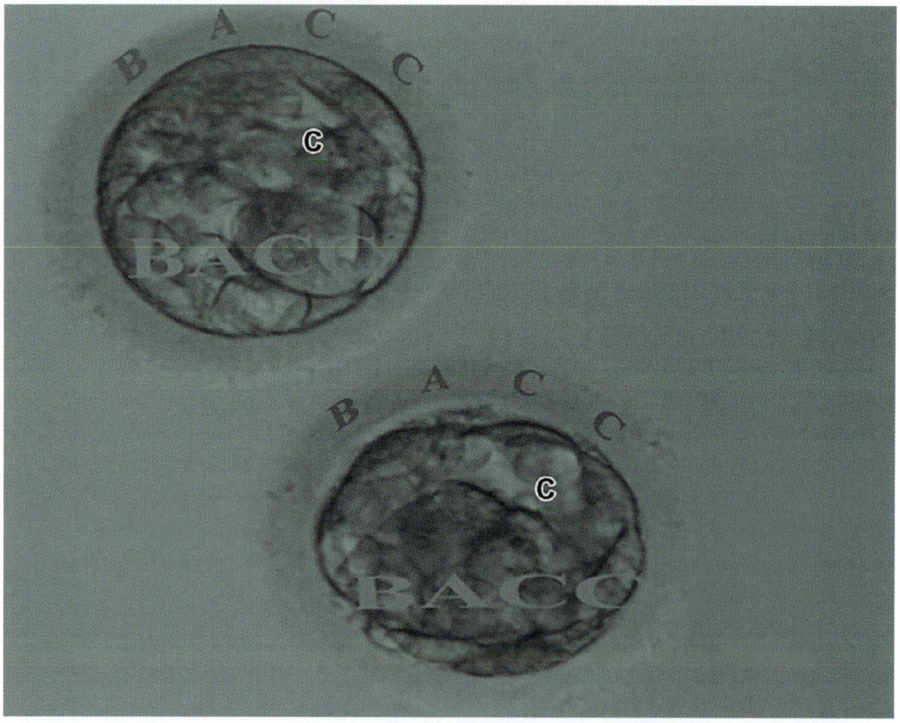

Fig. 8A: Cavitation "C" commencing in an early blastocyst, with indistinguishable cell types.

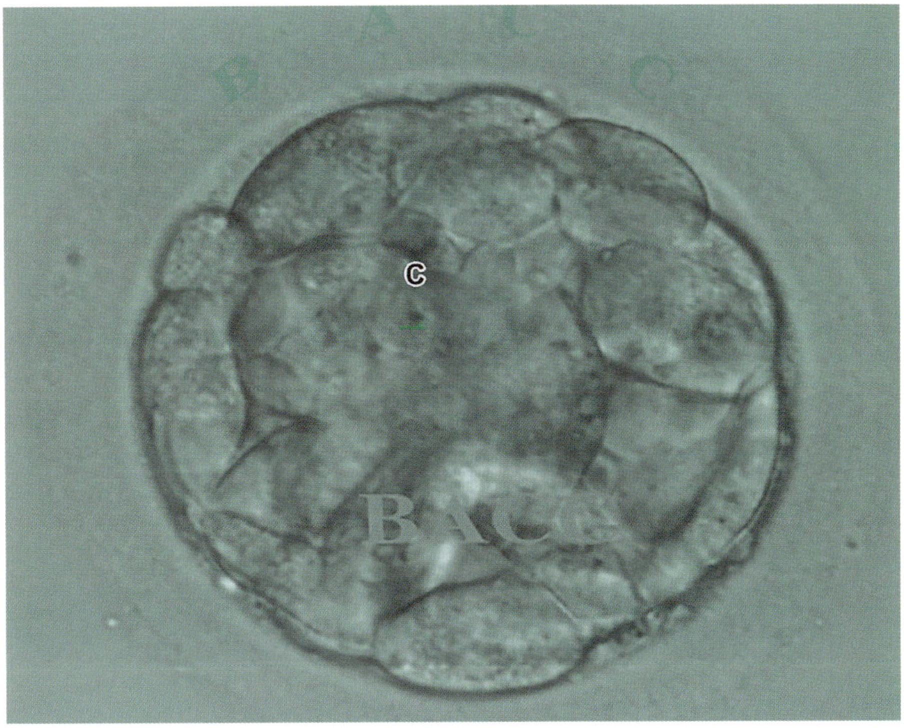

Fig. 8B: Mid-cavitating blastocyst with indistinguishable cell types.

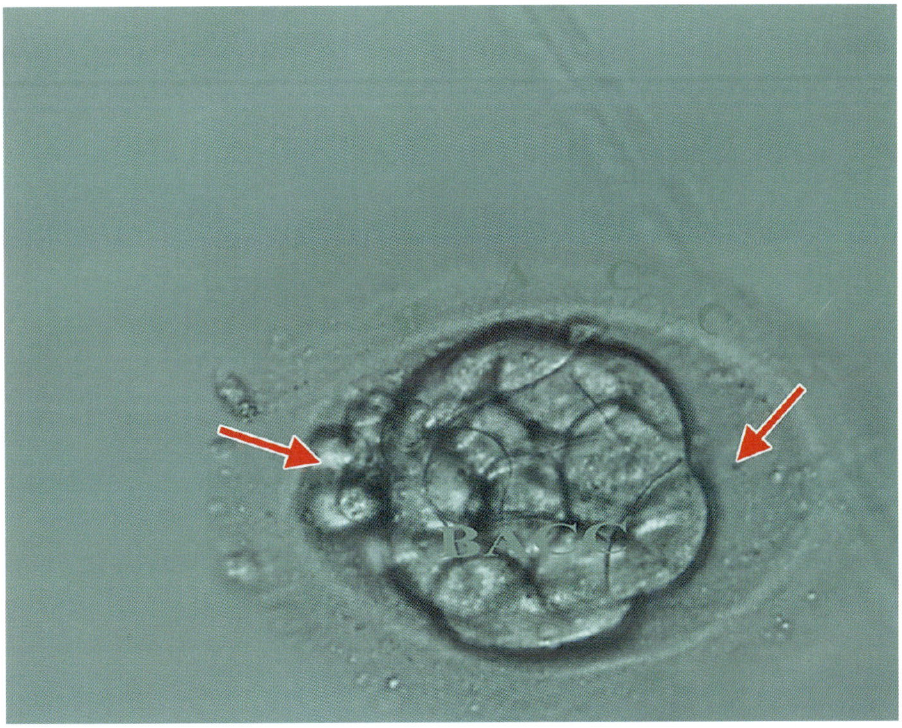

Fig. 8C: Early mid-cavitating blastocyst, with indistinguishable cell types. Note the fragmentation (arrow) and debris (arrow) in perivitelline space.

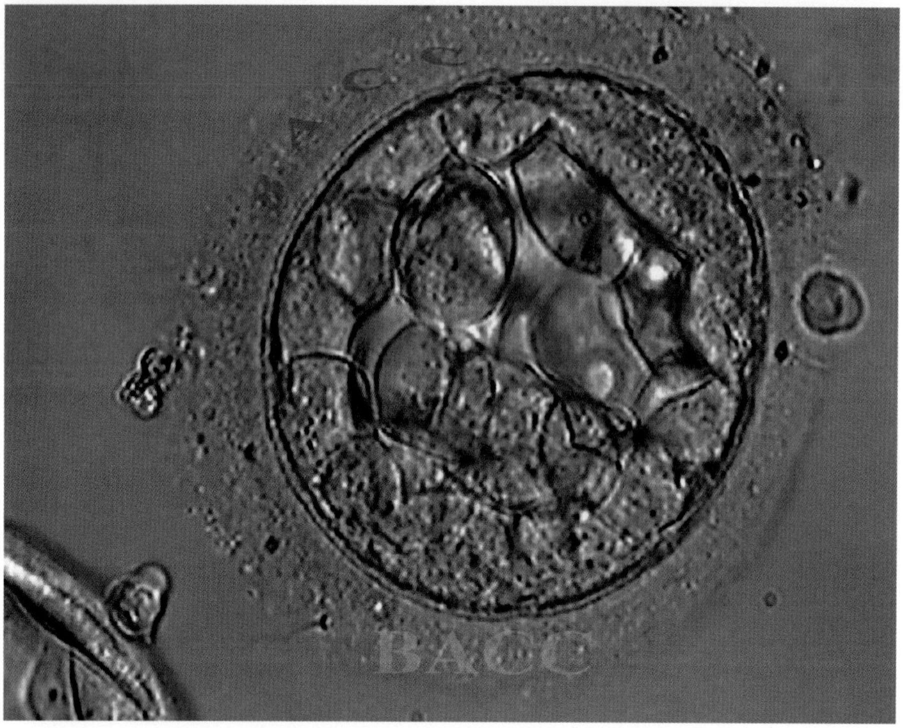

Fig. 8D: An early blastocyst with the cavity occupying more than 50% of the volume of the embryo. Note the flattened squamous-like trophectoderm cells lining left half of the cavity.

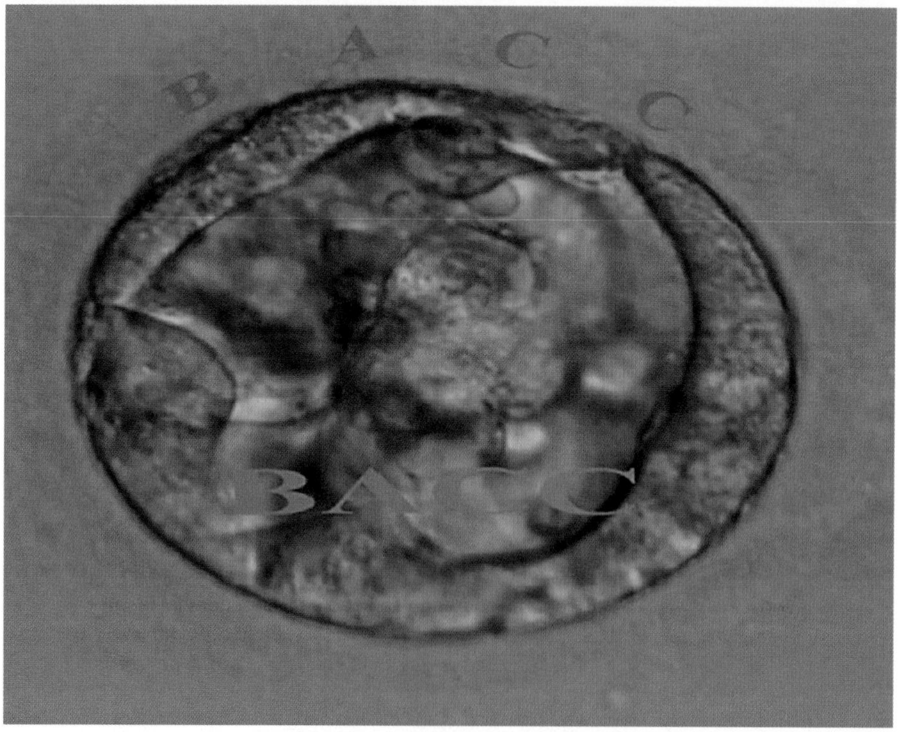

Fig. 8E: An early blastocyst with the cavity occupying more than 50% of the volume of the embryo. The overall volume of the blastocyst remains unchanged with thinning of the zona pellucida. Note the flattened squamous-like trophectoderm cells lining the cavity.

BLASTOCYST (FIGS. 9A AND B)

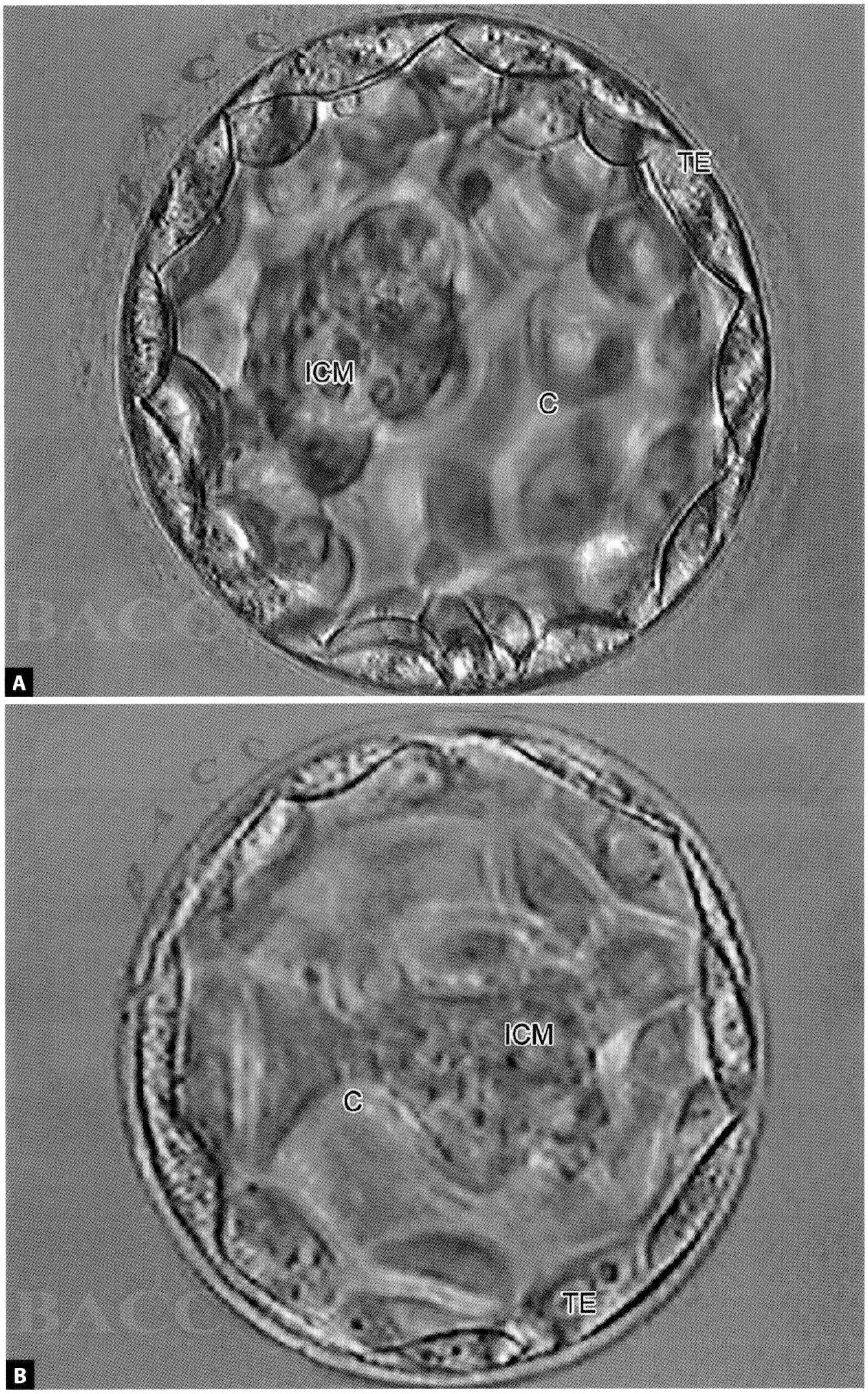

Figs. 9A and B: (A) Grade 3:1:1 showing, distinct compact inner cell mass (ICM) and trophectoderm (TE); (B) Grade 3:2:1 showing a cavity occupying the total volume of the embryo.

EXPANDED BLASTOCYST (FIGS. 10A TO E)

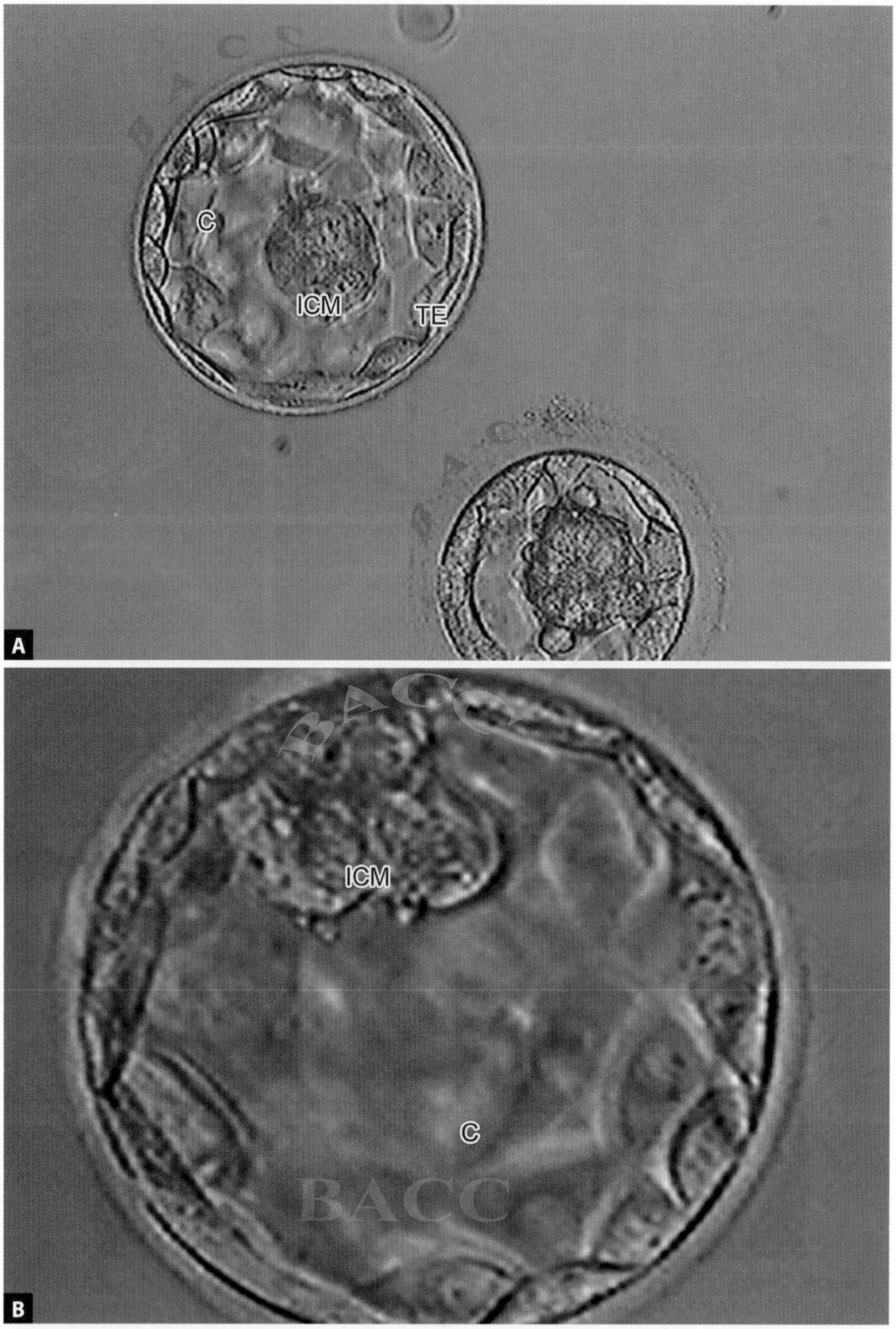

Figs. 10A and B: Expanded blastocyst. (A) Grade 3:1:1. The inner cell mas (ICM) cells are tightly compacted. The blastocele volume is now larger than the original volume of the embryo; (B) Grade 3:1:1. The ICM cells are tightly compacted. The blastocele volume is now larger than the original volume of the embryo.

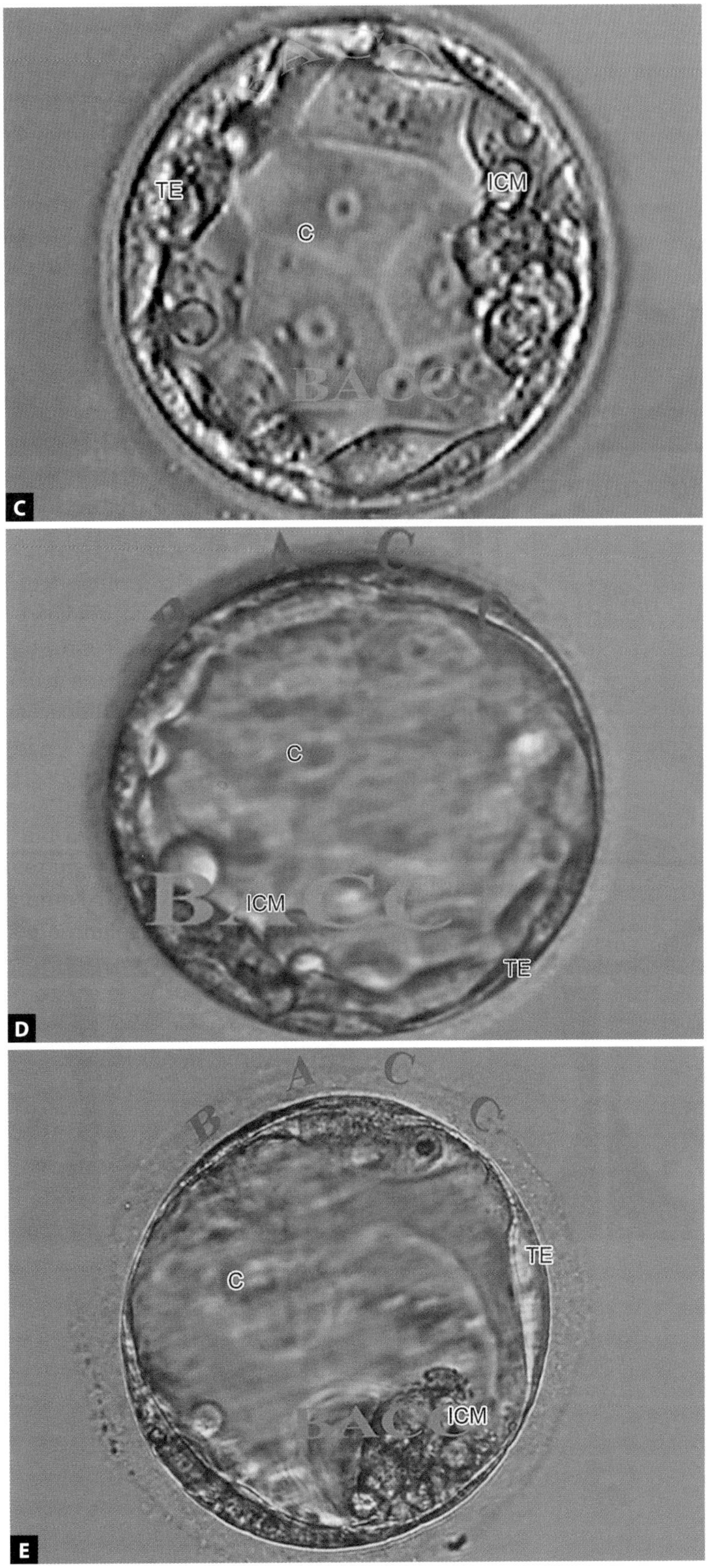

Figs. 10C to E: (C) Grade 3:3:2. The blastocyst volume is large. The inner cell mas (ICM) is difficult to discern with few cells, the trophectoderm (TE) cells are loosely attached and few in number; (D and E) Grade 3:3:3. The blastocyst volume is larger than the original volume. The ICM is difficult to discern with few cells. The TE cells are very few in number.

HATCHING BLASTOCYSTS (FIGS. 11A AND B)

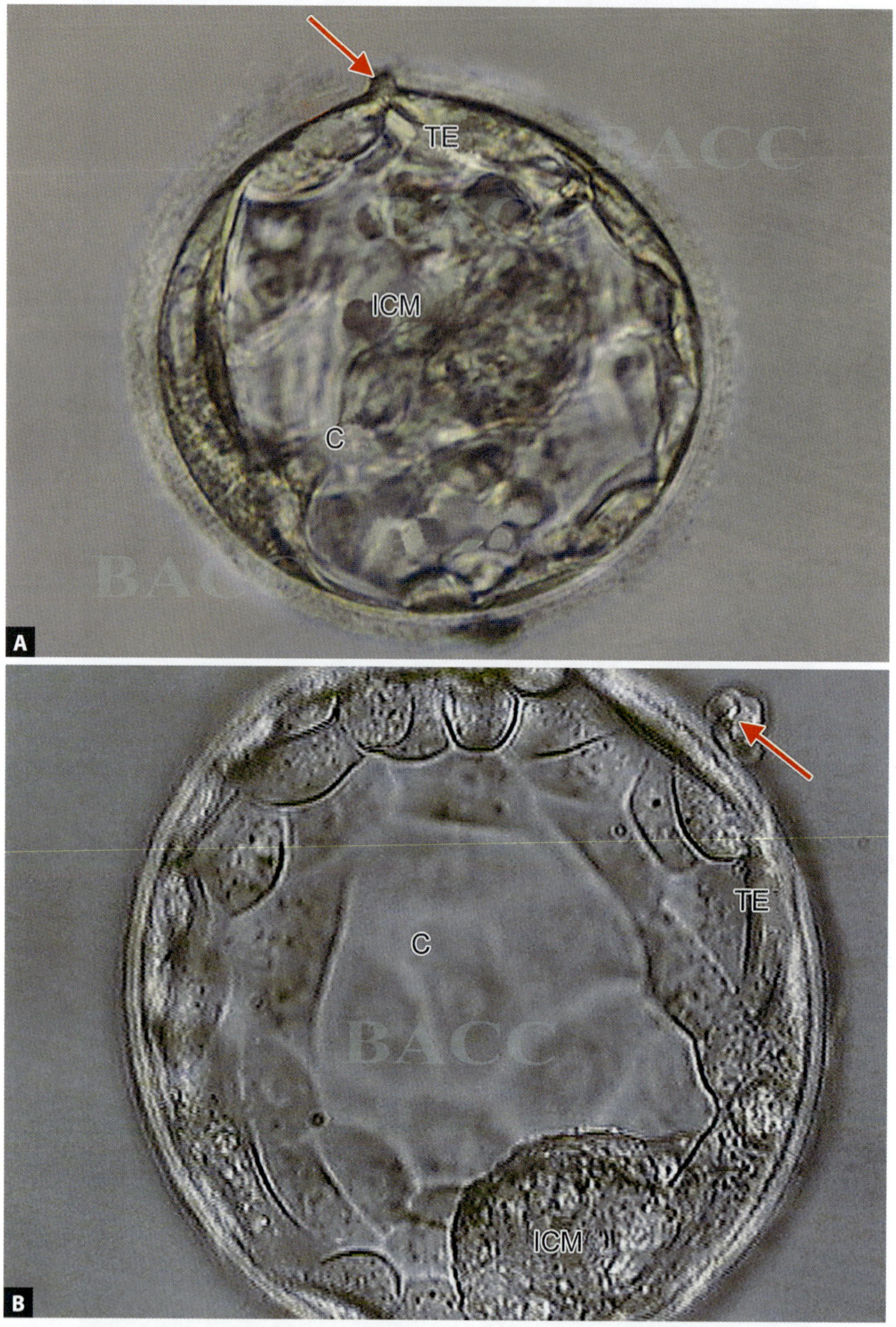

Figs. 11A and B: (A) Hatching blastocyst (Grade 4:2:2). The hatching blastocyst showing a large inner cell mass (ICM), with many cells that are loosely grouped together, trophectoderm (TE) cells are few in number with a loose epithelium. TE cells are herniating through a breach (arrow) in the thinned zona pellucida (ZP) at the 12 o'clock position; (B) Hatching blastocyst (Grade 4:1:1) showing a large, compact ICM at 5 o'clock position in this view. There are many TE cells of equivalent size lining the blastocele cavity and several TE cells are herniating through a breach (arrow) through the thinned ZP at 1 o'clock position.

HATCHED BLASTOCYSTS (FIGS. 12A AND B)

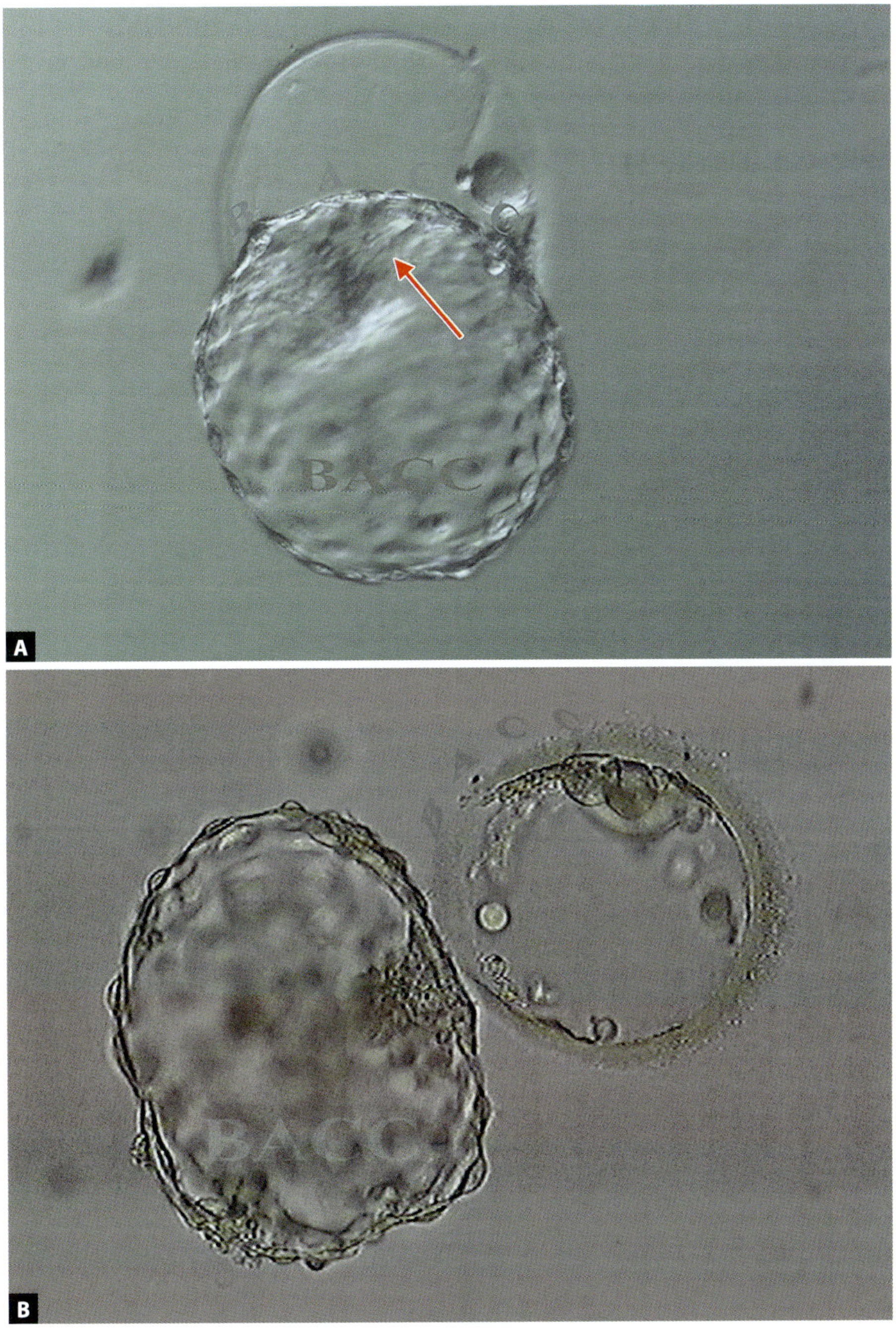

Figs. 12A and B: (A) Hatched blastocyst (Grade 4:1:1) showing a large, compact, crescent-shaped inner cell mass (ICM) retained within the zona pellucida (ZP) (arrow). There are many trophectoderm (TE) cells and almost 75% of the blastocyst has herniated out through a breach in the ZP; (B) completely hatched blastocyst (Grade 4:1:1) showing compact ICM and many TE cells.

MORPHOLOGY OF POOR QUALITY BLASTOCYSTS

These groups of blastocysts exhibit low cell numbers and higher degree of chromosomal aberrations. Poor quality blastocysts consists of various morphological subtypes namely blastocysts with excessive fragmentation, cytoplasmic strings, vacuoles, necrotic cells and trophoblast vesicles.

TROPHOBLAST VESICLE (FIG. 13)

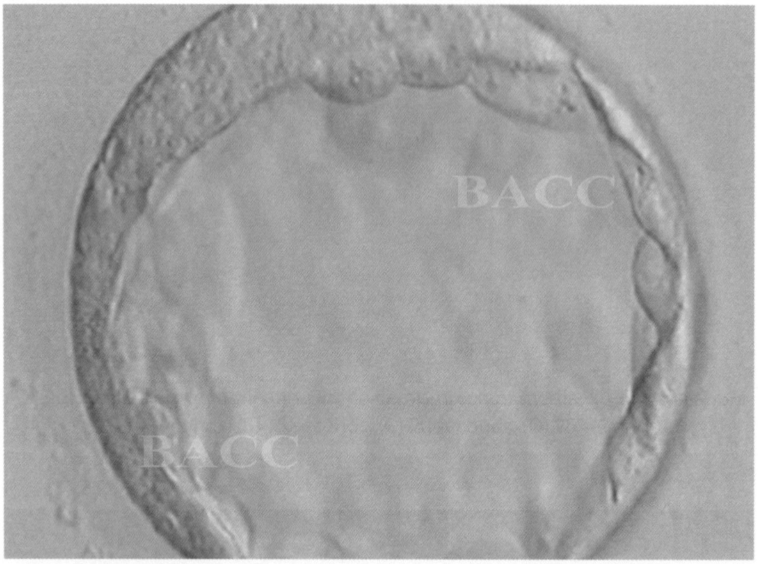

Fig. 13: Trophoblastic vesicle with a dominant blastocyst cavity. Blastocyst with no visible inner cell mass and a rudimentary trophectoderm.

NECROTIC FOCI (FIGS. 14A AND B)

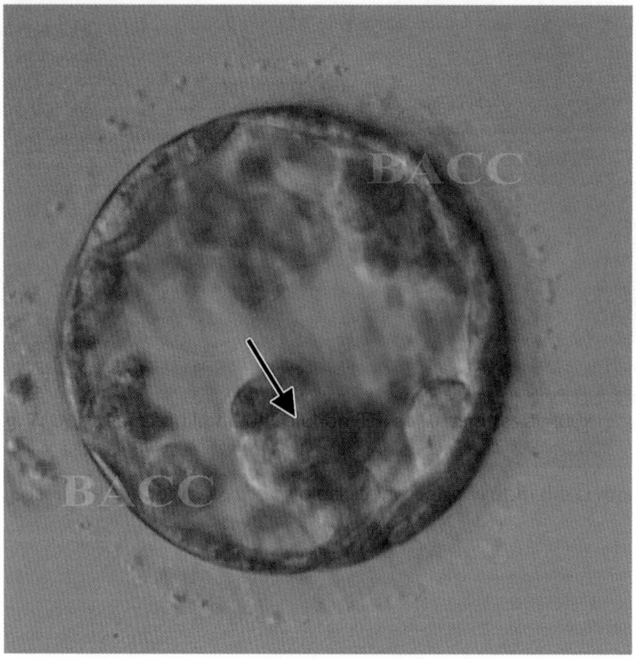

Fig. 14A: Early blastocyst showing dark, degenerative changes (arrow).

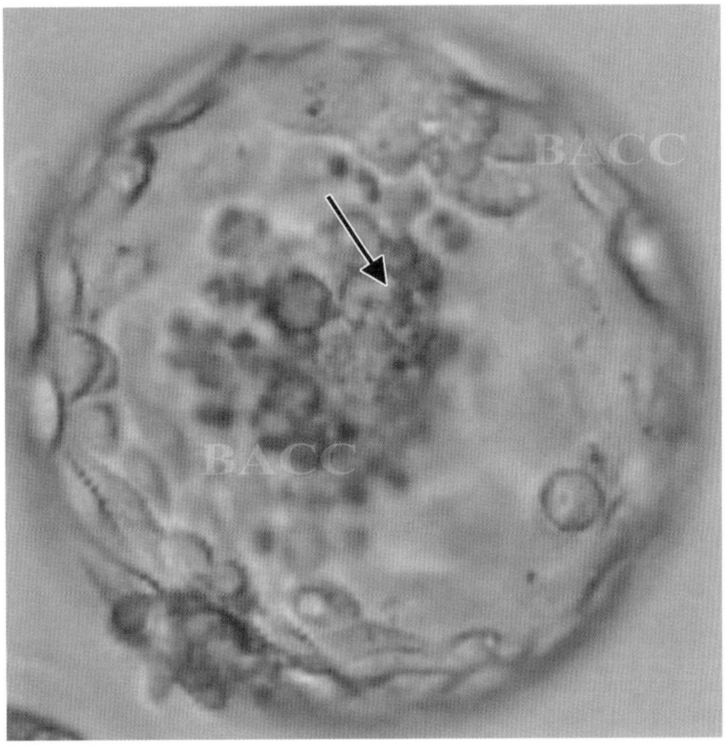

Fig. 14B: Hatching blastocyst showing necrotic foci (arrow).

VACUOLES (FIGS. 15A AND B)

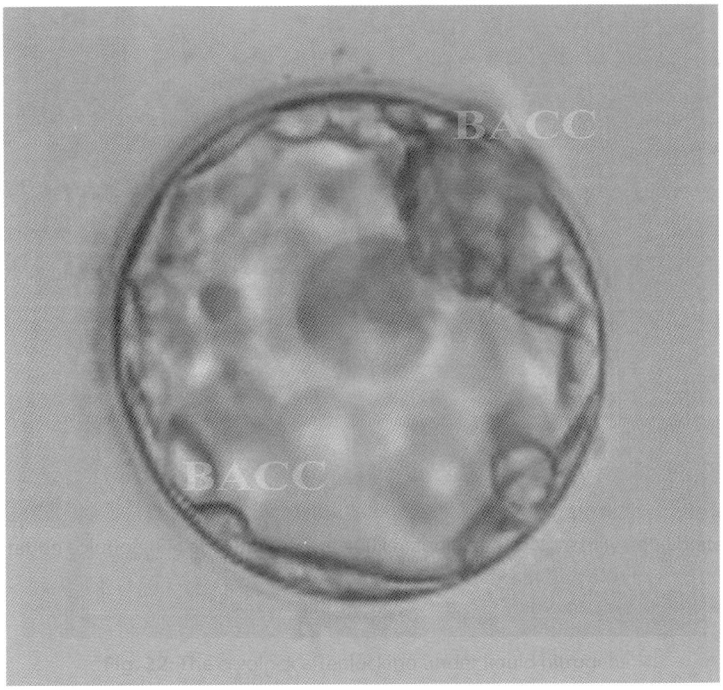

Fig. 15A: Expanded blastocyst in which a large vacuole can be seen in close proximity to ICM.

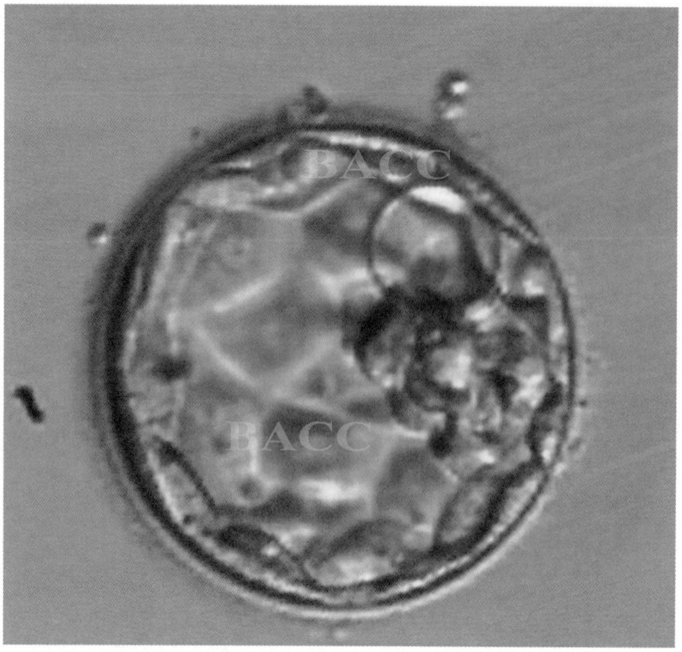

Fig. 15B: Late blastocyst showing vacuole in close vicinity to trophectoderm and ICM.

CYTOPLASMIC STRINGS (FIGS. 16A AND B)

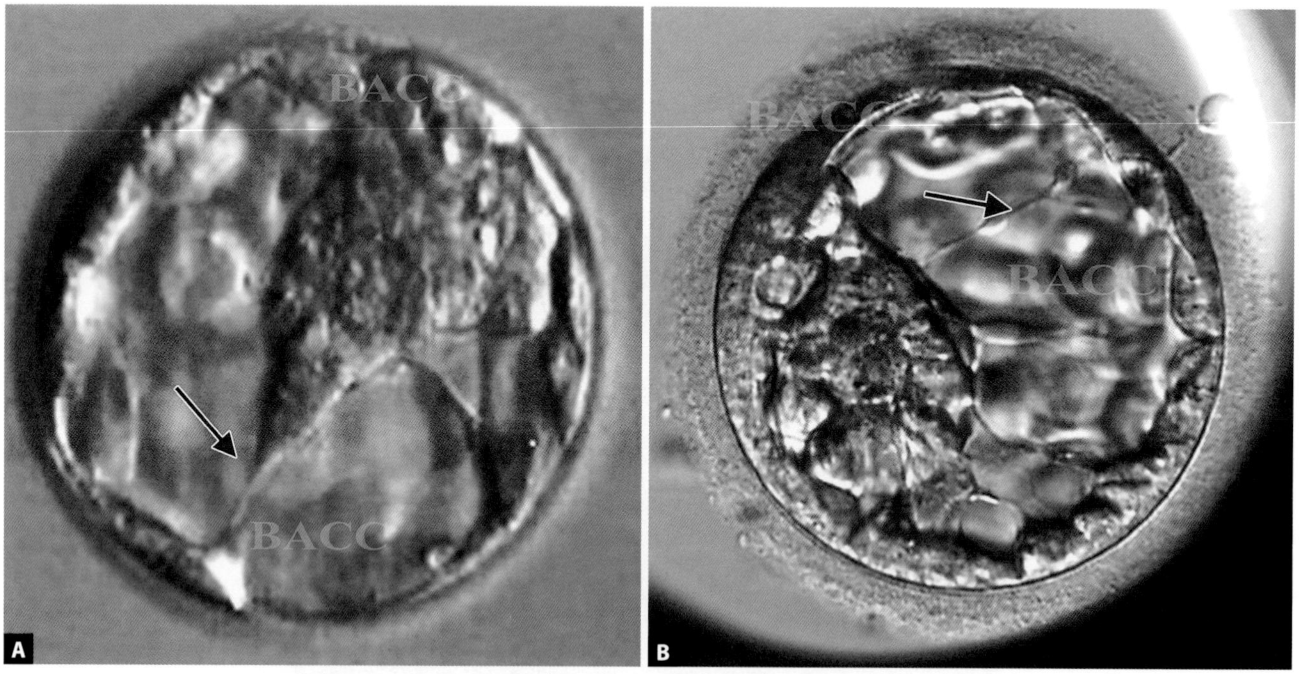

Figs. 16A and B: Blastocyst showing cytoplasmic strings (arrows) which represent polarized flow of cells from the polar to the mural trophectoderm which tend to withdraw as the cells reach their destination. When the cytoplasmic strings persist even in the expanded phase, it marks the developmental liability of the blastocysts.

REFERENCES

1. Alpha Scientists in Reproductive Medicine and ESHRE Special Interest Group Embryology. Istanbul consensus workshop on embryo assessment: proceedings of an expert meeting. Reprod Bio Med Online. 2011;22:632-46.
2. Gardner DK, Schoolcraft WB. In vitro culture of human blastocysts. In: Jansen R, Mortimer D (Eds). Towards Reproductive Certainty: Fertility and Genetics Beyond. London, UK: Parthenon Publishing; 1999. pp. 378-88.
3. Gardner DK, Schoolcraft WB. Culture and transfer of human blastocysts. Curr Opin Obstet Gynecol. 1999;11:307-11.

CHAPTER 133

In Vitro Fertilization/Intracytoplasmic Sperm Injection

Bezar Ghan VV, Divyashree PS

OOCYTE INSEMINATION IN IN VITRO FERTILIZATION

The mature oocytes are preincubated for 3–6 hours before insemination, as it is well known that an additional period of time is required for cytoplasmic maturation after extrusion of first polar body.

The standard insemination concentration is 100,000 (1 lakh) normal motile sperms per mL. 100 μL microdroplet with sperm suspension is prepared in 35 mm Petri dish with oil overlay.

After checking the oocyte cumulus complex (OCC), a single OCC is transferred into 100 μL of sperm droplet and kept inside the incubator **(Fig. 1)**.

After overnight incubation, cumulus and coronal cells are carefully removed. The cytoplasm of dissected oocyte is examined for the presence of pronuclei and two polar bodies for confirmation of fertilization.

INTRACYTOPLASMIC SPERM INJECTION

Intracytoplasmic sperm injection (ICSI) procedure entails the deposition of a single spermatozoon directly into the ooplasm, thus bypassing the zona and oolemma.

The procedure is carried out on an inverted microscope at 200–400× magnification, using multiple micromanipulation devices (micromanipulator, microinjectors and micropipettes) **(Fig. 2)**.

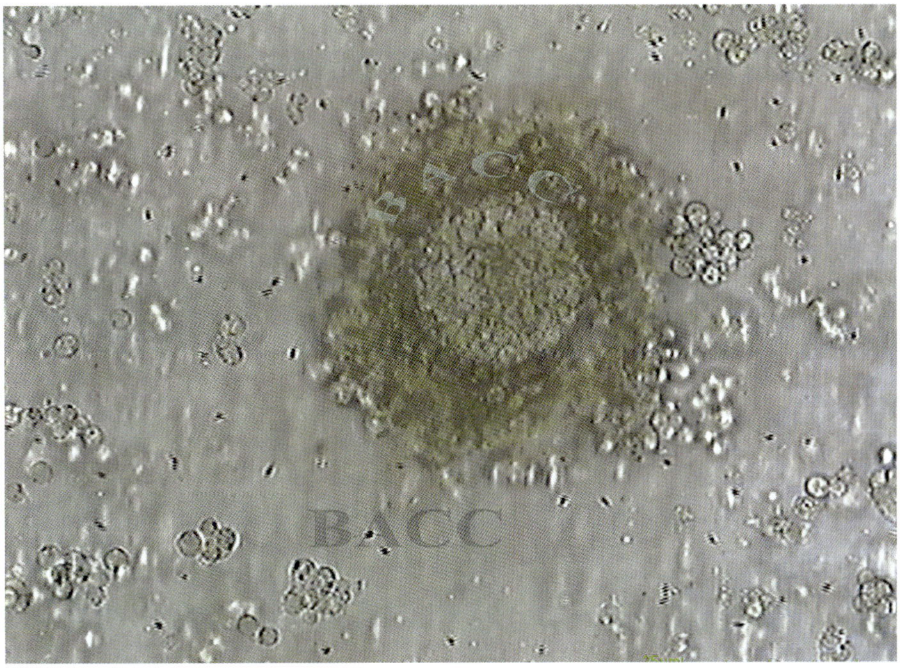

Fig. 1: Oocyte cumulus complex (OCC) charged with sperms for in vitro fertilization (IVF).

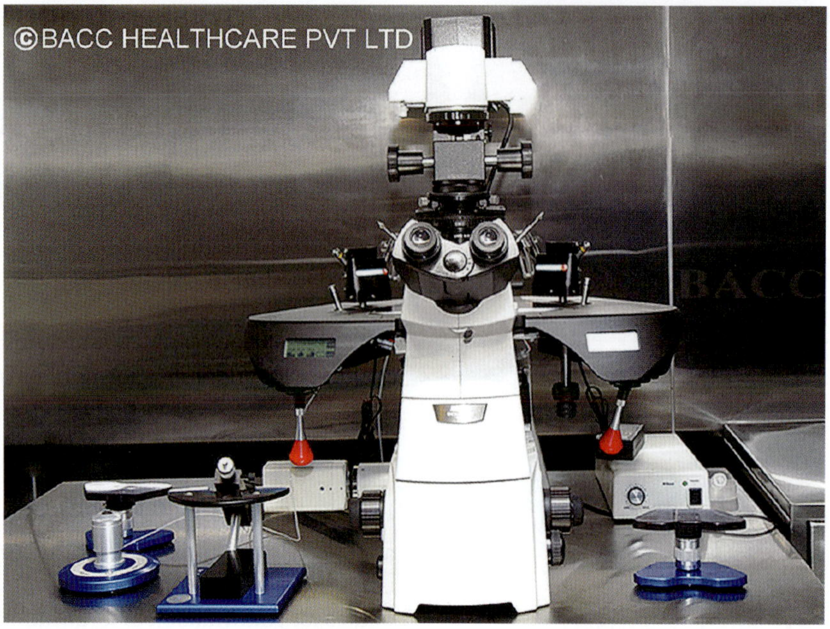

Fig. 2: Inverted microscope with micromanipulator research instrument (RI).

Intracytoplasmic sperm injection procedure involves following steps:

- Preparation of ICSI dish
- Semen/sperm preparation
- Preparation and evaluation of oocytes
- Alignment and equilibration of micropipettes
- Sperm immobilization
- Oocyte manipulation
- Microinjection of the oocyte.

Preparation of Intracytoplasmic Sperm Injection Dish (Fig. 3)

Central droplets of 5 μL of PVP (polyvinylpyrrolidone) solution.

At the periphery of PVP droplets, 5 μL droplets of HEPES/MOPS buffered media numbered from 1 to 7.

Sperms are suspended in the central PVP droplet, whereas each oocyte is placed in the surrounding HEPES/MOPS buffered droplets.

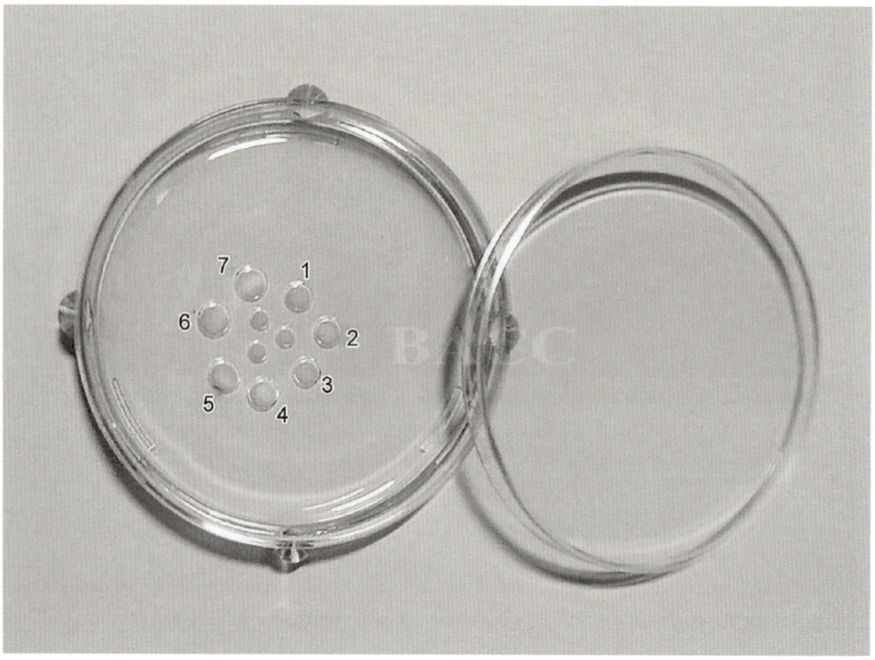

Fig. 3: Intracytoplasmic sperm injection dish.

These droplets are covered with light-weight oil.

Sperm and oocyte evaluation are discussed in detail in the initial chapters.

Alignment and Equilibration of Micropipettes

Proper alignment of micropipettes makes the micro-injection much easier.

Alignment of micropipettes is best done through microscope, initially under lesser magnification for coarse adjustment and then under higher magnification for fine adjustments.

After alignment both the pipettes should now be seen as shown in **Figures 4A and B**, like straight tools facing each other with their tips focused.

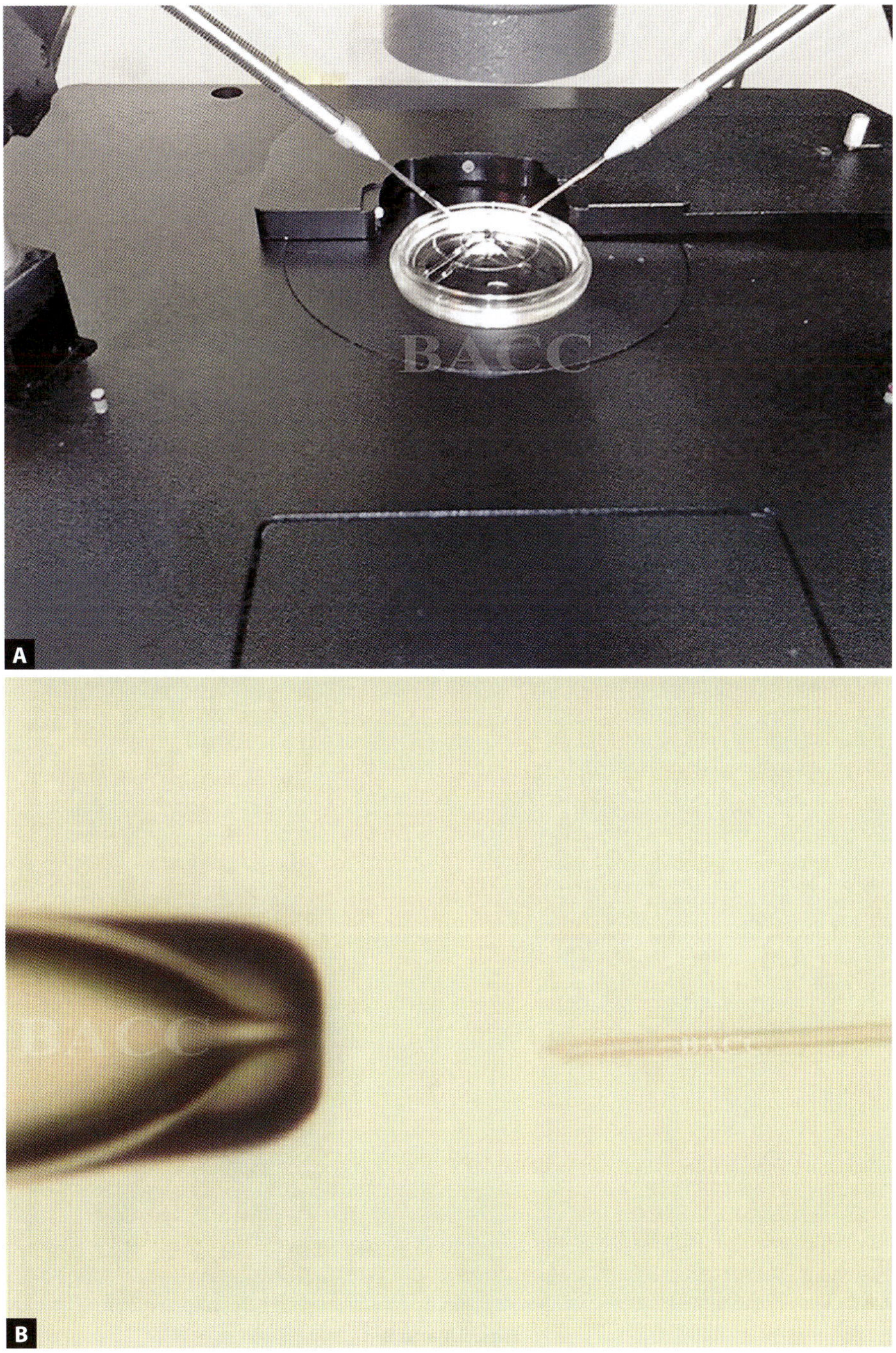

Figs. 4A and B: Properly aligned micropipettes through inverted microscope.

Sperm Immobilization

Sperm immobilization is one of the important steps during ICSI as it ensures release of oocyte activation factor into the ooplasm, thus favoring fertilization.

During this process, morphologically normal sperm is selected and it is immobilized either by touching or crushing the tail beyond the midpiece as shown in **Figure 5A**.

After immobilization, sperm is aspirated into injection pipette with its tail first **(Fig. 5B)**. **Figure 5C** showing sperm inside the injection pipette before ICSI.

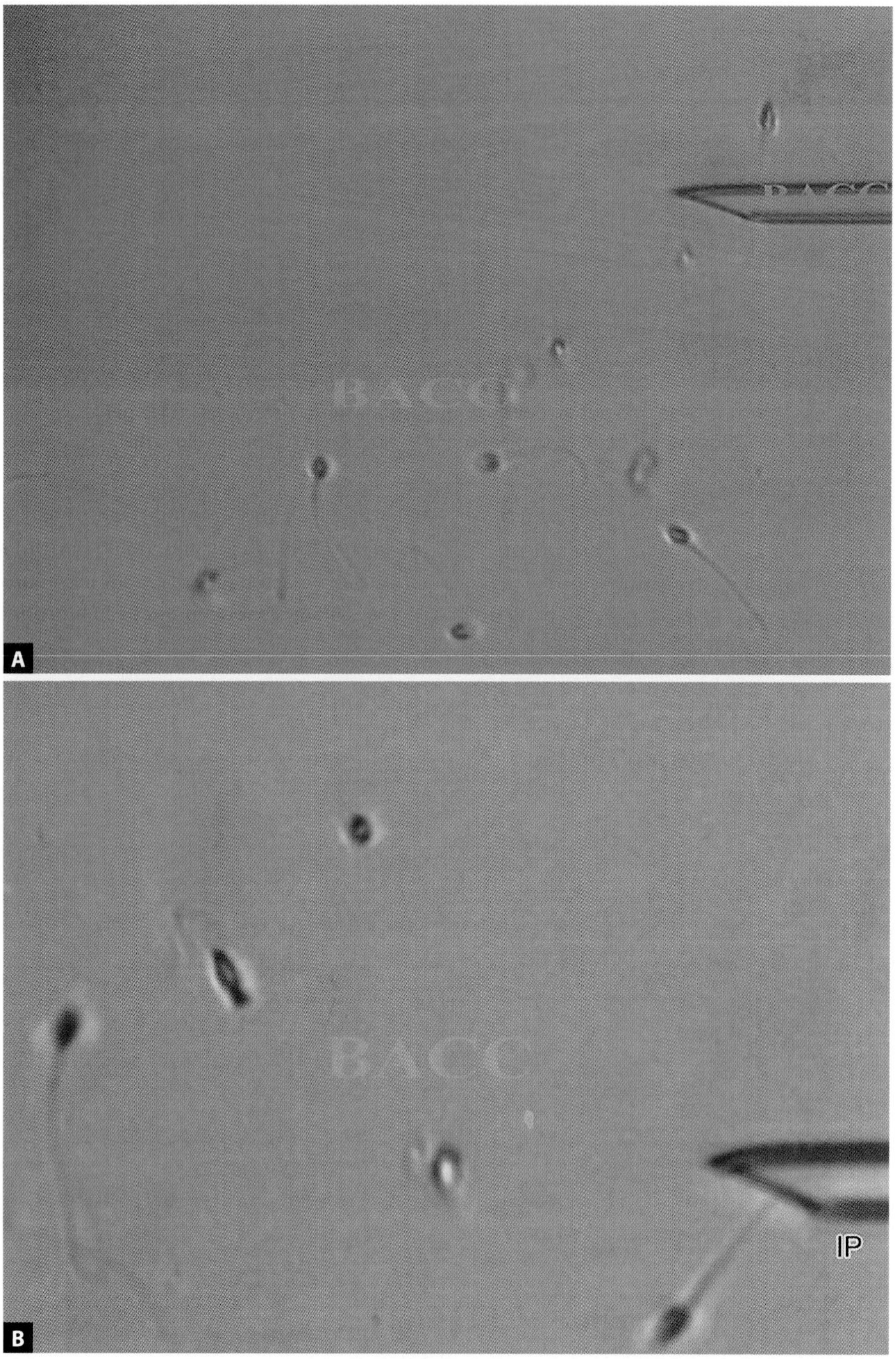

Figs. 5A and B

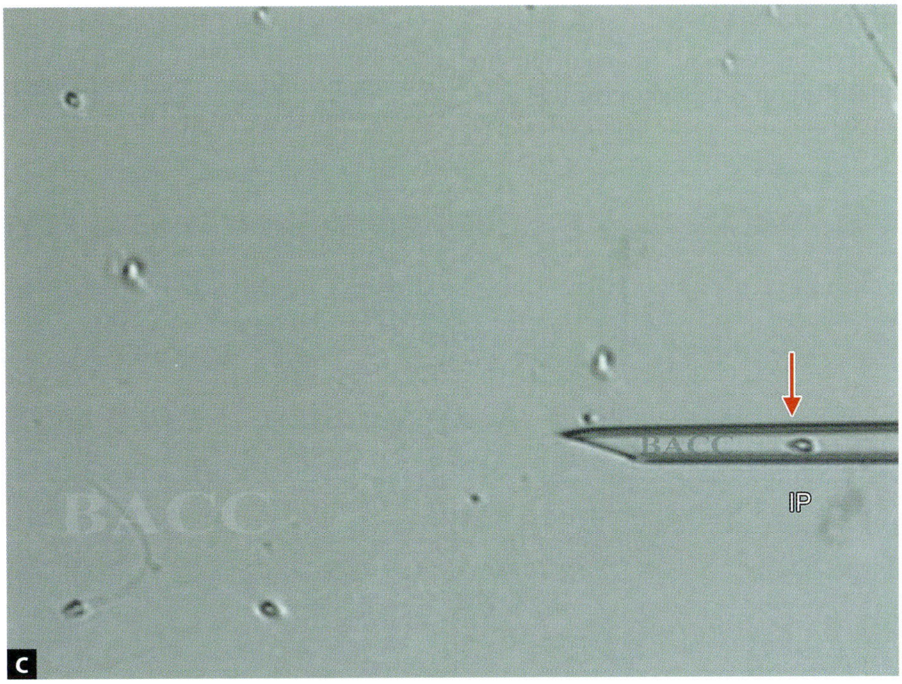

Figs. 5A to C: Sperm immobilization.

Oocyte Manipulation

Oocyte manipulation should be very gentle.

Two points to be kept in mind during oocyte manipulation. (1) Oocyte holding with adequate pressure to aid microinjection, not too high which can damage the oocyte and not too less which can cause slippage during microinjection. (2) The polar body should be positioned in 6 or 12 o'clock position, as shown in **Figure 6**, to avoid damage to the spindle apparatus.

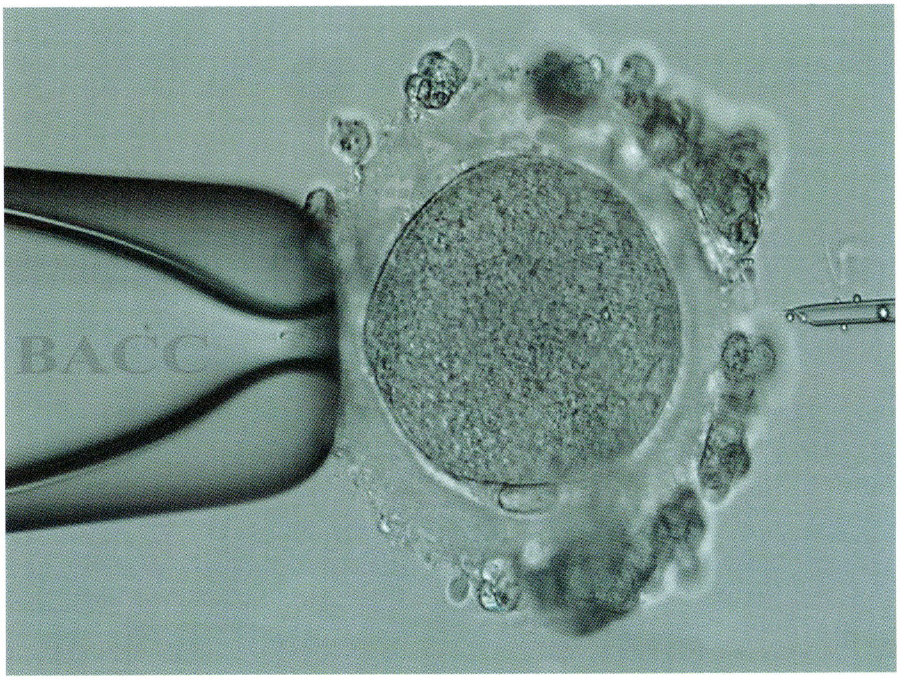

Fig. 6: Oocyte holding and positioning of polar body. Metaphase II oocyte held with holding pipette with polar body at 6 o'clock position.

Microinjection of the Oocyte

After holding the oocyte in position, injection pipette containing immobilized sperm is brought near the zona. Sperm is stabilized in the injection pipette before advancing the injection pipette into the ooplasm. Injection pipette is now gently pushed into the ooplasm, past ZP and oolemma, leaving behind the point of indentation at the site of penetration **(Figs. 7A and B)**.

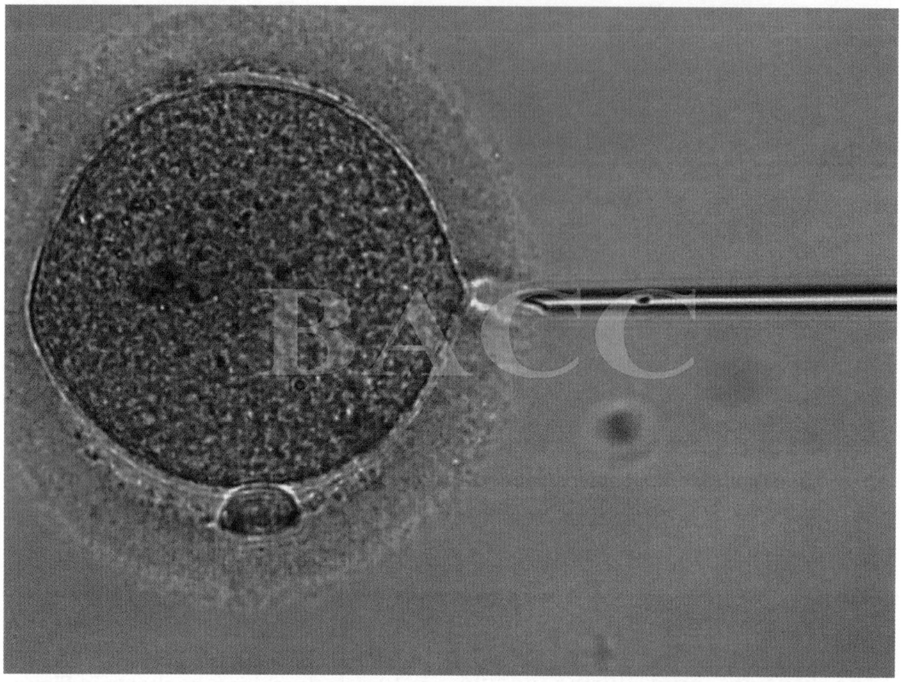

Fig. 7A: The micropipettes and the oocyte in position before intracytoplasmic sperm injection (ICSI).

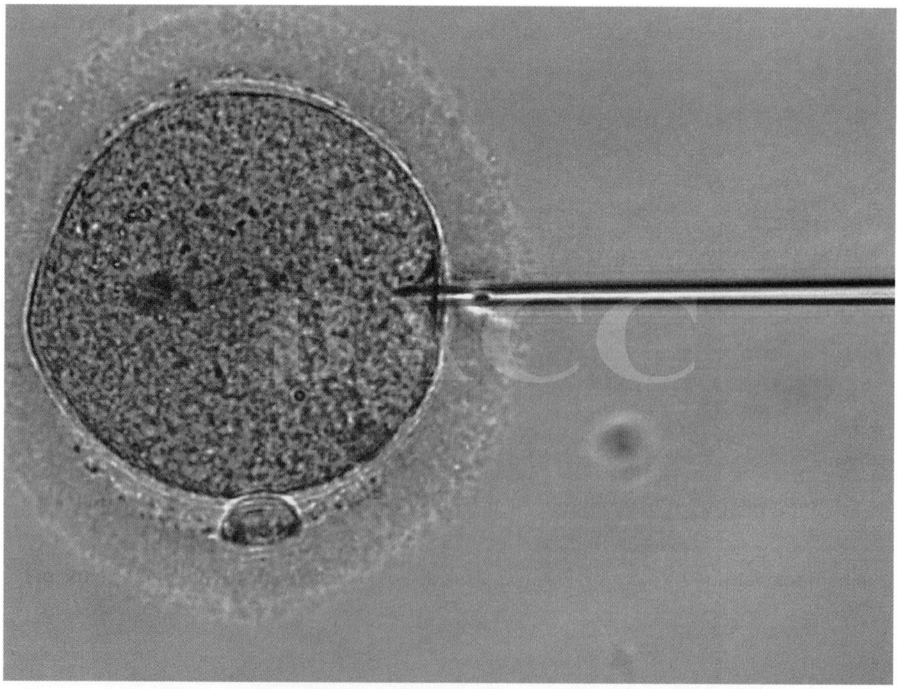

Fig. 7B: The injection pipette holding sperm inside, piercing the oolemma.

After piercing the oolemma, ooplasm is gently aspirated into injection pipette until oolemma is broken and the cytoplasmic contents mixed with sperm is released back into the ooplasm **(Figs. 7C to E)**.

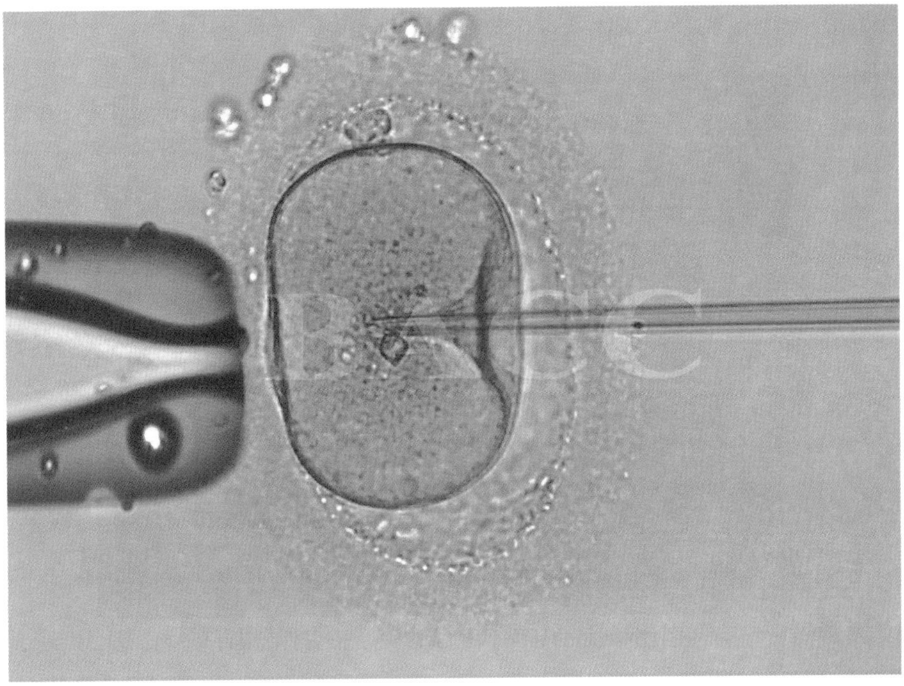

Fig. 7C: Injecting pipette penetrating into the oocyte.

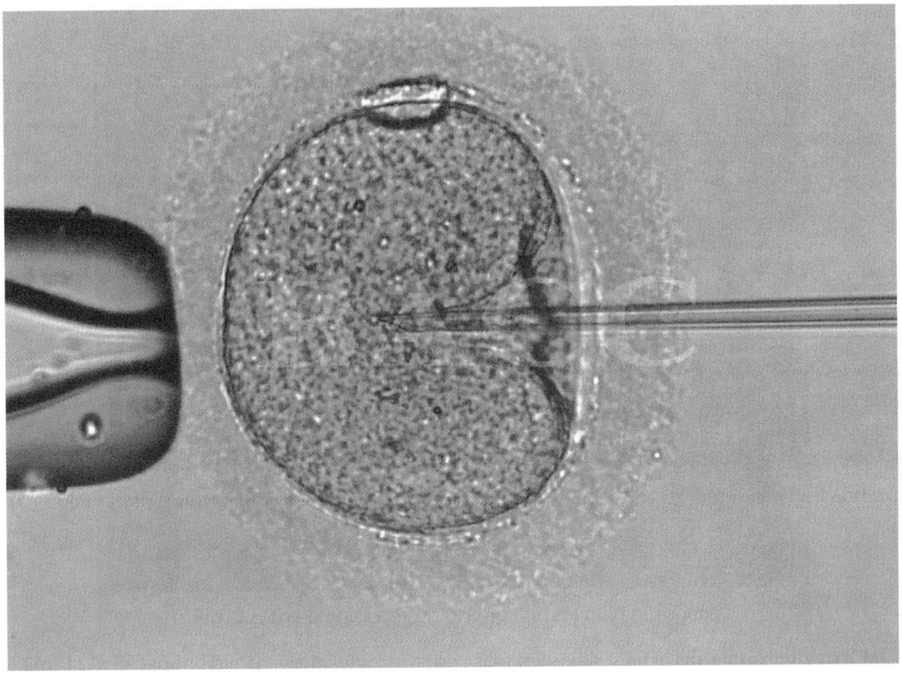

Fig. 7D: Sperm and cytoplasmic contents are gently expelled into the oocyte.

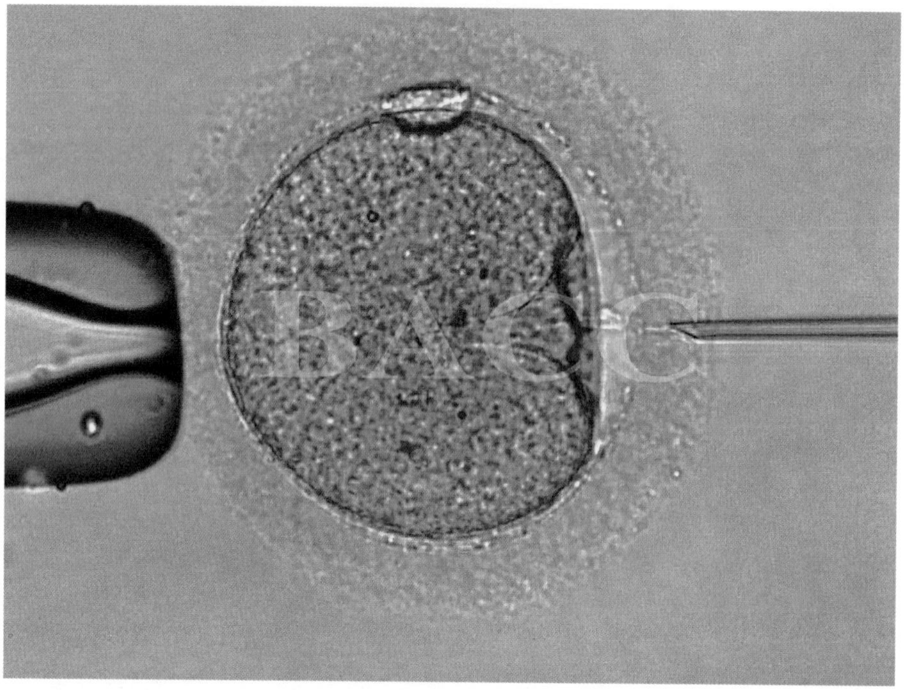

Fig. 7E: Metaphase II (MII) oocyte, immediate postintracytoplasmic sperm injection (ICSI) (note the funneling of the ooplasm).

CHAPTER 134

Advanced Techniques

Anitha S Kumari K, Bezar Ghan VV, Divyashree PS, Dileep Kumar R, Anu Kottur, Kamini A Rao, Mohammed Ashraf C

PHYSIOLOGICAL INTRACYTOPLASMIC SPERM INJECTION

Anitha S Kumari K, Bezar Ghan VV, Divyashree PS, Mohammed Ashraf C

INTRODUCTION

Physiological intracytoplasmic sperm injection (PICSI) is an advanced method of sperm selection, before intracytoplasmic sperm injection (ICSI) **(Figs. 1A and B)**. PICSI represents a physiologic alternative for slowing sperm motility before ICSI, avoiding any potential damaging effect of synthetic polyvinylpyrrolidone (PVP).[1]

In the natural human fertilization process, hyaluronic acid (HA) seems to play a pivotal role in physiological sperm selection. Spermatozoa that are able to bind permanently to HA in vitro are mature and have completed the spermiogenetic process of plasma membrane remodeling, cytoplasmic extrusion and nuclear maturity.[2] These mature spermatozoa have a high density of HA receptors.

Sperms are added to the dot of hyaluronan and within minutes the bound sperms are attached by their acrosome to the surface of the dot **(Figs. 2A and B)**.

An ICSI microtool is used to select the HA bound sperm, which will be used for ICSI **(Fig. 3)**.

PHYSIOLOGICAL INTRACYTOPLASMIC SPERM INJECTION DISH

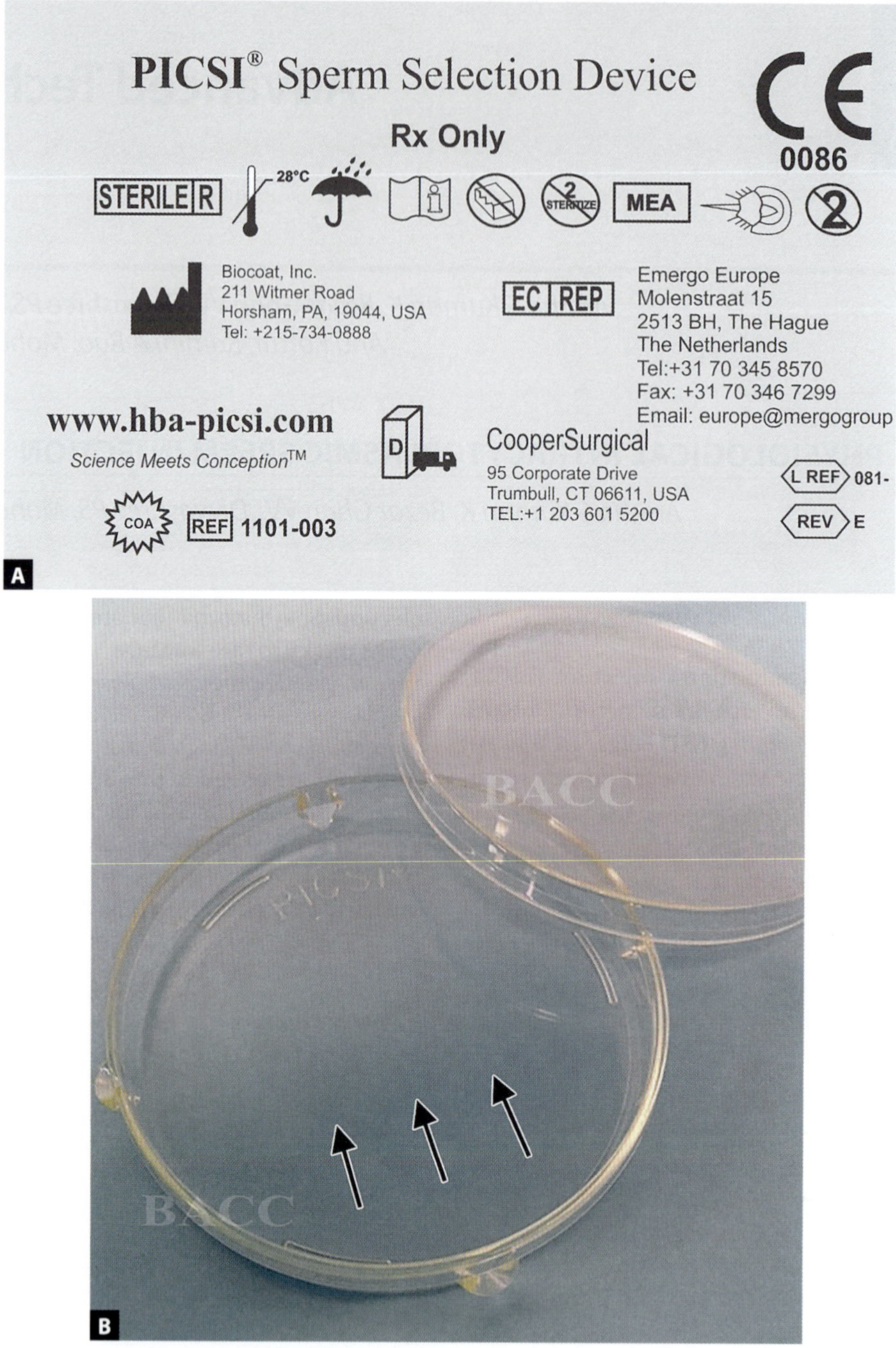

Figs. 1A and B: Physiological intracytoplasmic sperm injection (PICSI) dish.

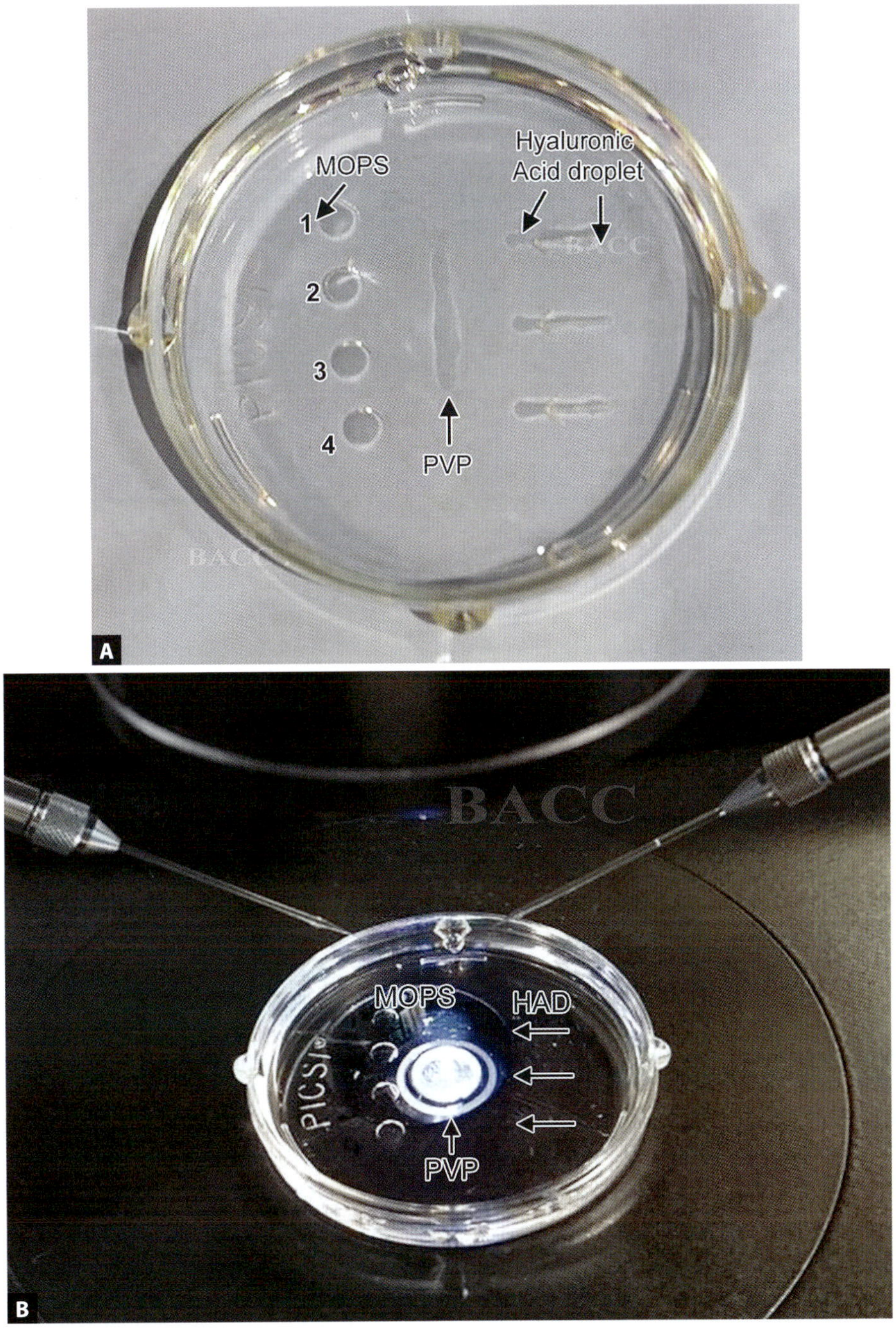

Figs. 2A and B: Physiological intracytoplasmic sperm injection (PICSI) dish with MOPS, PVP, and hyaluronan microdroplets. (HAD: hyaluronic acid droplet; MOPS: (3-(N-Morpholino) propane sulfonic acid; PVP: polyvinylpyrrolidone)

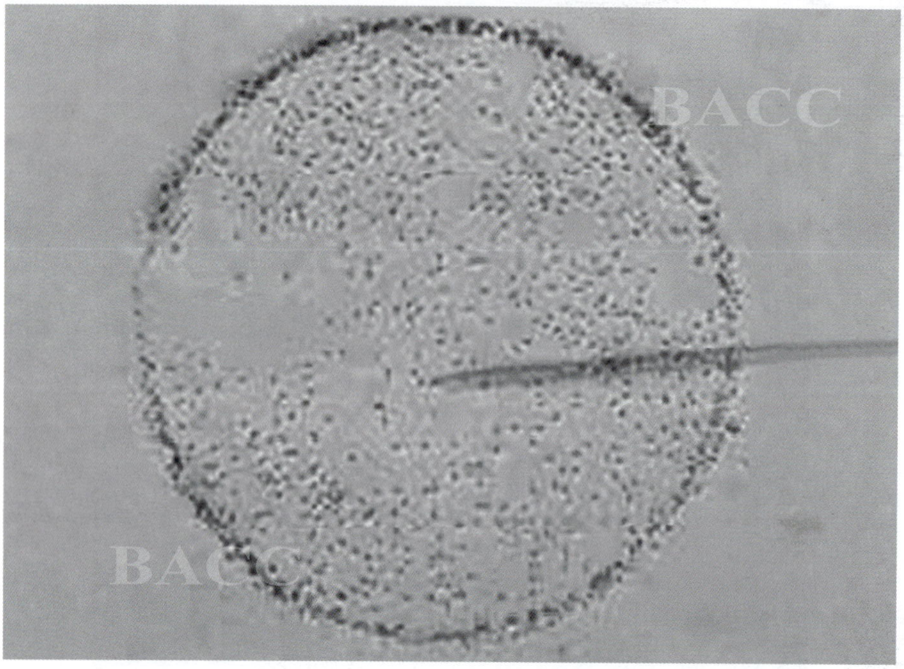

Fig. 3: Selection of hyaluronic acid (HA) bound sperms with injection pipette.

INTRACYTOPLASMIC MORPHOLOGICALLY SELECTED SPERM INJECTION

Bezar Ghan VV, Dileep Kumar R, Anitha S Kumari K, Divyashree PS

INTRODUCTION

Intracytoplasmic sperm injection is usually performed at an optical magnification of 400×, since this magnification allows identification of only major morphological defects of the sperm; minor morphological defects of the sperms, which seem to be related to ICSI outcome, can be missed.[3]

Methods of advance sperm selection include motile sperm organelle morphology examination (MOSME; magnification 6,600×) and intracytoplasmic morphologically selected sperm injection (IMSI).

Motile sperm organelle morphology examination is an unstained cytological technique; its incorporation together with micromanipulation system has resulted in evolution of IMSI.

Intracytoplasmic morphologically selected sperm injection is a real-time method in which the sperm structure is visualized at a magnification of 6,600× **(Figs. 4A to N)**.

The meta-analysis by Souza Setti et al. concludes that IMSI not only significantly improves the percentage of top-quality embryos, implantation and pregnancy rates, but also significantly reduces miscarriage rates as compared with ICSI.[4]

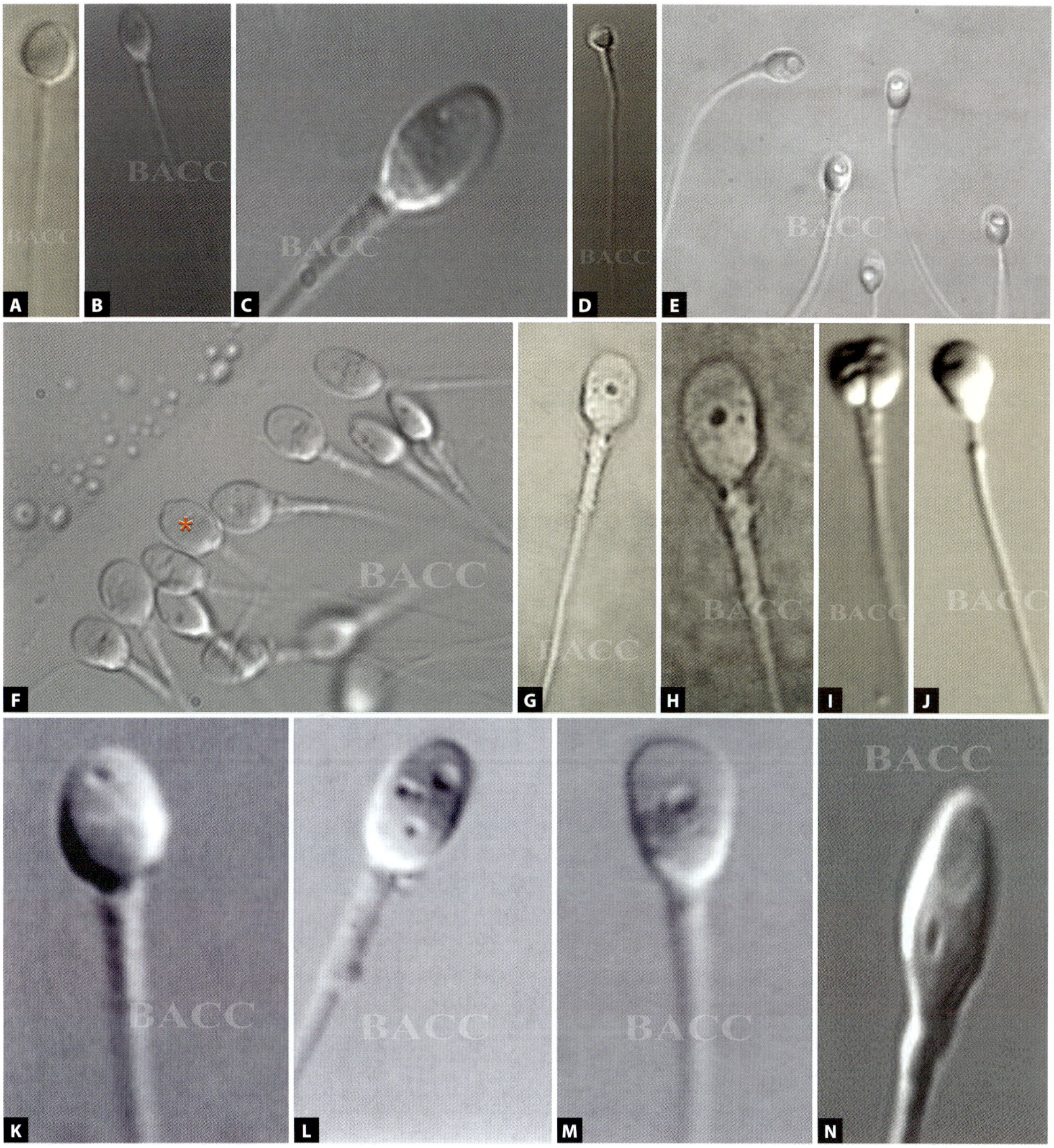

Figs. 4A to N: (A to C) Sperms with normal morphology; (D) Sperm head showing vacuole with normal mid-piece and tail; (E) Sperms under 6,600x magnification showing vacuoles; (F) All sperms showing vacuoles except one (*) showing extrusion; (G to N) Morphologically abnormal sperms under 6,600x magnification; (G and H) Sperms with vesicles; (I) Double-headed sperm with vesicles; (J) Pear-shaped head with vesicle and beaded mid-piece; (K) Round-headed sperm with vesicle; (L) Sperm head with multiple vesicles; (M and N) Sperms with abnormal head shape, containing vesicle.

POLOSCOPY

Divyashree PS, Bezar Ghan VV, Anu Kottur

INTRODUCTION

The important role of meiotic spindle during oogenesis and fertilization need not be overemphasized. The developmental competence of a mature oocyte can be obtained by the detection and analysis of meiotic spindle.

Polarized light microscopy (poloscopy) helps to visualize the meiotic spindle noninvasively and in a dynamic fashion **(Figs. 5 to 9)**.

PRINCIPLE OF POLOSCOPY

The highly orderly structure of spindle microtubules generates the phenomenon of birefringence, which consists of the decomposition of a single incident beam of polarized light into two orthogonal rays. This creates a difference in contrast between the spindle and the rest of the cell which may be detected by imaging methods (e.g., the poloscope) that digitally amplify birefringence signals and after computational manipulations, make quantifiable the degree of microtubule orientation within living cells.

Several studies have confirmed that the absence of the spindle compromises the ability of the oocyte to fertilize and undergo normal preimplantation development.[5-7]

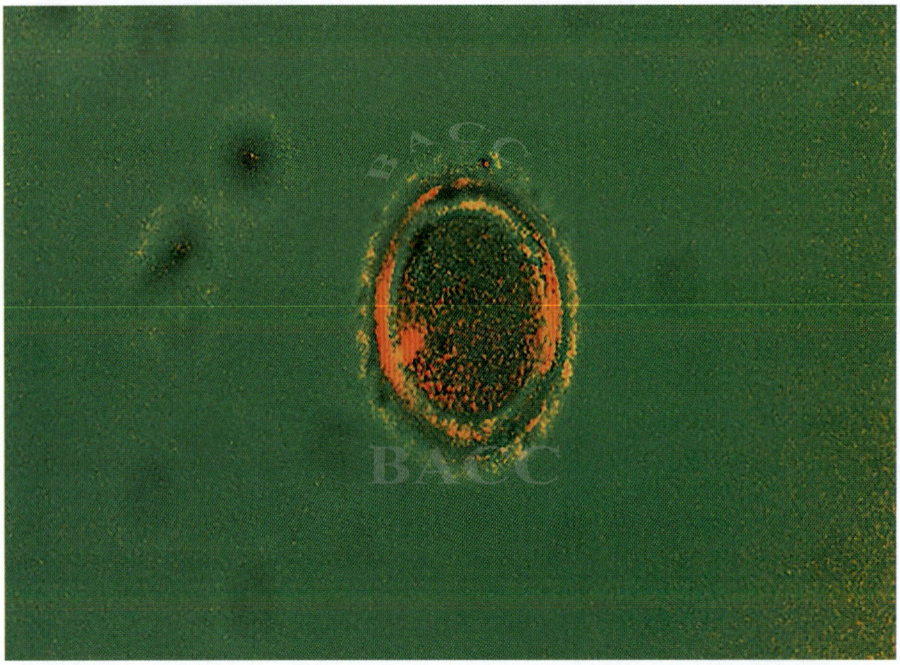

Fig. 5: Telophase I oocyte visualized using polarized light microscopy. The meiotic spindle (MS) can be seen at 8 o'clock position and first polar body (IPB) at 6 o'clock position.

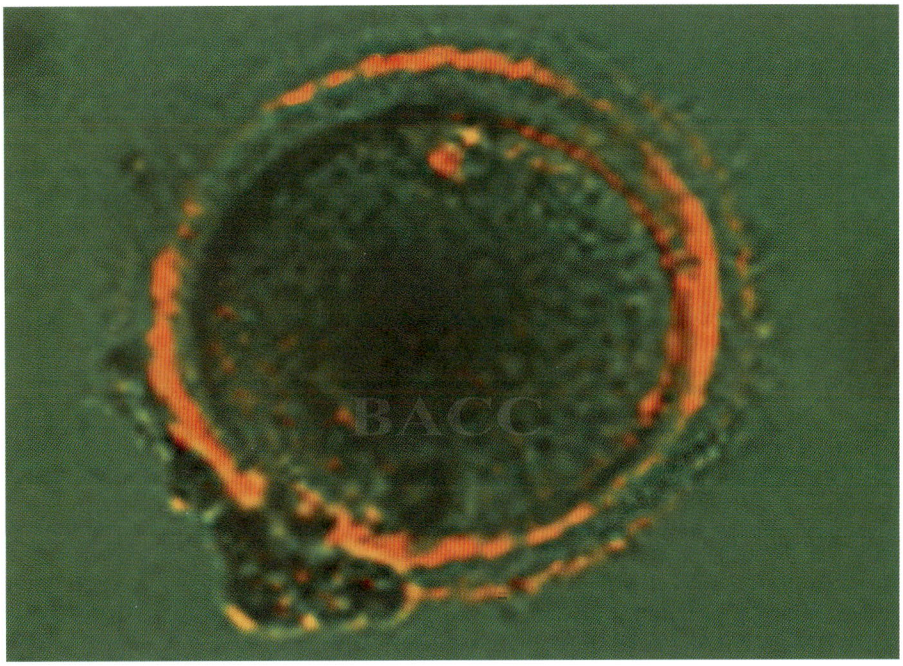

Fig. 6: Metaphase II (MII) oocyte visualized using polarized light microscopy. The meiotic is visible along with the polar body at 12 o'clock position, indicating the first meiotic division is not complete.

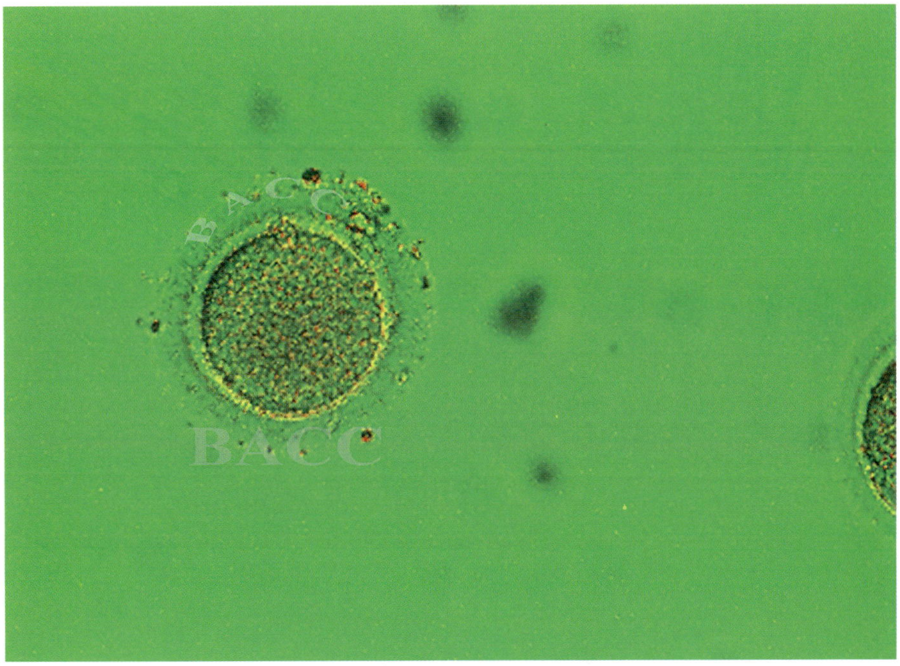

Fig. 7: Metaphase II (MII) oocyte visualized using polarized light microscopy. The meiotic spindle of the second meiotic division is absent.

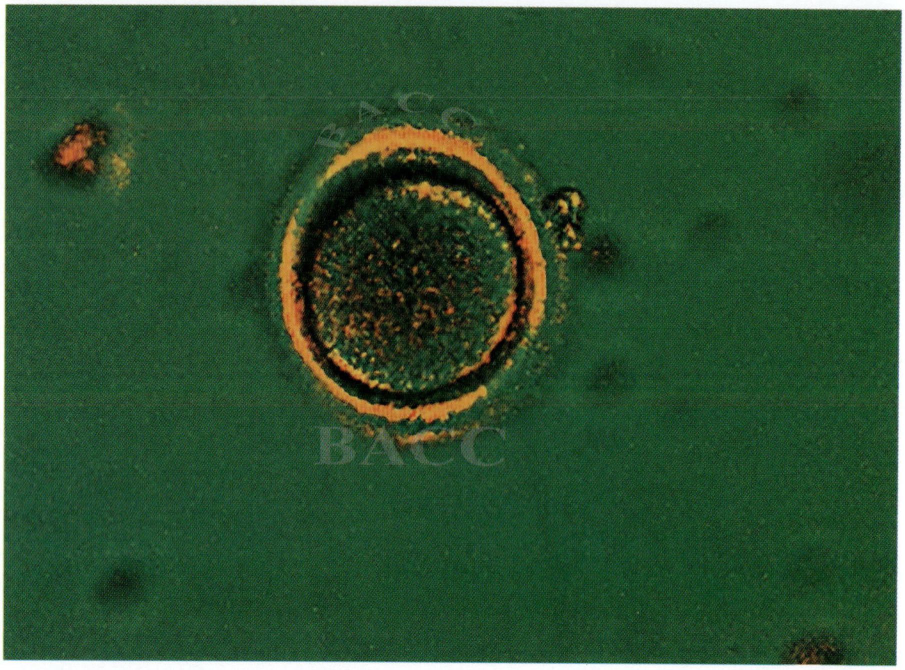

Fig. 8: Metaphase I (MI) oocyte visualized using polarized light microscopy. Note the absence of meiotic spindle and polar body.

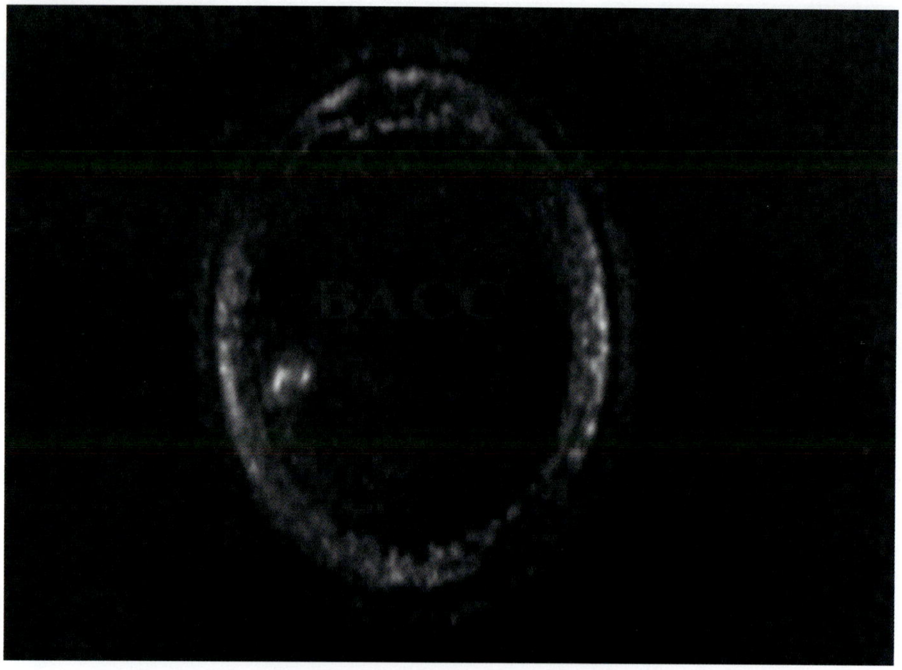

Fig. 9: Metaphase II (MII) oocyte visualized using polarized light microscopy.
Note the meiotic spindle at 9 o'clock position and polar body at 11 o'clock position.

TIME-LAPSE IMAGING

Divyashree PS, Anitha S Kumari K, Mohammed Ashraf C, Bezar Ghan VV

INTRODUCTION

Time-lapse imaging (TLI) is a powerful tool for the study of early embryo development. It offers many advantages over traditional time-point microscopy. Using time-lapse microscopy (TLM) **(Fig. 10)**, biological samples are cultured directly on an imaging device that captures images at defined intervals over a specific period of time. Individual captured images can then be processed into a time-lapse sequence, and from the video sequence, morphological, dynamic and quantitative data can be extracted. In contrast, traditional time-point microscopy acquires images at distinct time points. Such time points are often selected for user convenience rather than biological relevance, and they are acquired at a significantly lower frequency than TLI sequences **(Figs. 11 to 17)**. For example, in embryo grading and embryo research, images may be collected daily, while TLI enables images to be captured at 20-minute, 5-minute or even 10-s frequencies.[8,9]

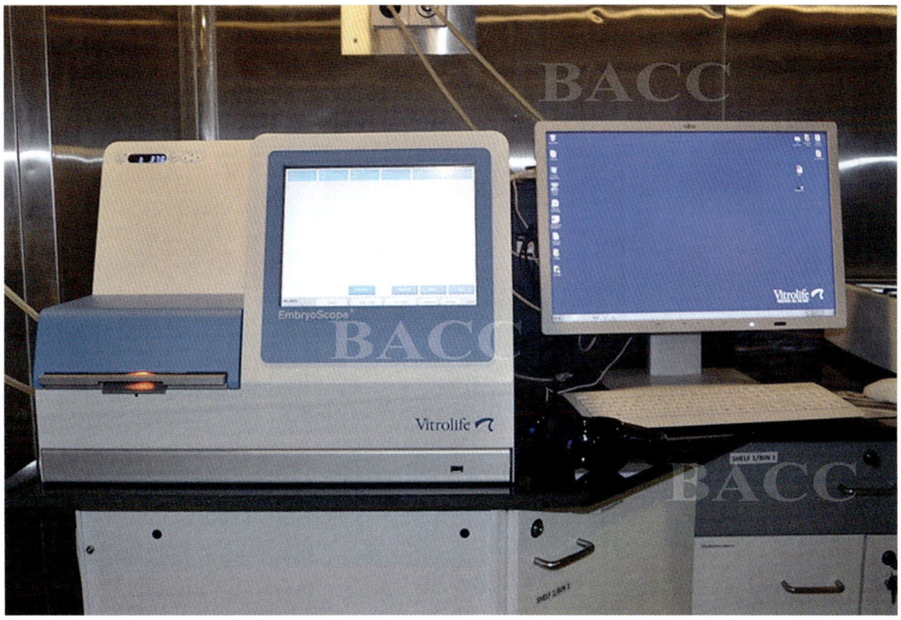

Fig. 10: Embryoscope (Time lapse system).

1 PRONUCLEI

The asynchrony in Pronuclei (PN) formation or PN fusion during fertilization can lead to the presence of 1 pronuclei. This results in the possibility of oocytes having a diploid set of chromosomes and two polar bodies. Transfer of such oocytes can be considered but the possibility of aneuploidy is higher **(Figs. 11A to H)**.

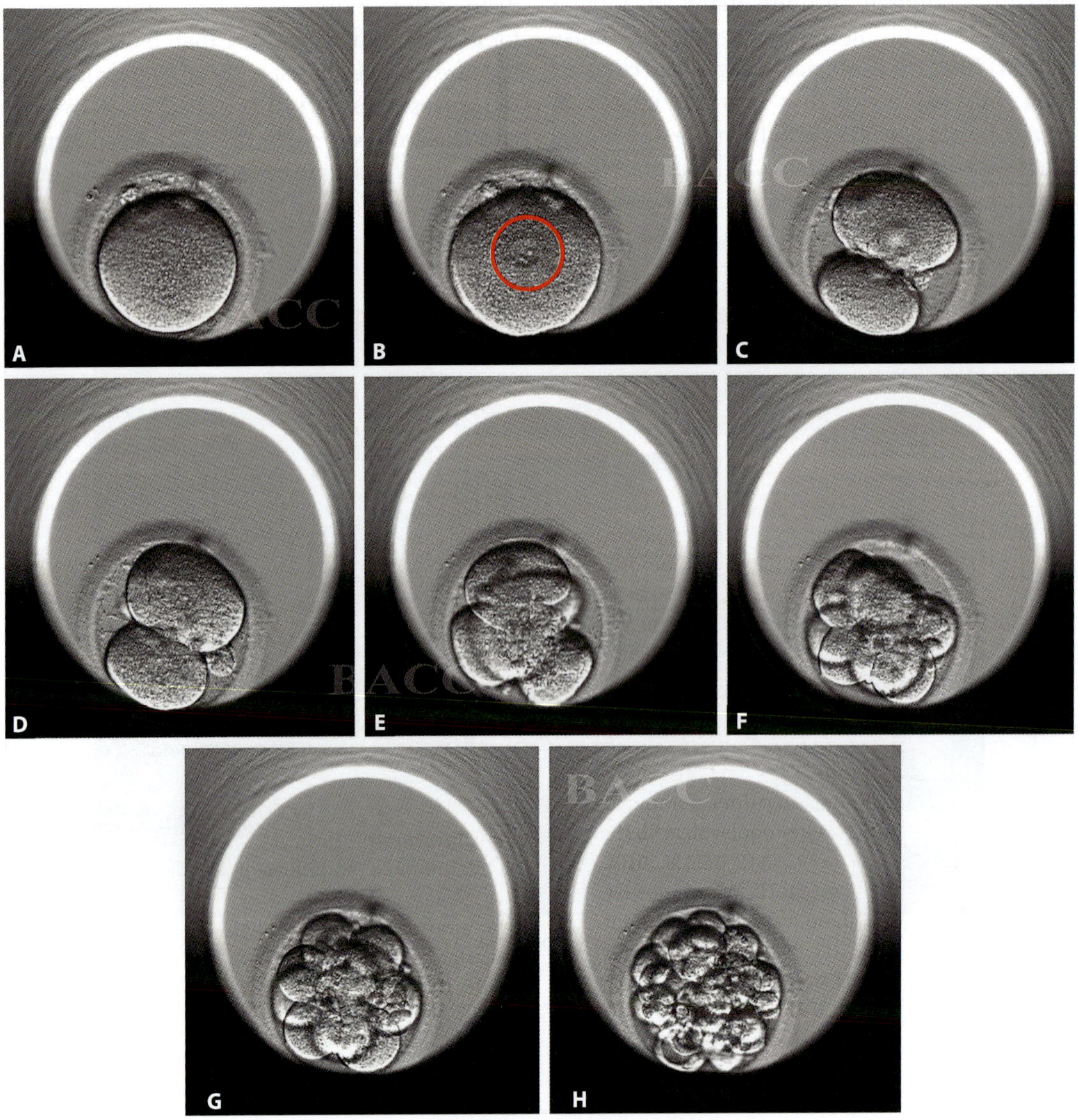

Figs. 11A to H: A time-lapse imaging (TLI) showing the formation of a 1 Pronuclei (1PN) (abnormal fertilization) resulting in the development of an embryo.

3 PRONUCLEUS

The pictures depict the formation of triploid zygote with the injection of a single sperm. In this case, it is believed that the oocyte did not complete meiosis and has retained half of the female genetic material that should be discarded in the second polar body. These oocytes will have two maternal and one paternal pronuclei. An embryo is considered anomalous if it has more than two pronucleus regardless of the source of the extra nucleus **(Figs. 12A to M)**.

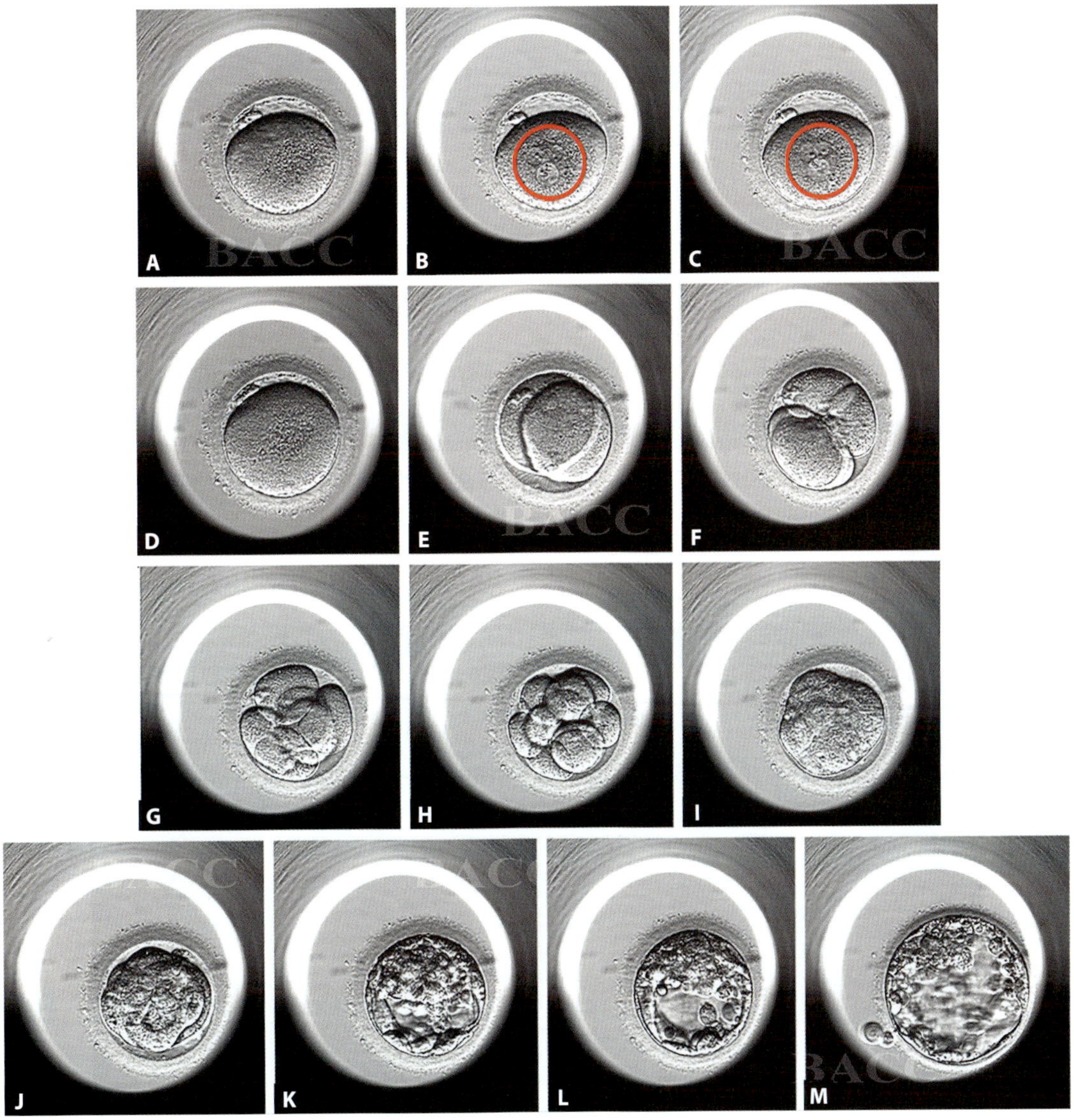

Figs. 12A to M: Time-lapse imaging (TLI) showing the formation of a 3PN (abnormal fertilization) resulting in the development of a blastocyst (anomalous embryo).

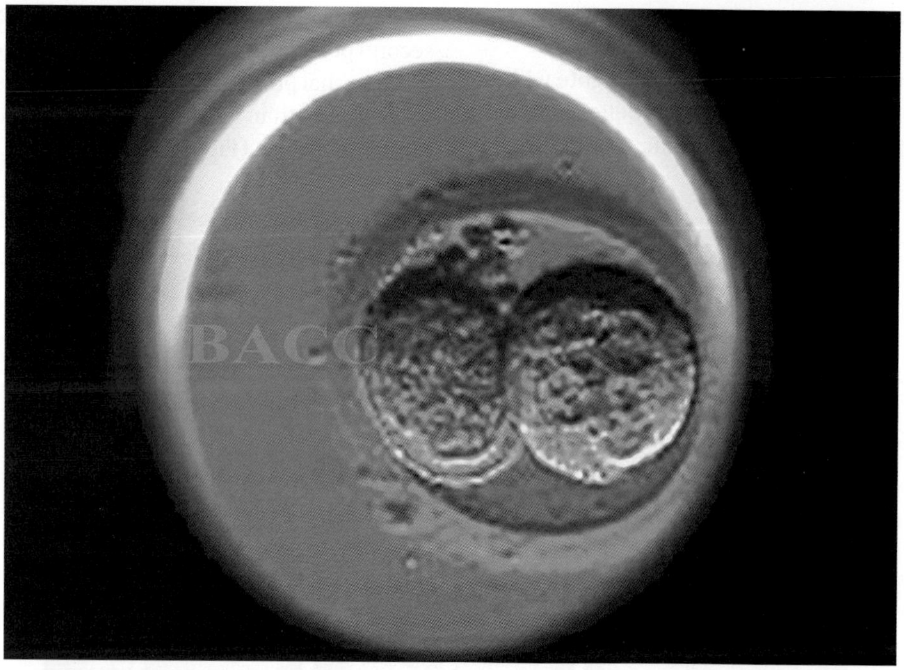

Fig. 13: An early cleavage embryo seen at two-cell stage, 25 hours postinsemination. Fragmentation at 12 o'clock position.

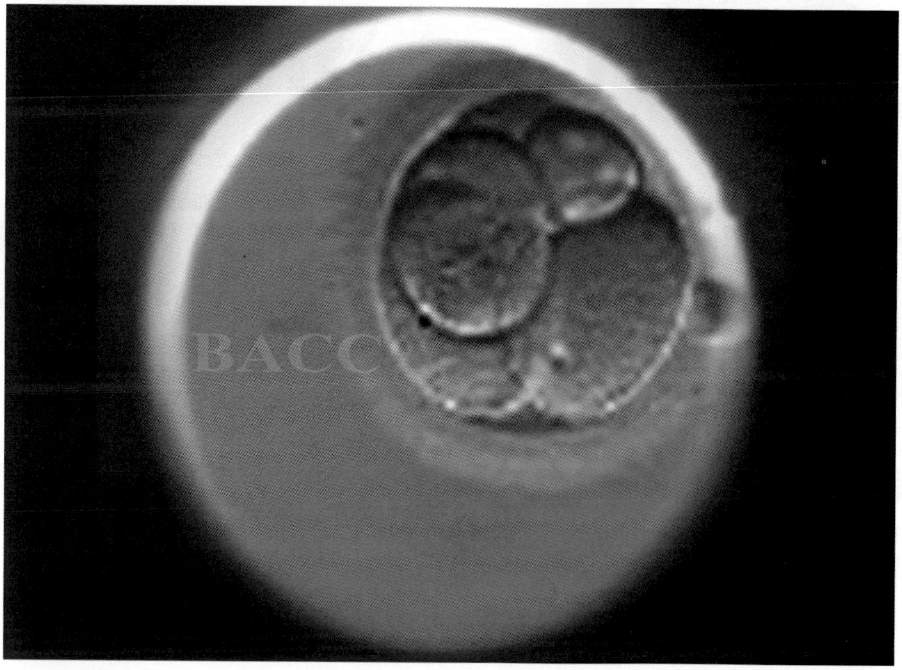

Fig. 14: Time-lapse imaging (TLI) at 44 hours postinsemination showing five-celled embryo. The division is earlier in one of the blastomeres resulting in a five-celled embryo at 34 hours.

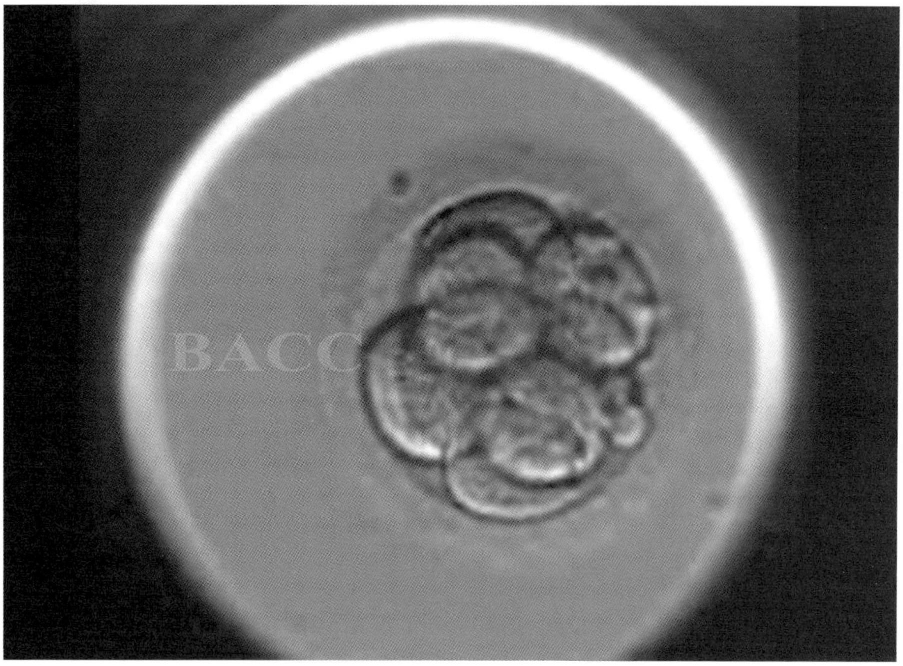

Fig. 15: Time-lapse imaging (TLI) at 68 hours postinsemination showing eight-celled embryo.

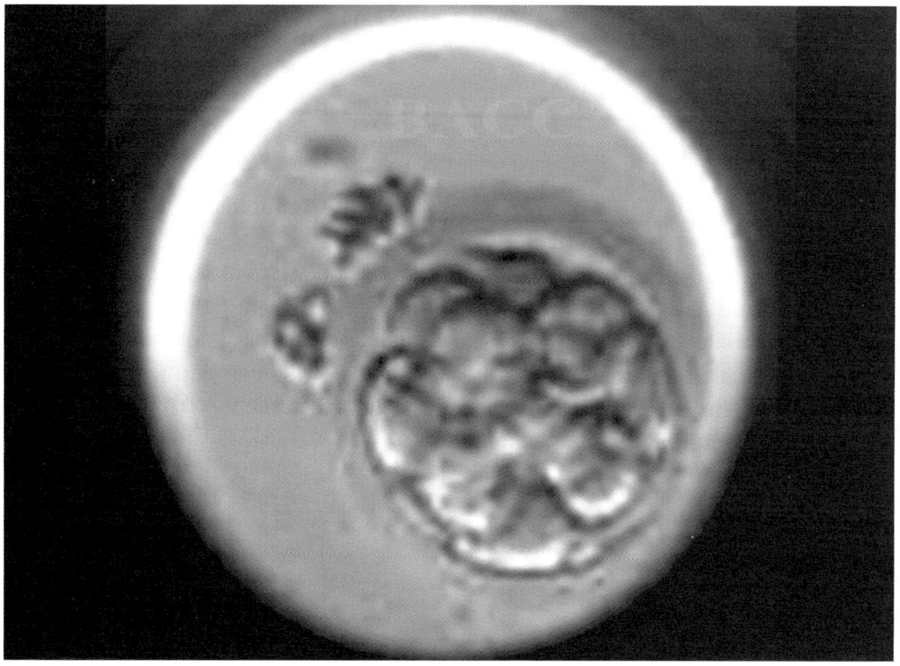

Fig. 16: Time-lapse imaging (TLI) at 95 hours postinsemination showing embryo entering into the stage of morula.
Note: Fragment formation and fragment uptake of an embryo that can occur at different stages of cell division is an example of the dynamic cellular division (note the presence of fragmentation in Figure 15 and fragmentation uptake in Figure 16).

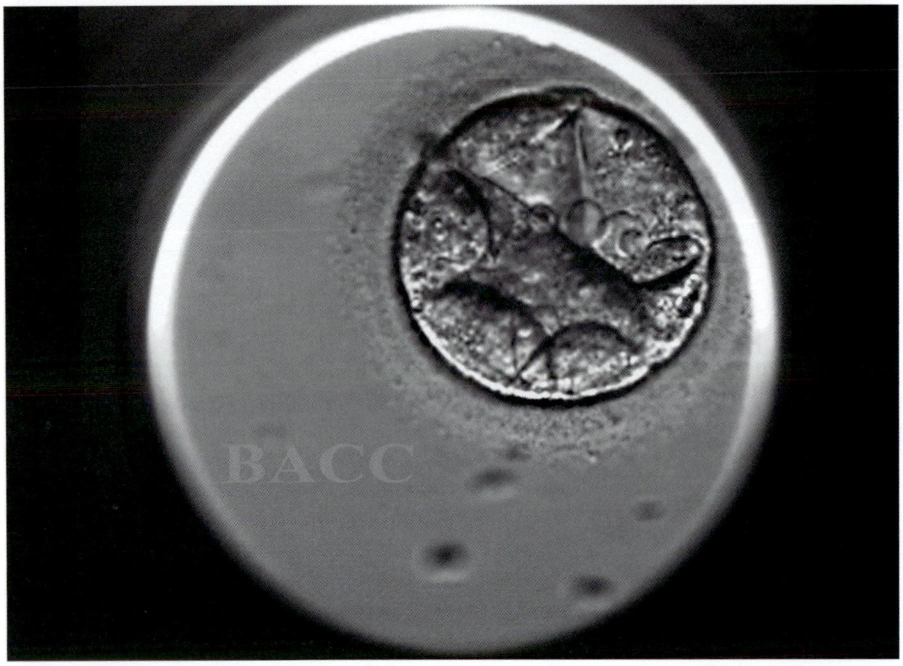

Fig. 17: Time-lapse imaging (TLI) at 105 hours postinsemination showing embryo in the early blastocyst stage.

LASER-ASSISTED HATCHING

Bezar Ghan VV, Divyashree PS, Kamini A Rao

INTRODUCTION

For the trophectoderm cells to interact with endometrial cells, blastocyst should get out of the zona pellucida (ZP) (hatching). It has been postulated that during in vitro culture of human embryos, zona hardening can occur and as a consequence hatching can be inhibited.[10]

Recent systematic review and meta-analysis by Martins et al.[11] conclude that assisted hatching (AH) was related with increased clinical pregnancy and multiple pregnancy rates in women with previous repeated failure or in frozen-thawed embryo transfer.

The procedure is performed on a microscope slide, and the embryo is placed in a drop of medium covered with paraffin oil. The embryo is held with a holding pipette and the laser is delivered through a microscopic laser glass fiber, fitted to the manipulator by a pipette holder, in direct contact with the ZP. Several pulses are necessary to penetrate the ZP. Because each laser pulse removes only small portions of the ZP, the fiber tip has to be continuously readjusted to guarantee close contact with the remaining zona **(Figs. 18 to 21)**.

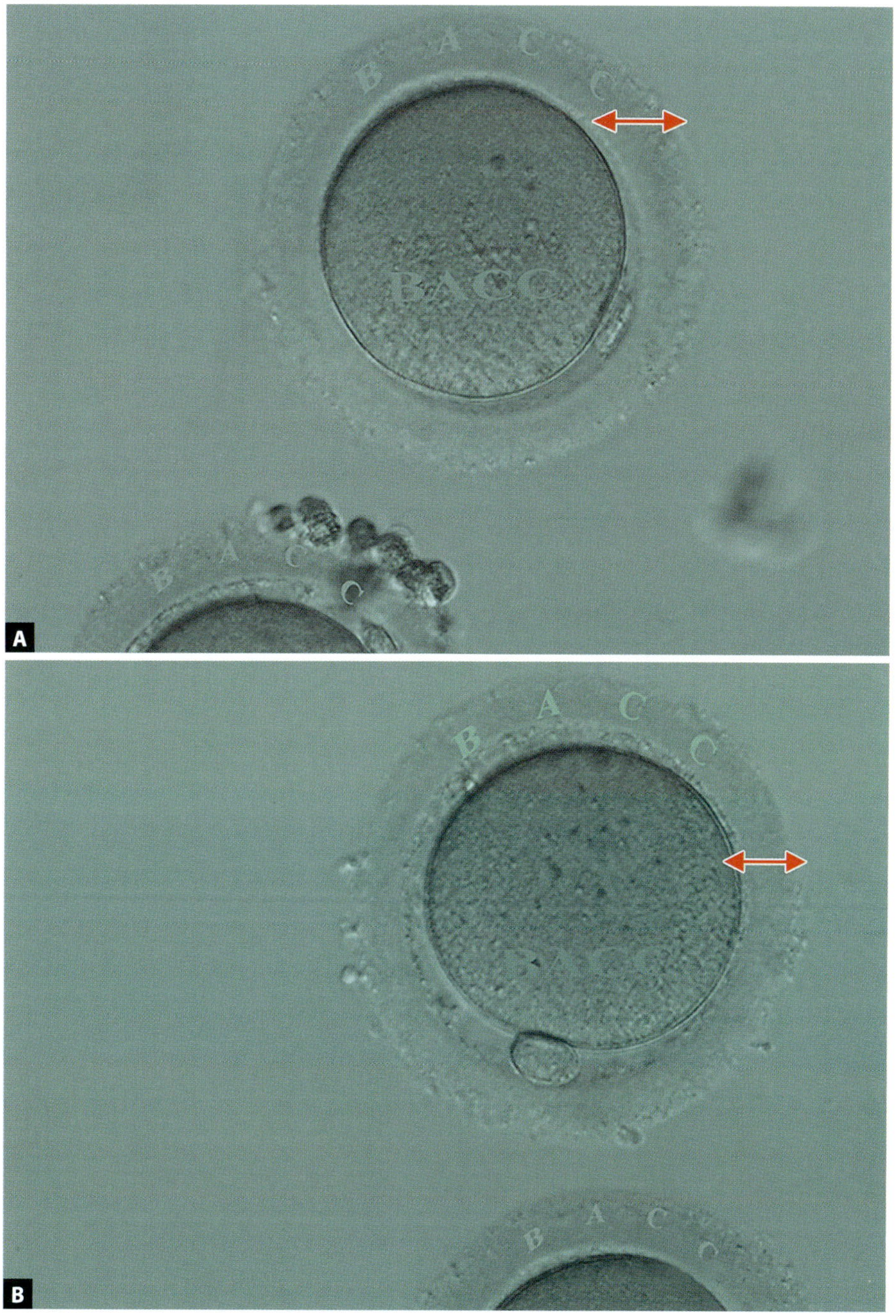

Figs. 18A and B: Denuded mature oocytes showing thick zona.

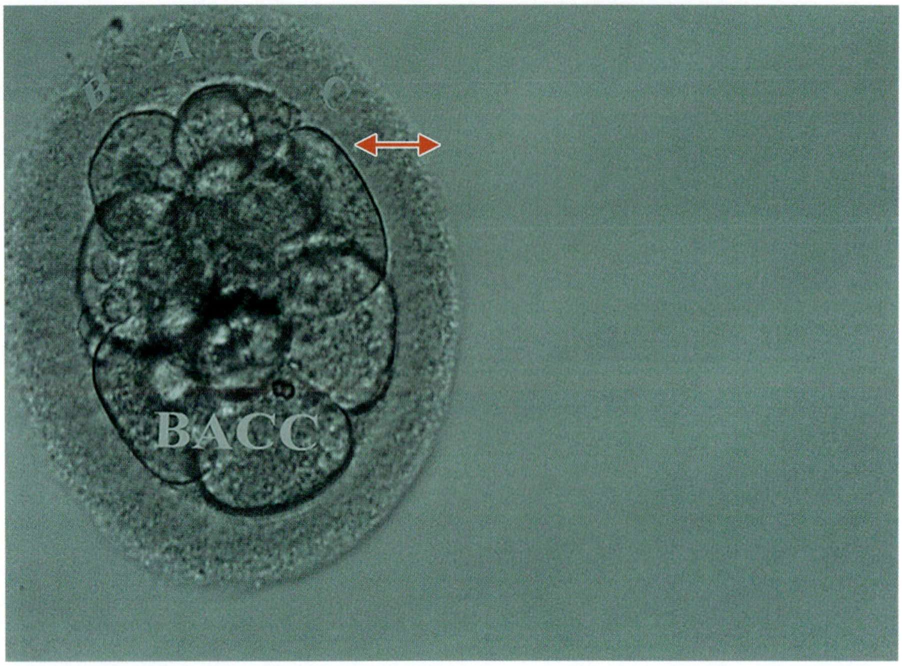

Fig. 19: Eight-celled human embryo showing thick zona before laser-assisted hatching (LAH).

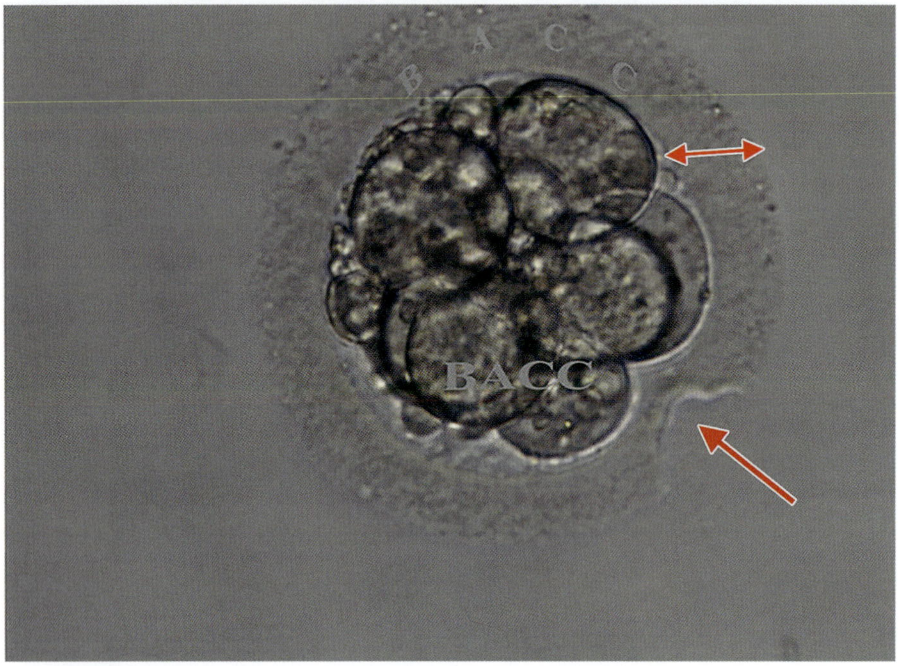

Fig. 20: Eight-celled human embryo after laser-assisted hatching (LAH) at 4 o'clock position.

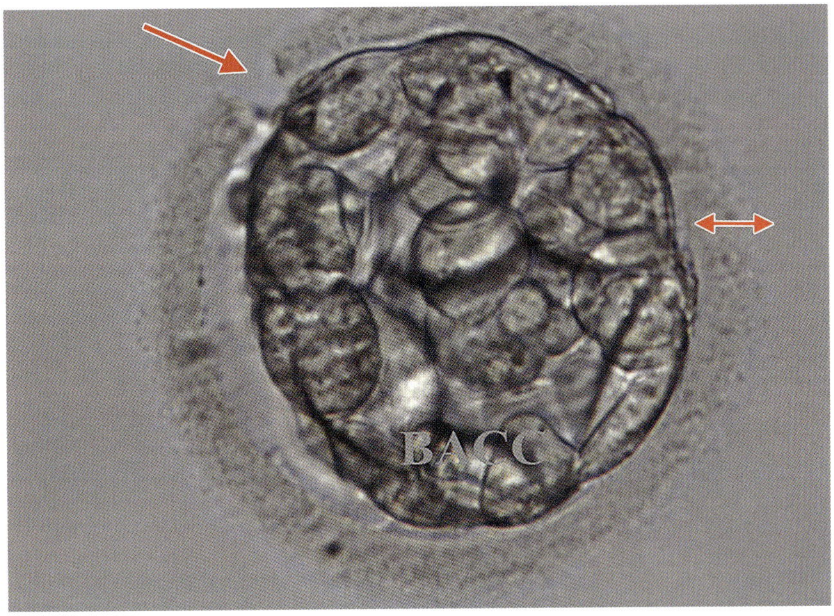

Fig. 21: Human blastocyst after laser-assisted hatching (LAH) at 11 o'clock position.

MAGNETIC-ACTIVATED CELL SORTING (MACS) OF HUMAN SPERMATOZOA

Mohammed Ashraf C

The sperm cell membrane plays a vital role in sperm survival. MACS was introduced as a technique that separates apoptotic spermatozoa from nonapoptotic ones **(Fig. 22)**. In an abnormal sperm, the phosphatidyl serine located in the inner leaflet of the lipid bilayer of the plasma membrane moves to the outer leaflet (apoptotic marker).

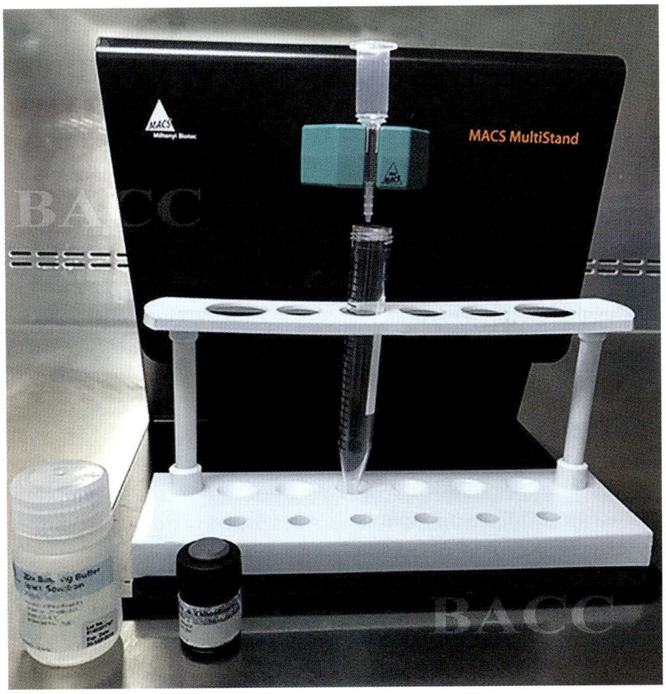

Fig. 22: Magnetic-activated cell sorting.

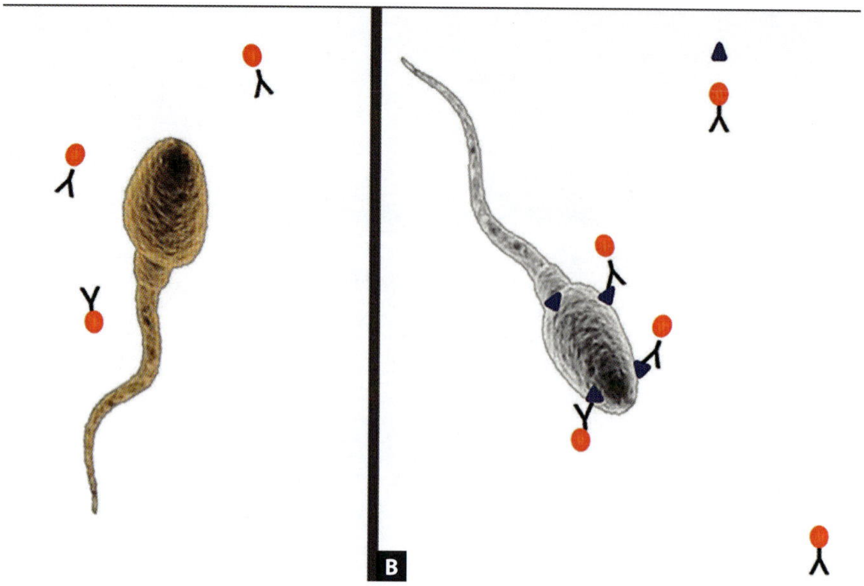

Figs. 23A and B: (A) Normal sperm (viable spermatozoa) Annexin V negative: no annexin V binding; (B) Abnormal sperm (apoptotic) Annexin V positive: annexin V binding.

Image denotes Annexin V Microbead.

The isolation of sperm cells with exposed phosphatidyl serine is performed using Annexin V-coated microbeads **(Figs. 23A and B)**.

In MACS technique, spermatozoa are incubated with a buffer containing Annexin V-conjugated microbeads and are then exposed to a magnetic field in an affinity column which separates apoptotic sperms.[12]

REFERENCES

1. Jean M, Mirallie S, Boudineau M, et al. Intracytoplasmic sperm injection with polyvinylpyrrolidone: a potential risk. Fertil Steril. 2001;76:419-20.
2. Huszar G, Celik-Ozenci C, Cayli S, et al. Hyaluronic acid binding by human sperm indicates cellular maturity, viability, and unreacted acrosomal status. Fertil Steril. 2003;79(Suppl 3):1616-24.
3. Berkovitz A, Eltes F, Soffer Y, et al. ART success and in vivo sperm cell selection depend on the ultramorphological status of spermatozoa. Andrologia. 1999;31:1-8.
4. Souza Setti A, Ferreira RC, Paes de Almeida Ferreira Braga D, et al. Intracytoplasmic sperm injection outcome versus intracytoplasmic morphologically selected sperm injection outcome: a meta-analysis. Reprod Biomed Online. 2010; 21:450-5.
5. Rama Raju GA, Prakash GJ, Krishna KM, et al. Meiotic spindle and zona pellucida characteristics as predictors of embryonic development: a preliminary study using PolScope imaging. Reprod Biomed Online. 2007;14:166-74.
6. Madaschi C, de Souza Bonetti TC, de Almeida Ferreira Braga DP, et al. Spindle imaging: a marker for embryo development and implantation. Fertil Steril. 2008;90:194-8.
7. Cooke S, Tyler JP, Driscoll GL. Meiotic spindle location and identification and its effect on embryonic cleavage plane and early development. Hum Reprod. 2003;18:2397-405.
8. Wong CC, Loewke KE, Bossert NL, et al. Non-invasive imaging of human embryos before embryonic genome activation predicts development to the blastocyst stage. Nat Biotechnol. 2010;28:1115-21.
9. Meseguer M, Herrero J, Tejera A, et al. The use of morphokinetics as a predictor of embryo implantation. Hum Reprod. 2011;26:2658-71.
10. Cohen J, Elsner C, Kort H, et al. Impairment of the hatching process following IVF in the human and improvement of implantation by assisted hatching using micromanipulation. Hum Reprod. 1990;5:7-13.
11. Martins WP, Rocha IA, Ferriani RA, et al. Assisted hatching of human embryos: a systematic review and meta-analysis of randomized controlled trials. Hum Reprod Update. 2011;17:438-53.
12. Said TM, Grunewald S, Paasch U, et al. Advantage of combining magnetic cell separation with sperm preparation techniques. Reprod Biomed Online. 2005;10(6):740-6.

CHAPTER

135 Cryopreservation

Bezar Ghan VV, Anitha S Kumari K, Divyashree PS, Mohammed Ashraf C

INTRODUCTION

The main principle of cryopreservation for mammalian oocytes and embryos is to reduce damage caused by intracellular ice formation. Two basic techniques have been developed: (1) controlled slow rate freezing protocols, and (2) rapid freezing protocols such as vitrification.

There are various studies comparing the effectiveness between slow freezing and vitrification. Eventually, the overwhelming comparative evidence has made it clear to everybody that in developmental stages, vitrification produces better survival and more competent oocytes/embryos than traditional freezing.[1]

In this chapter, we summarize the basic steps of vitrification along with the morphological changes during vitrification and warming.

CRYOPRESERVATION OF OOCYTES

Materials

Vitrification of oocytes contains two solutions: (1) equilibration solution (ES), (2) vitrification solution (VS).

Equilibration solution: It is a 3-(N-morpholino) propanesulfonic acid (MOPS) buffered solution of modified human tubal fluid (HTF) containing nonessential and essential amino acids, gentamicin sulfate (10 mg/L), 7.5% (v/v) each of dimethyl sulfoxide (DMSO) and ethylene glycol and 12 mg/mL human serum albumin **(Figs. 1 to 9)**.

Vitrification solution: It is a MOPS buffered solution of modified HTF containing nonessential and essential amino acids, gentamicin sulfate (10 mg/L), 15% (v/v) each of DMSO and ethylene glycol, 12 mg/mL human serum albumin and 0.6 M sucrose **(Figs. 10 to 13)**.

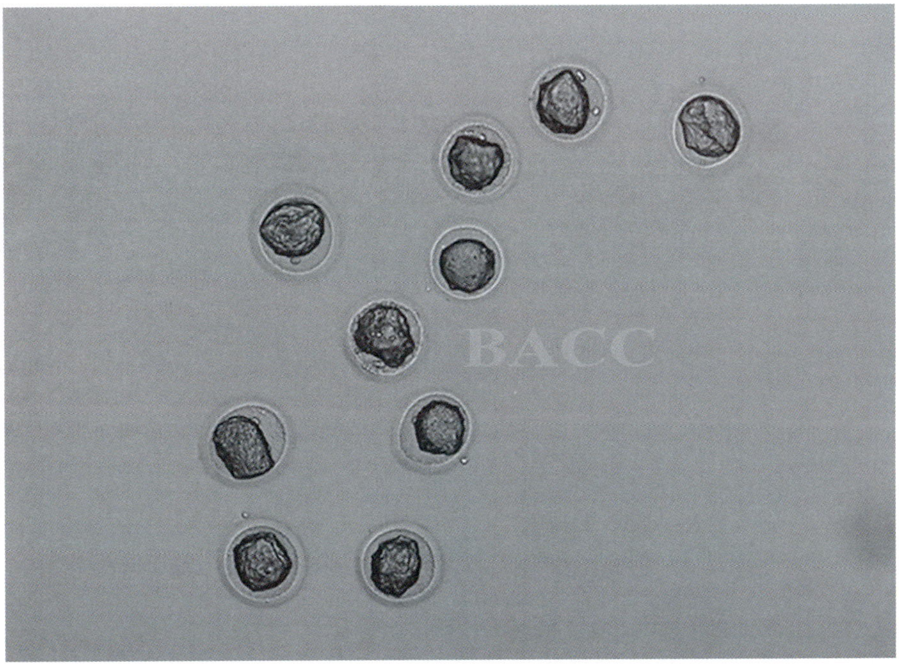

Fig. 1: Oocytes in equilibration solution (ES) at 30 seconds. Oocytes beginning to shrink.

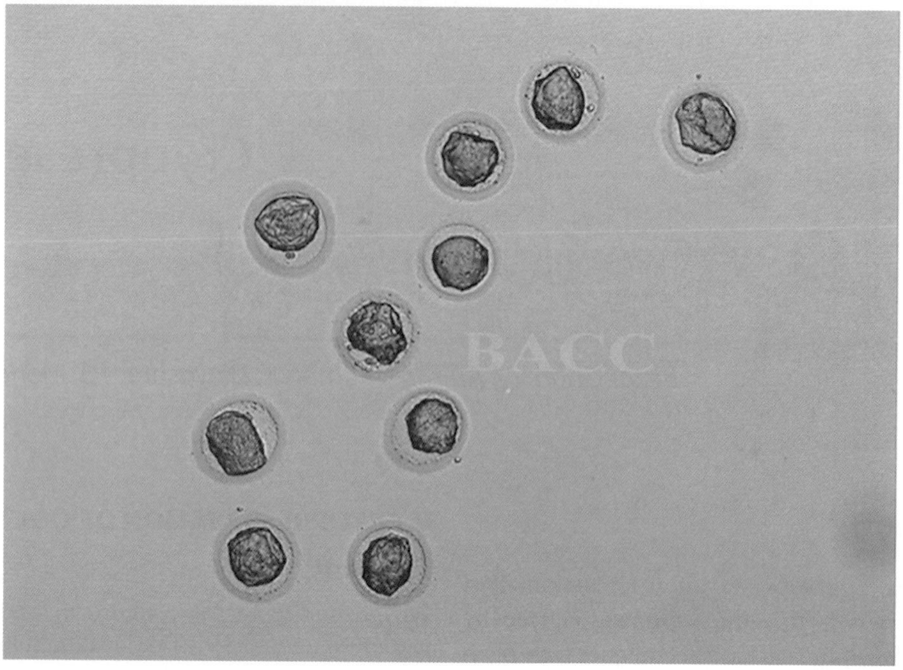

Fig. 2: Oocytes in equilibration solution (ES) at 1 minute at 10x magnification. Note further shrinkage of oocytes.

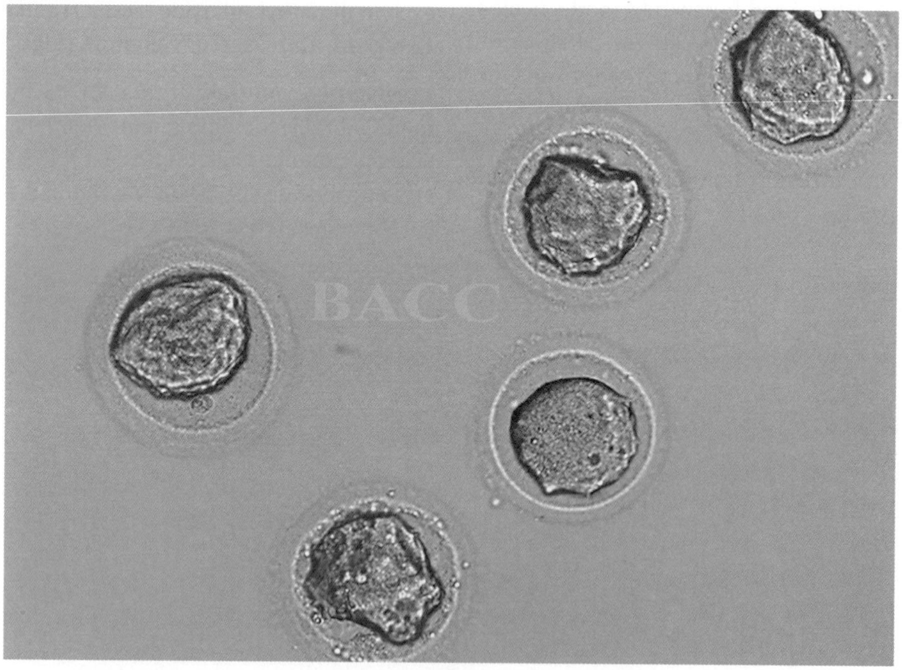

Fig. 3: Oocytes in equilibration solution (ES) at 1 minute at 200x magnification.

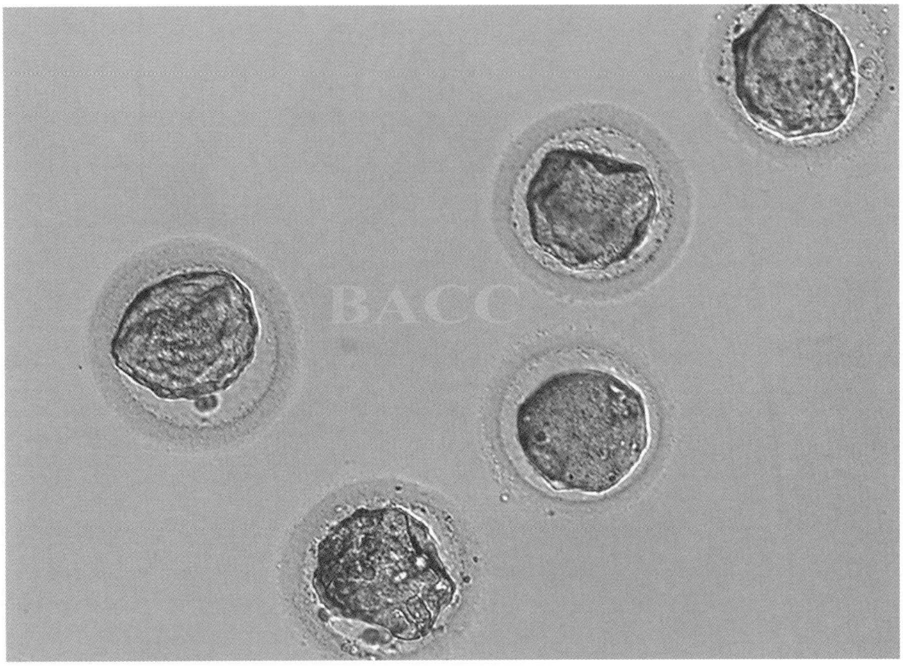

Fig. 4: Oocytes in equilibration solution (ES) at 2 minutes at 200x magnification.

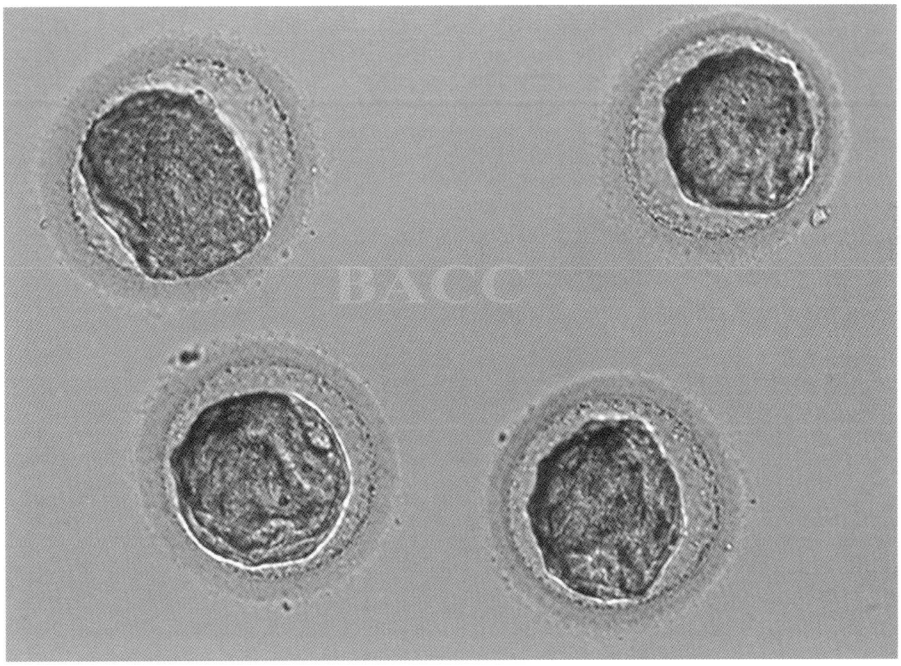

Fig. 5: Oocytes in equilibration solution (ES) at 3 minutes at 200x magnification.

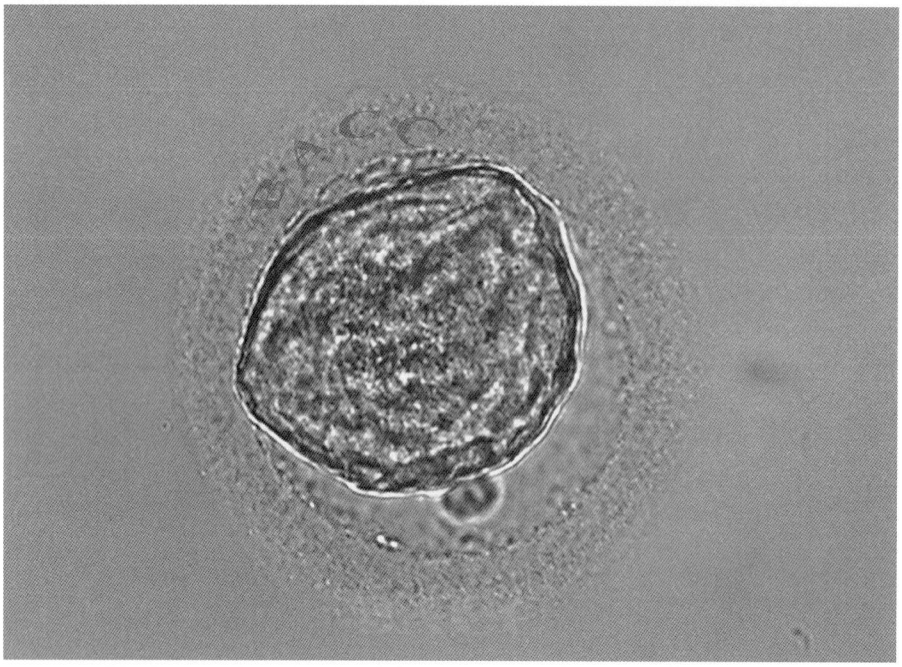

Fig. 6: Oocytes in equilibration solution (ES) at 3 minutes at 400x magnification.

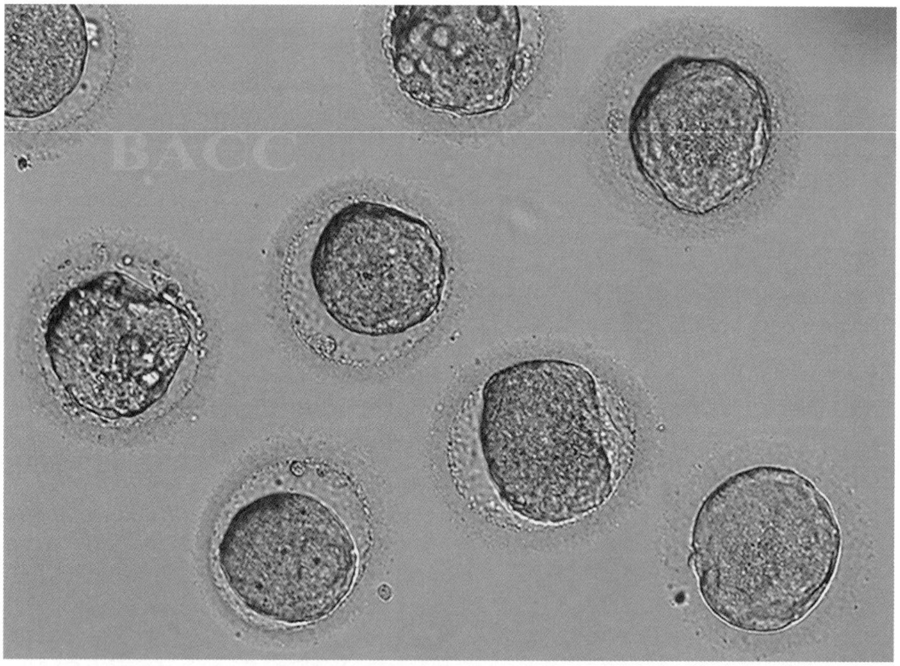

Fig. 7: Oocytes in equilibration solution (ES) at 10 minutes at 200x magnification.

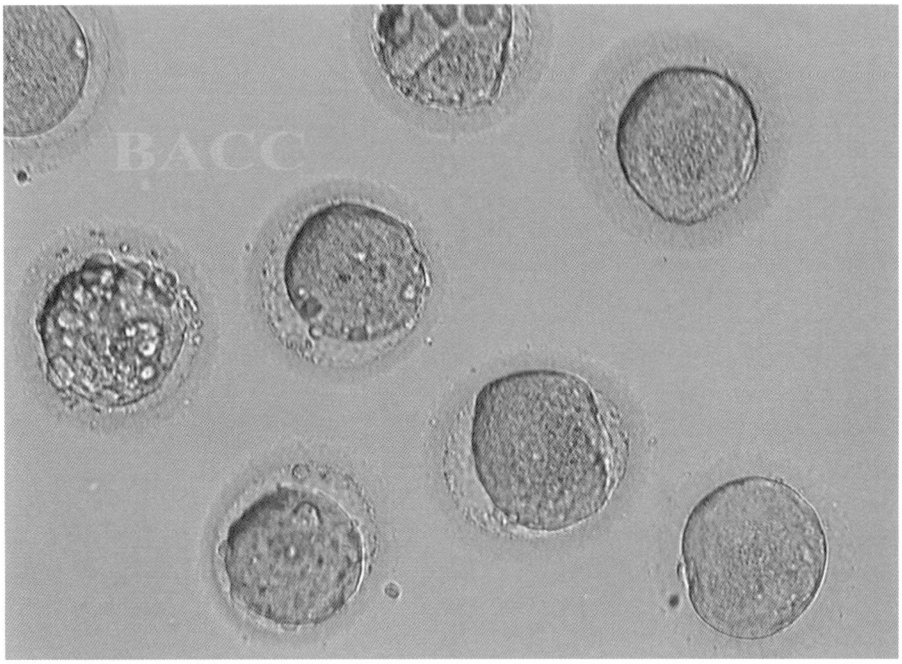

Fig. 8: Oocytes in equilibration solution (ES) at 15 minutes at 200x magnification.

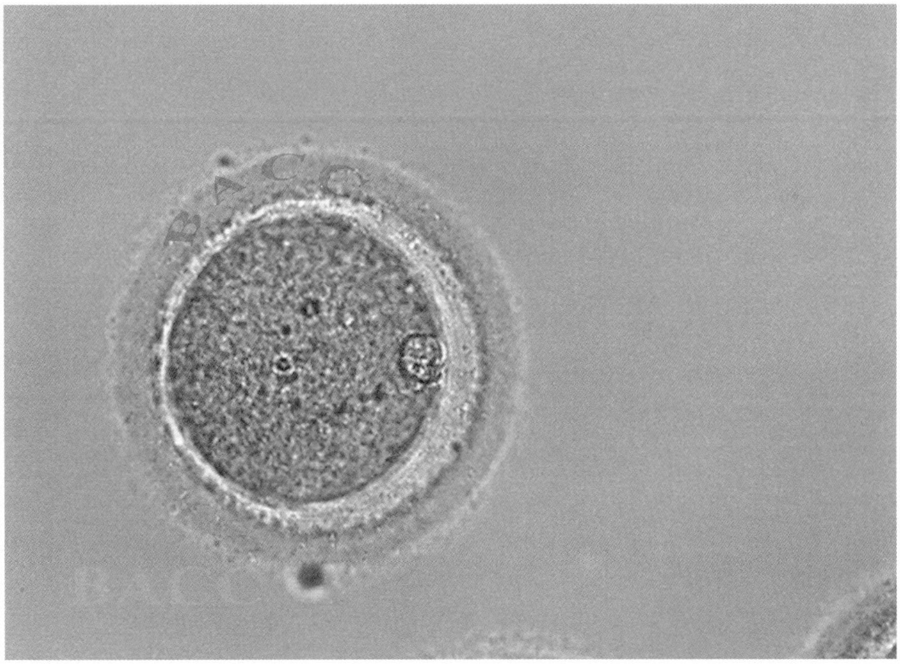

Fig. 9: Oocytes in equilibration solution (ES) at 15 minutes at 400x magnification. Note fully equilibrated and expanded oocyte.

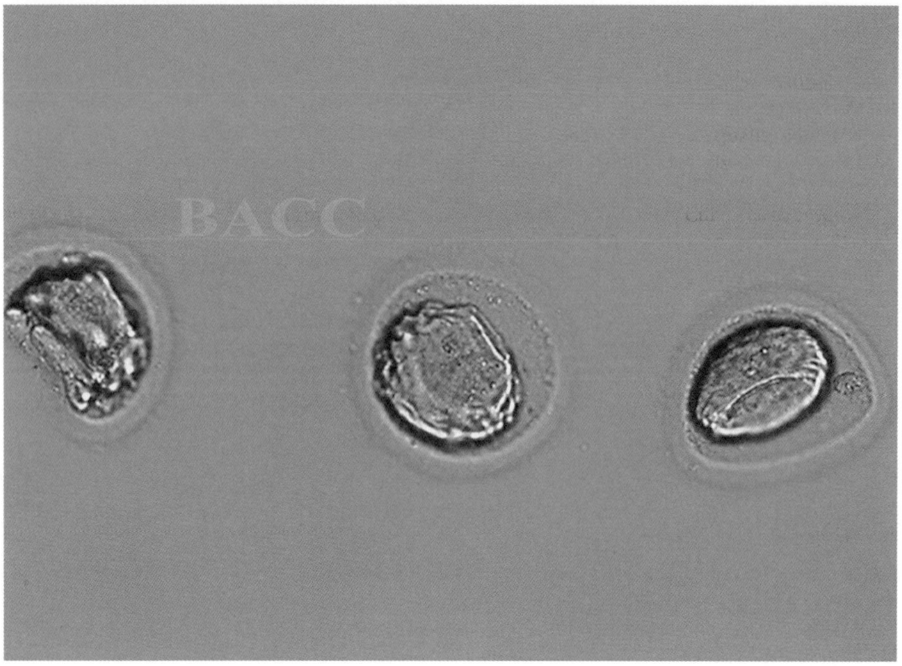

Fig. 10: Oocytes in vitrification solution (VS) at 10 seconds at 200x magnification. Oocytes beginning to shrink again.

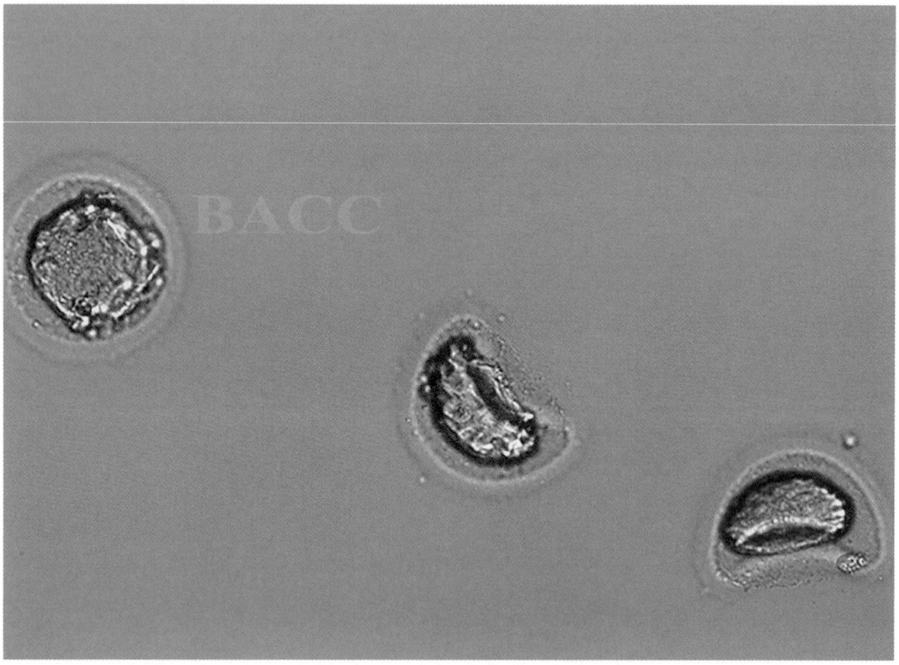

Fig. 11: Oocytes in vitrification solution (VS) at 30 seconds at 200x magnification. Note further shrinkage of oocyte.

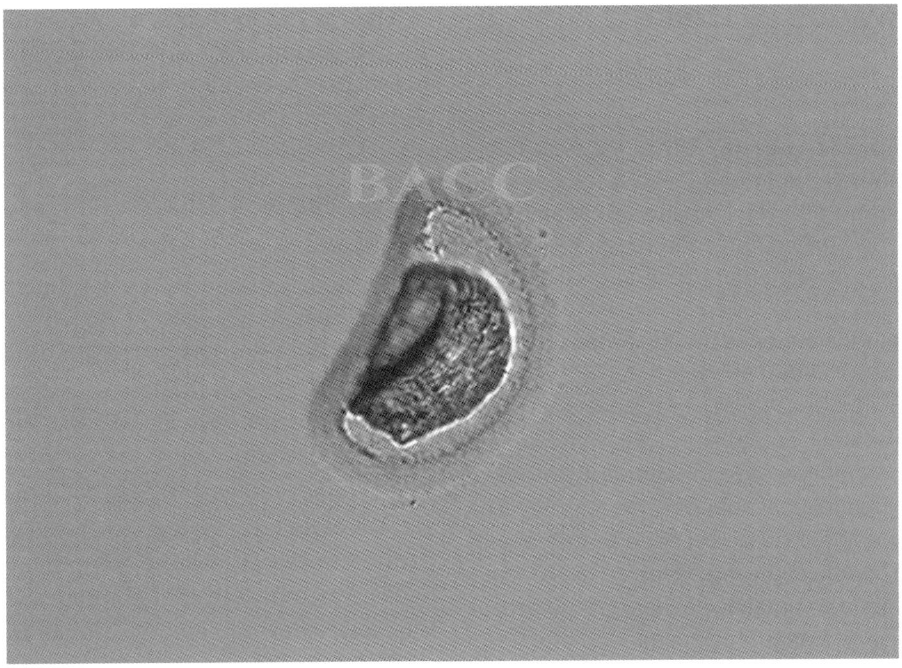

Fig. 12: Oocytes in vitrification solution (VS) at 90 seconds at 200x magnification. Note fully shrunken kidney-shaped oocyte.

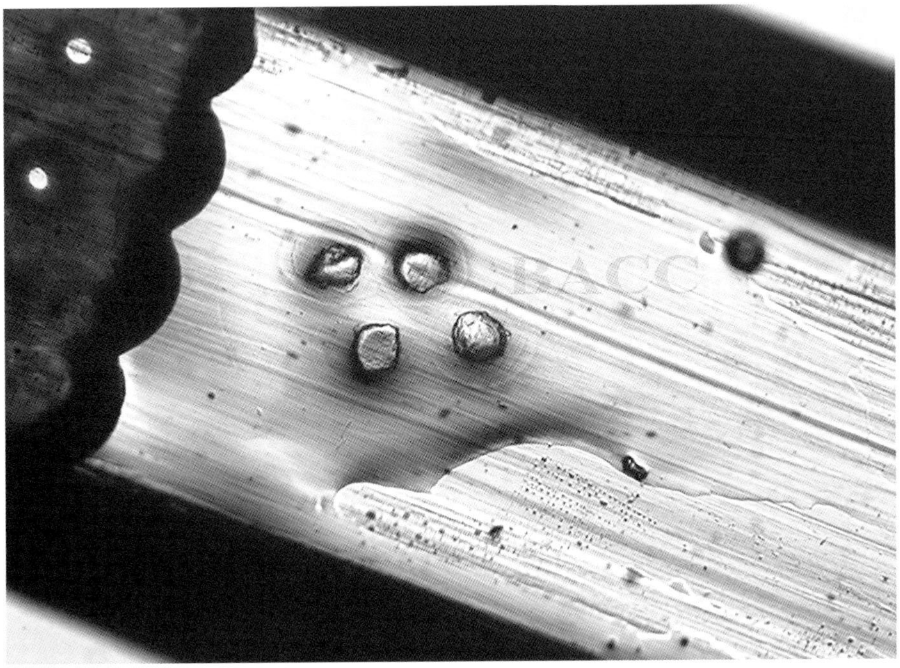

Fig. 13: Vitrified oocytes loaded on a cryodevice before immersion into liquid nitrogen.

CRYOPRESERVATION OF EMBRYOS

Vitrification

Materials

Vitrification of embryos contains three solutions: (1) equilibration solution (ES): contains no cryoprotectant, (2) vitrification solution 1 (VS1): contains ethylene glycol as cryoprotectant; (3) vitrification solution 2 (VS2): contains ethylene glycol, propanediol, ficoll and sucrose as cryoprotectants.

Equilibration solution contains no cryoprotectant. The embryos are kept in this solution for a minimum of 5 minutes to a maximum of 10 minutes **(Fig. 14)**.

Vitrification solution 1 contains ethylene glycol as a cryoprotectant. The embryos are transferred from ES to VS1. The embryos remain in this solution for 2 minutes. The embryos tend to float to the surface; if so collect them and replace them to the bottom of the dish **(Figs. 15 to 18)**.

Vitrification solution 2 contains ethylene glycol, propanediol, ficoll and sucrose as cryoprotectants.

Transfer the embryos from VS1 to VS2 and let the embryos remain in VS2 for 30 seconds.

Figures 19A to D show eight-celled embryos floating in the media containing ethylene glycol, propanediol, ficoll and sucrose as cryoprotectants at 10, 15, 20 and 25 seconds respectively.

Warming

Materials

- *Warming solution 1 (WS1):* Contains sucrose as cryoprotectant
- *Warming solution 2 (WS2):* Contains sucrose as cryoprotectant
- *Warming solution 3 (WS3):* Contains sucrose as cryoprotectant
- *Warming solution 4 (WS4):* Contains no cryoprotectant.

In a cryodewer, bring the cryodevice containing the vitrified embryos close to the prepared wells **(Figs. 20 to 22)**. Place the vitrified embryos quickly into the WS1 **(Fig. 23)**. Allow the embryos to fall from the cryodevice and sink to the bottom. Leave for 10–30 seconds **(Fig. 24)**.

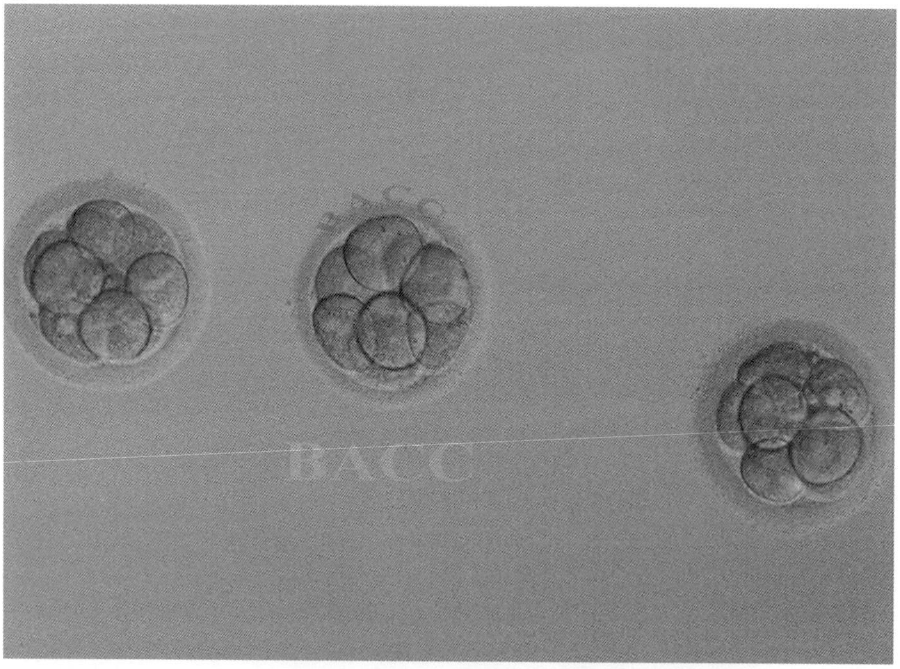

Fig. 14: Eight-celled embryos in equilibration solution kept for 5–10 minutes at 37°C.

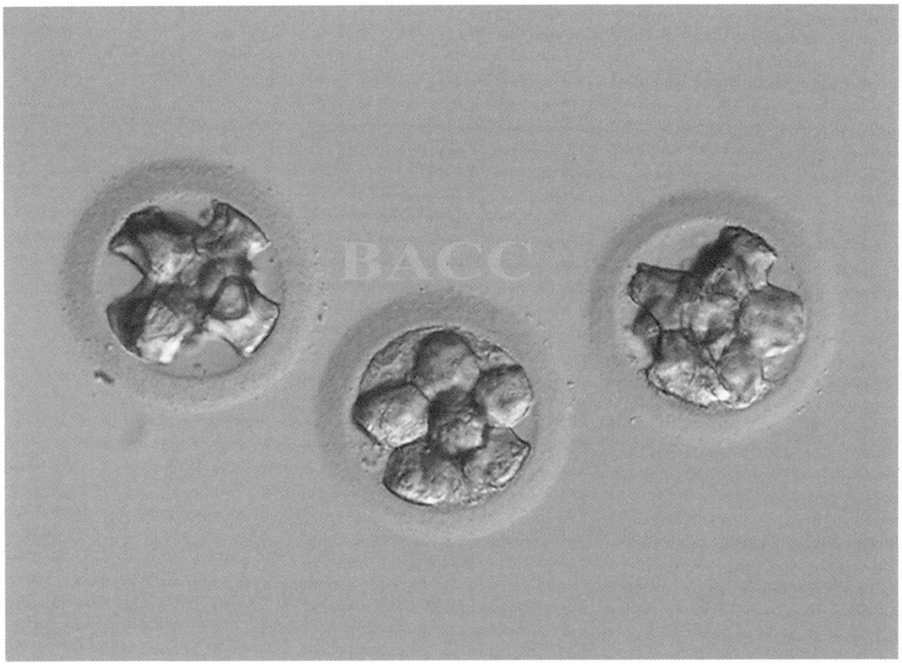

Fig. 15: Eight-celled embryos in vitrification solution 1 (VS1), containing ethylene glycol as a cryoprotectant at 15 seconds. Note the blastomere shrinkage.

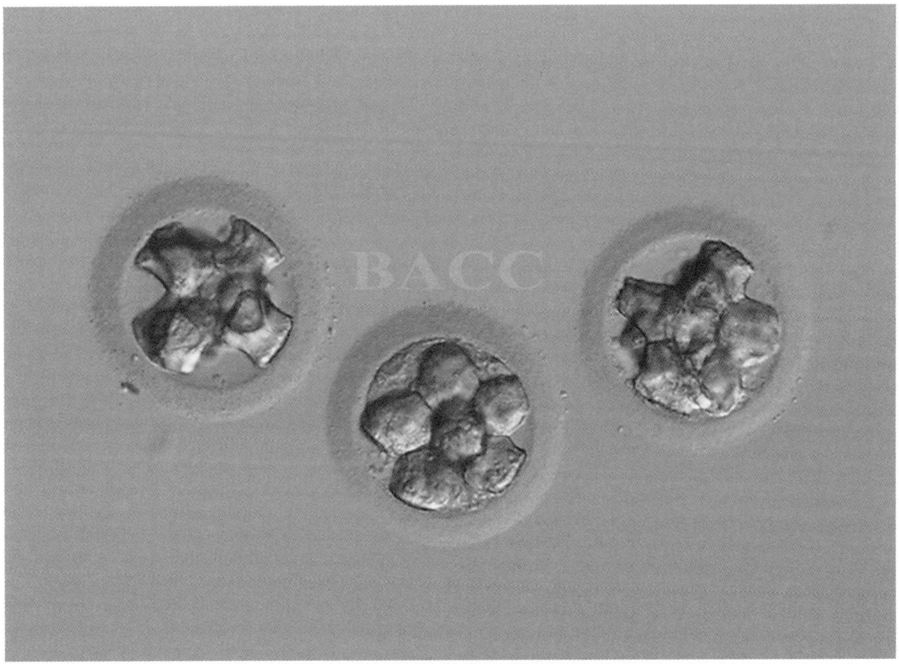

Fig. 16: Eight-celled embryos in vitrification solution 1 (VS1) containing ethylene glycol as a cryoprotectant at 30 seconds. Note the blastomere shrinkage.

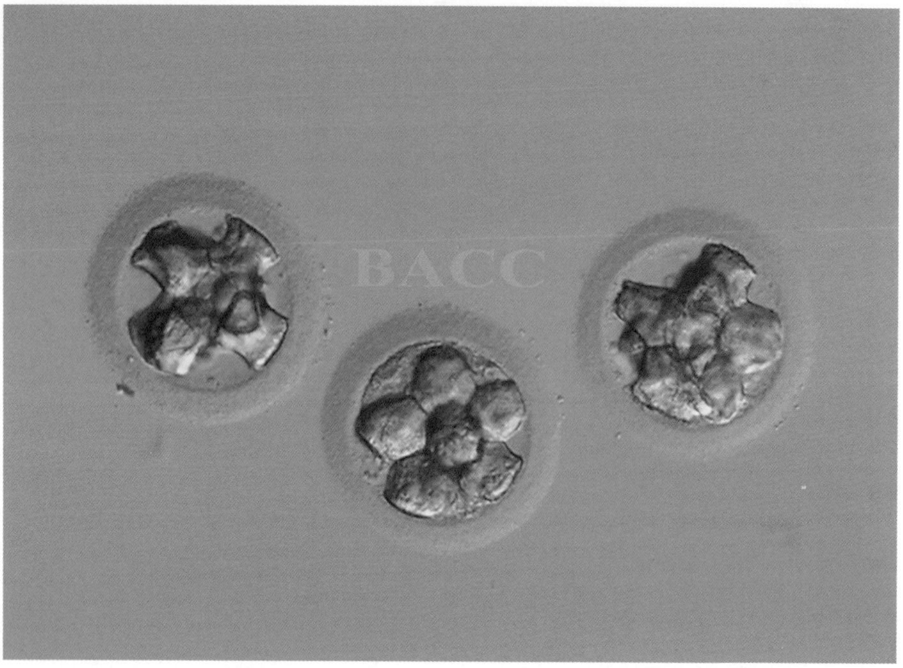

Fig. 17: Eight-celled embryos in vitrification solution 1 (VS1) containing ethylene glycol as a cryoprotectant at 60 seconds. Note the blastomere shrinkage.

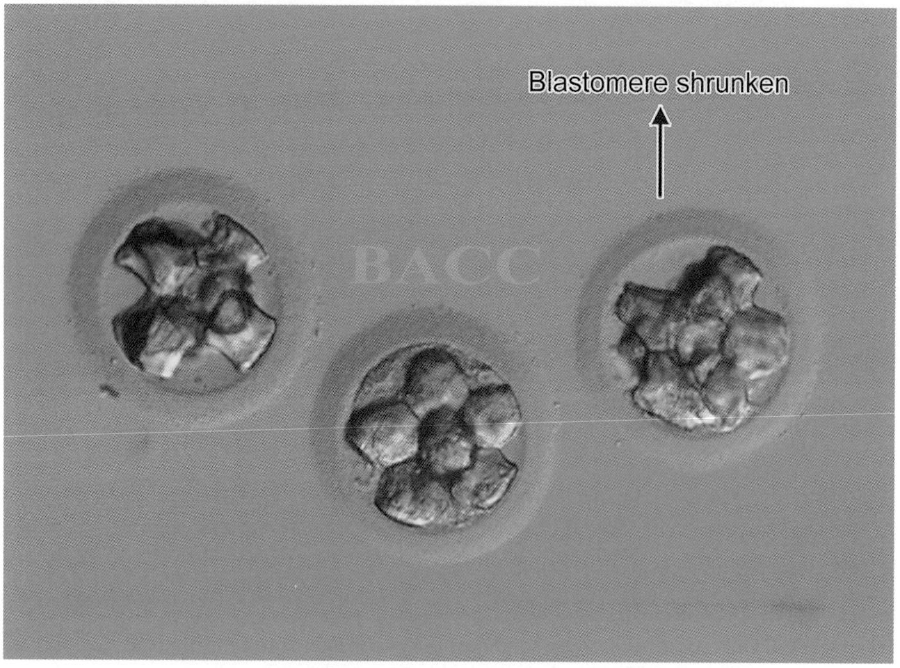

Fig. 18: Eight-celled embryos in vitrification solution 1 (VS1) containing ethylene glycol as a cryoprotectant at 90 seconds. Note the degree of blastomere shrinkage.

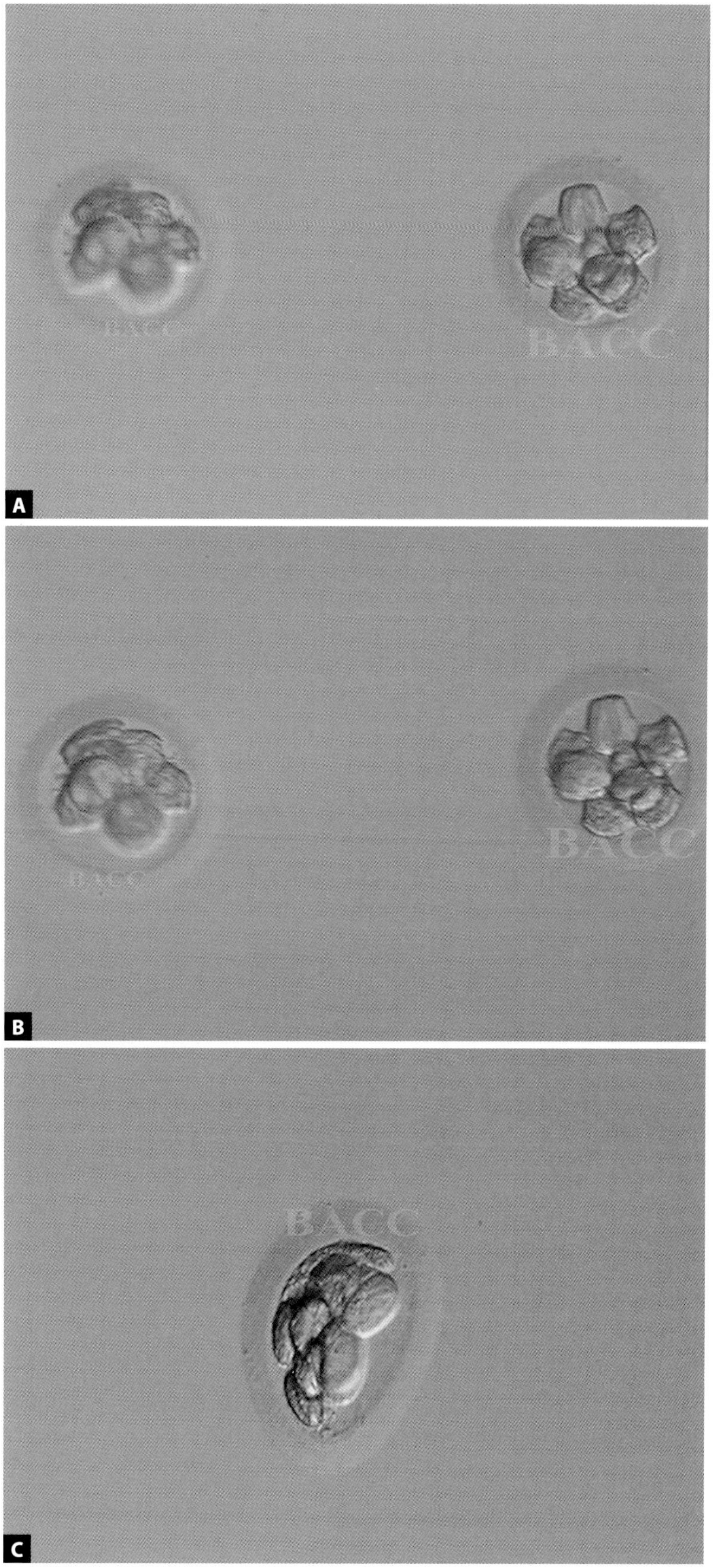

Figs. 19A to C

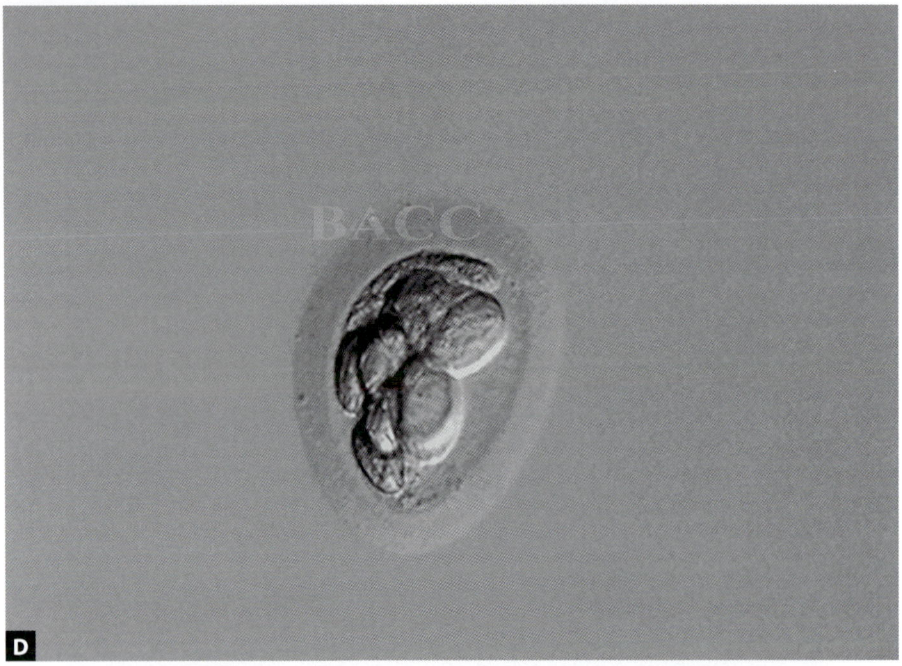

Figs. 19A to D: Eight-celled embryos floating in the cryoprotectant media vitrification solution 2 (VS2) at (A) 10 seconds; (B) 15 seconds; (C) 20 seconds; (D) 25 seconds.

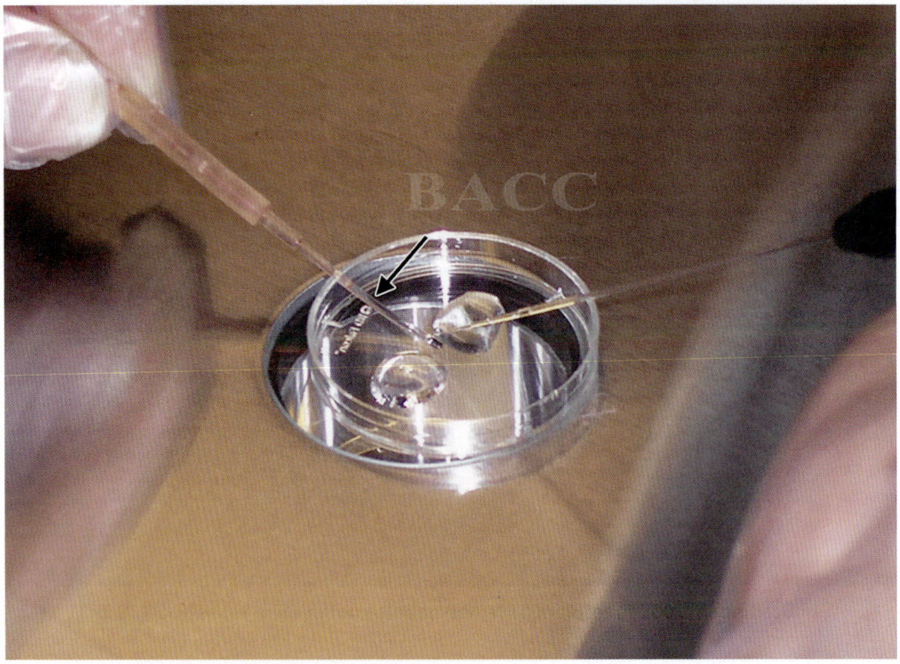

Fig. 20: Loading the embryos to the cryolock device (arrow) from the cryoprotectant media.

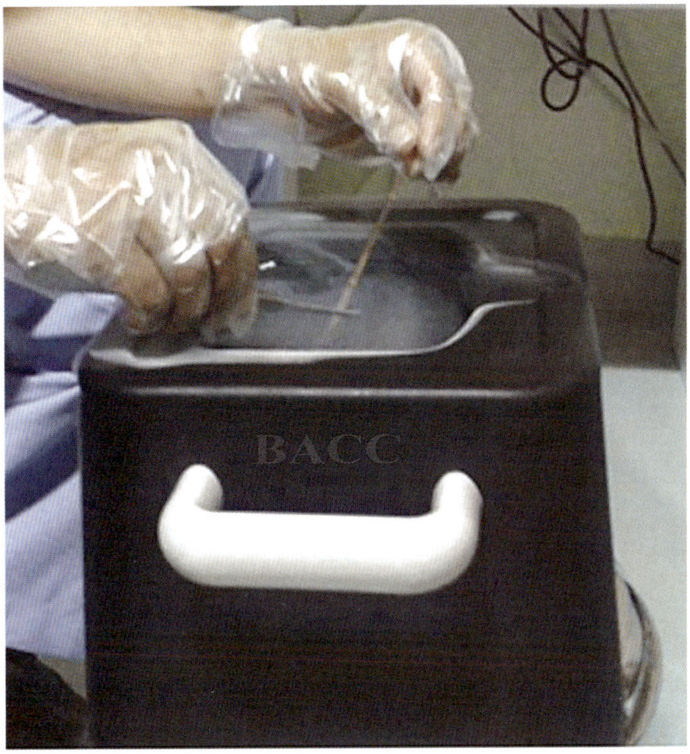

Fig. 21: Locking the cryolock under liquid nitrogen.

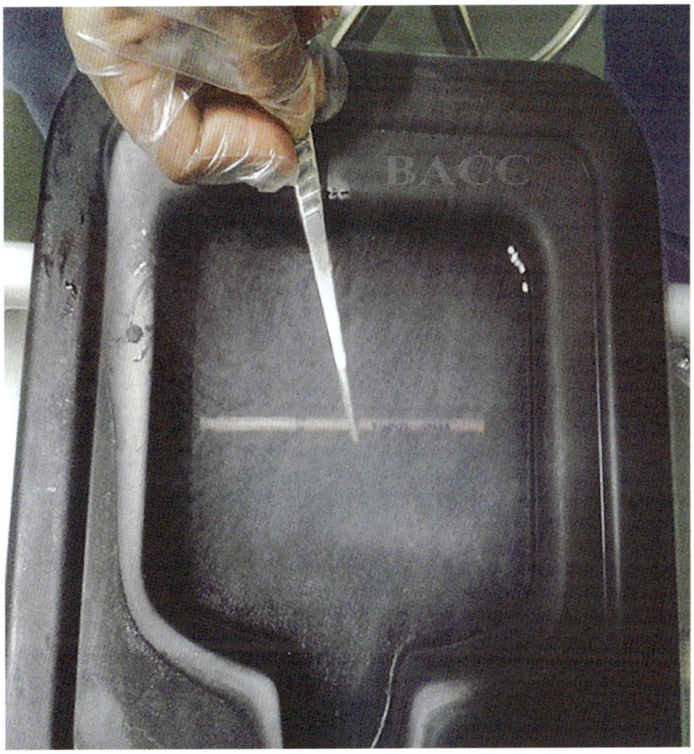

Fig. 22: The cryolock after locking under liquid nitrogen.

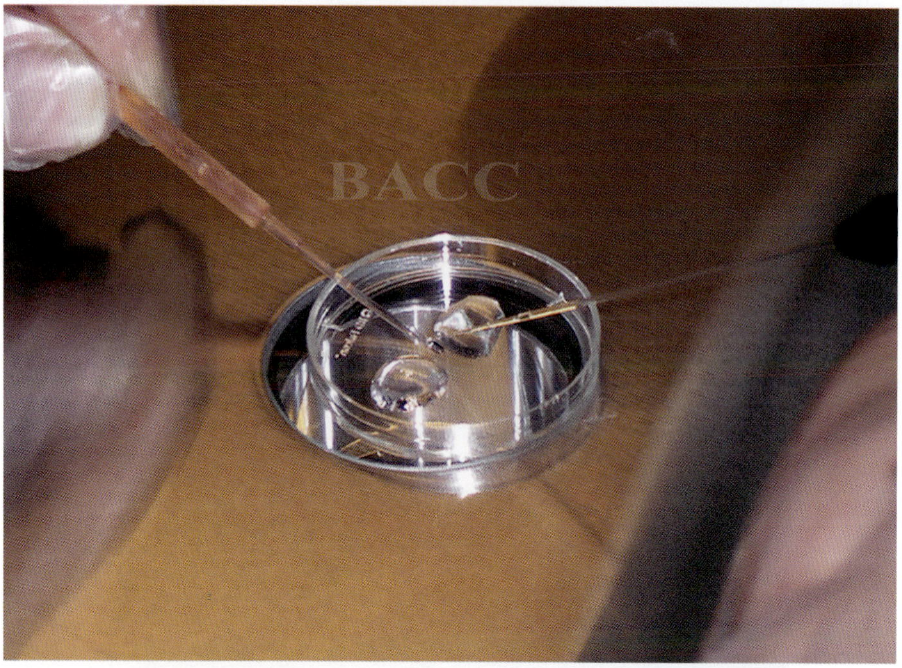

Fig. 23: The cryodevice is immersed into the warming solution 1 (WS1) for the embryos to fall in the media.

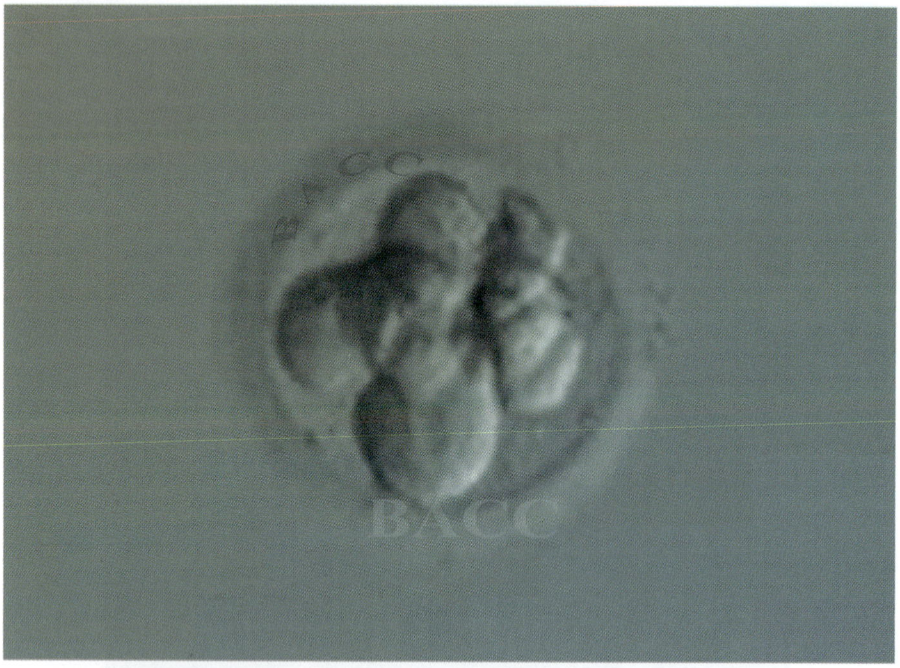

Fig. 24: The eight-celled embryos in warming solution 1 (WS1) kept for 30 seconds.

Warming solution 2: Transfer the embryos to WS2 and let the embryos remain in the solution for 1 minute **(Fig. 25)**.

Warming solution 3: Transfer the embryos to WS3 and let the embryos remain for 2 minutes **(Fig. 26)**.

Warming solution 4: Transfer the embryos into WS4 and let the embryos remain in the solution for 5 minutes **(Fig. 27)**.

Rinse the embryos in culture media several times and continue with embryo transfer or continued culture.

BLASTOCYST CRYOPRESERVATION

Materials

Vitrification of blastocysts contains three solutions: (1) *equilibration solution:* Contains no cryoprotectants **(Fig. 28)**, (2) *vitrification solution 1* **(Figs. 29 and 30)**: Contains ethylene glycol and propanediol as cryoprotectants; (3) *vitrification solution 2:* Contains ethylene glycol, propanediol and ficoll as cryoprotectants **(Fig. 31)**.

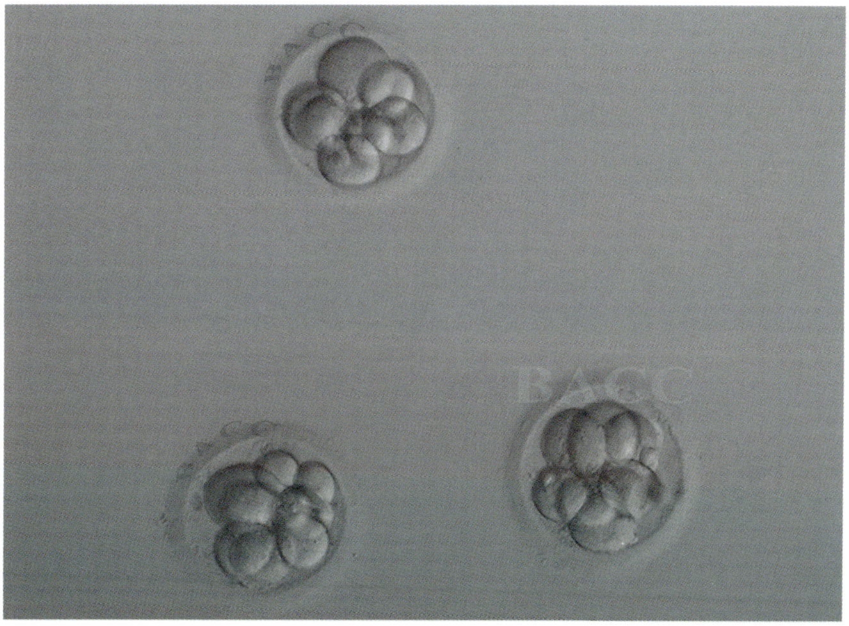

Fig. 25: Eight-celled embryos in warming solution 2 (WS2). Note the blastomere expansion.

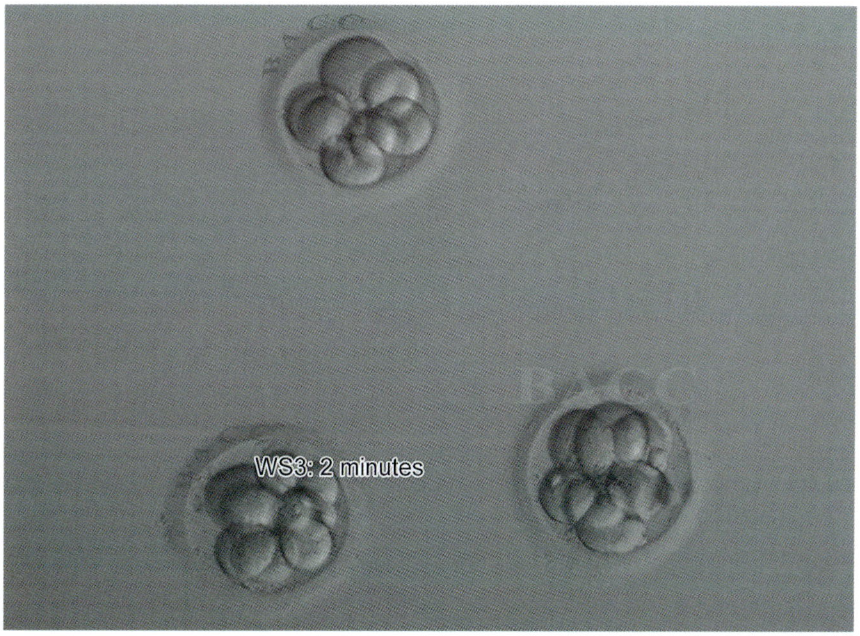

Fig. 26: Eight-celled embryos in warming solution 3 (WS3). Note the blastomere expansion.

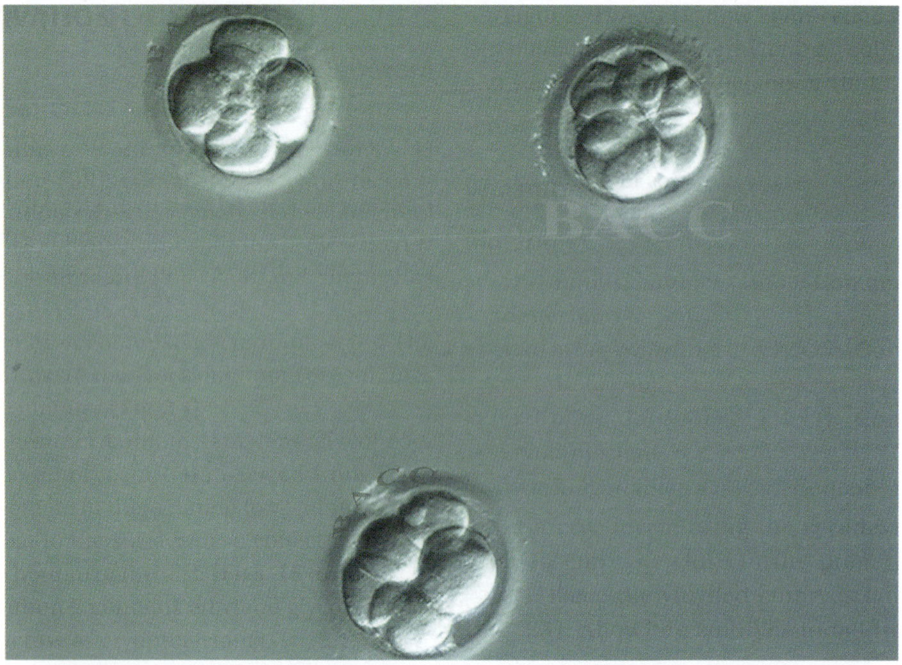

Fig. 27: Eight-celled embryos in warming solution 4 (WS4). Note the blastomeres having regained the cell contents/blastomeres are completely expanded.

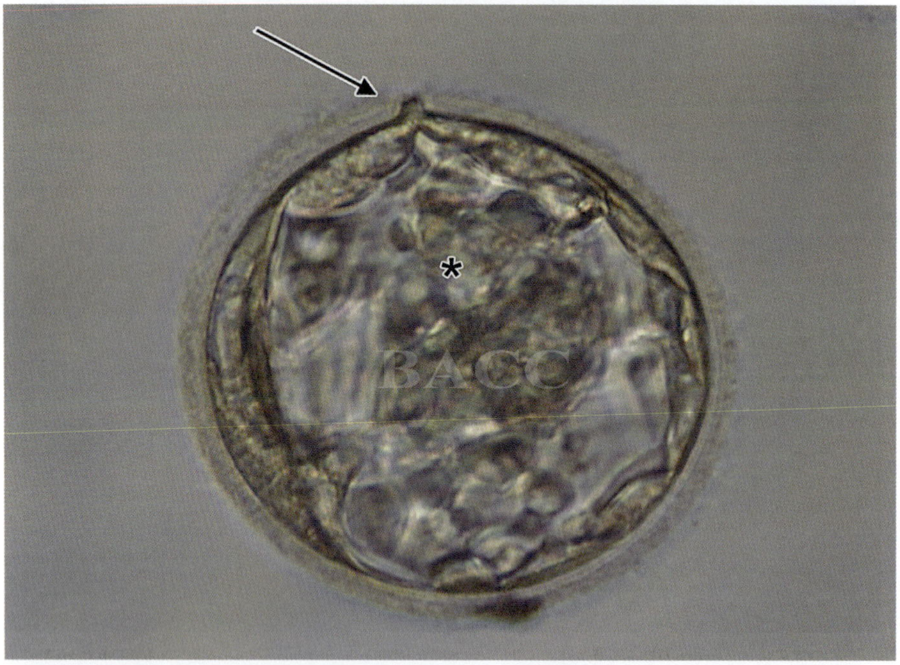

Fig. 28: Collapsed blastocyst in equilibration solution (ES). Arrow indicates the laser pulse given between two trophectoderm cells to bring about artificial shrinkage in the blastocyst and (*) indicates the collapsed inner cell mass. An octax laser was used and a single opening was created using a single laser pulse.

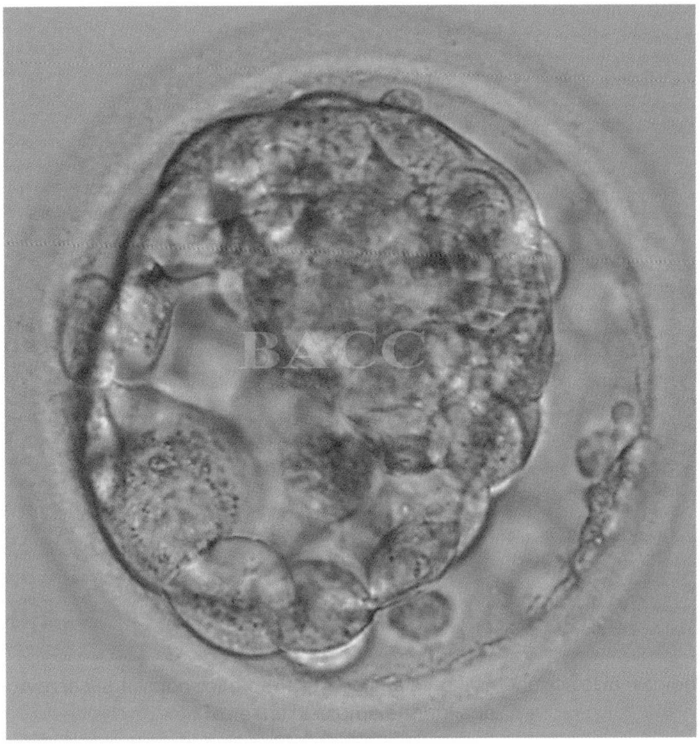

Fig. 29: Blastocyst in vitrification solution 1 (VS1) at the end of 1 minute.

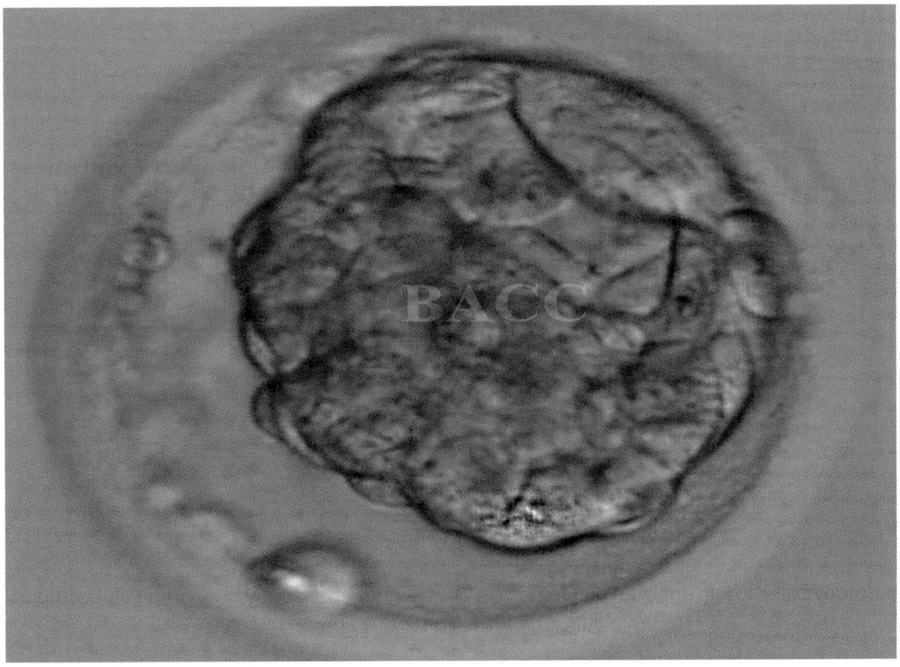

Fig. 30: Blastocyst in vitrification solution 1 (VS1) at the end of 2 minutes. Note the shrinkage of the blastocyst.

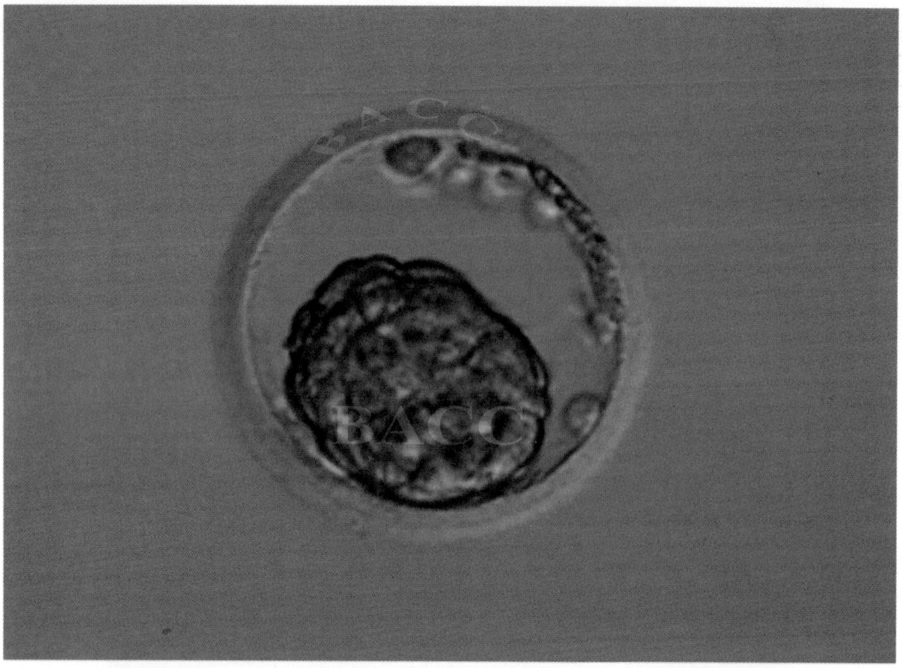

Fig. 31: Blastocyst in vitrification solution 2 (VS2) at the end of 45 seconds. Note fully shrunken blastocyst ready to be loaded on to the cryodevice.

Blastocele cavity has to be collapsed with laser-assisted hatching (LAH) shot (arrow) before placing the embryos in ES. Note the collapsed inner cell mass (ICM) (*) in this blastocyst when placed in ES at the end of 10 minutes (***see* Fig. 28**).

BLASTOCYST WARMING

Materials

- *Warming solution 1*: Contains sucrose as cryoprotectant.
- *Warming solution 2:* Contains sucrose as cryoprotectant.
- *Warming solution 3:* Contains no cryoprotectant.

Vitrified blastocysts are placed in WS1 immediately after removing from the cryodevice. Note the shrunken blastocyst within the zona **(Figs. 32 and 33)**.

Figures 34 and 35 show blastocyst in WS2 at 2 minutes and 3 minutes, respectively. Note the gradual expansion of

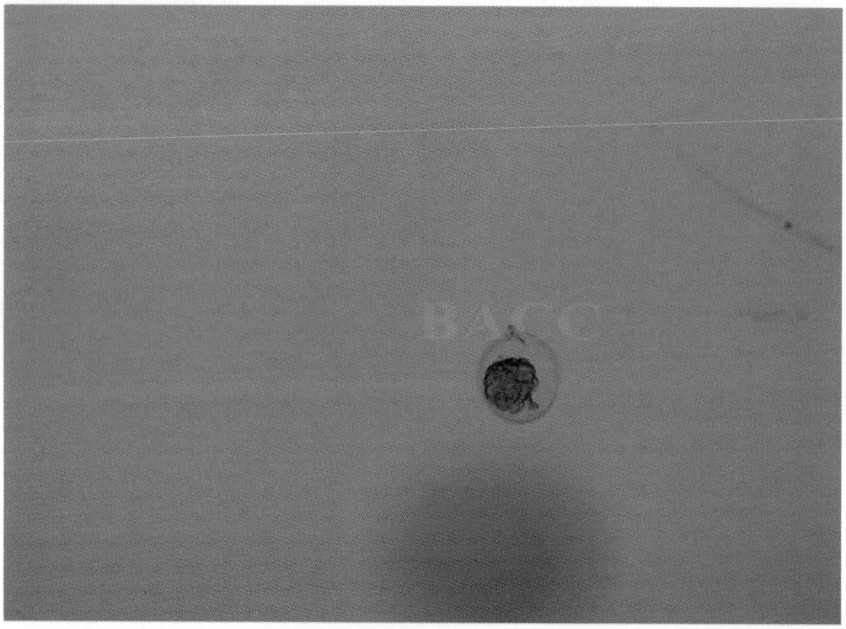

Fig. 32: Vitrified blastocyst in warming solution 1 (WS1) at 30 seconds.

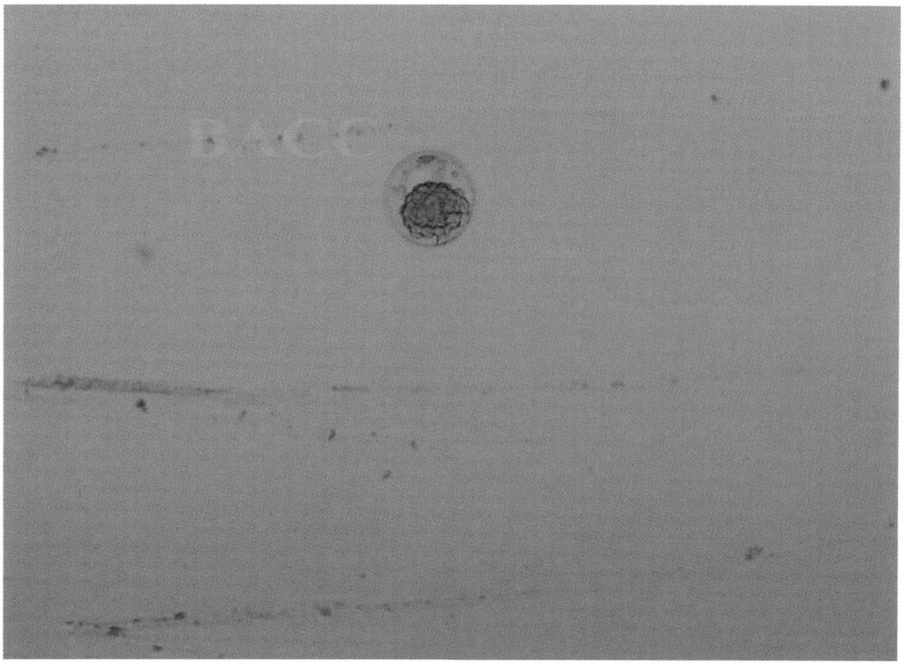

Fig. 33: Vitrified blastocyst in warming solution 1 (WS1) at 1 minute. Note the gradual expansion of blastocyst with in the zona.

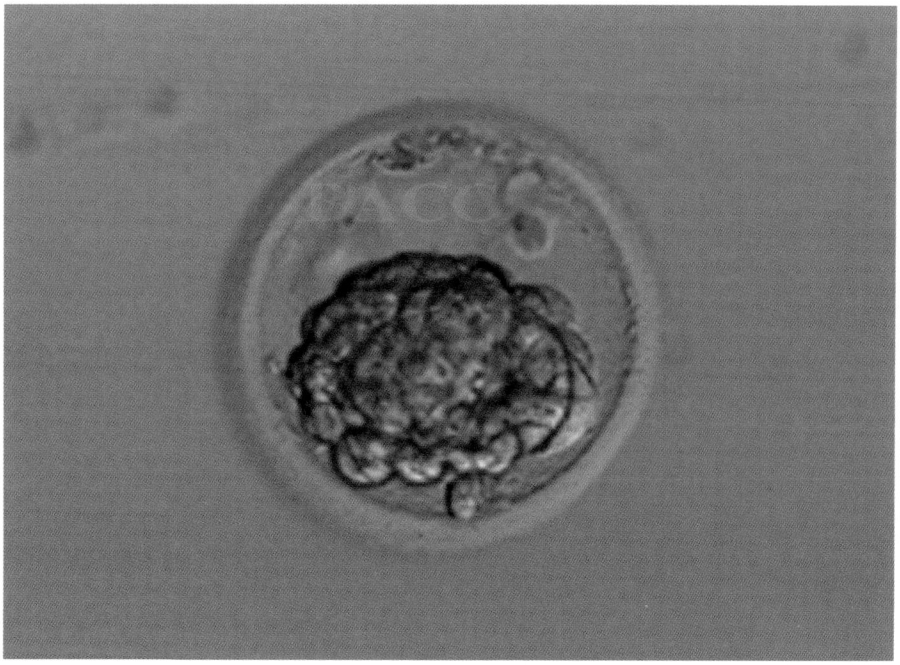

Fig. 34: Blastocyst in warming solution 2 (WS2) at 2 minutes.

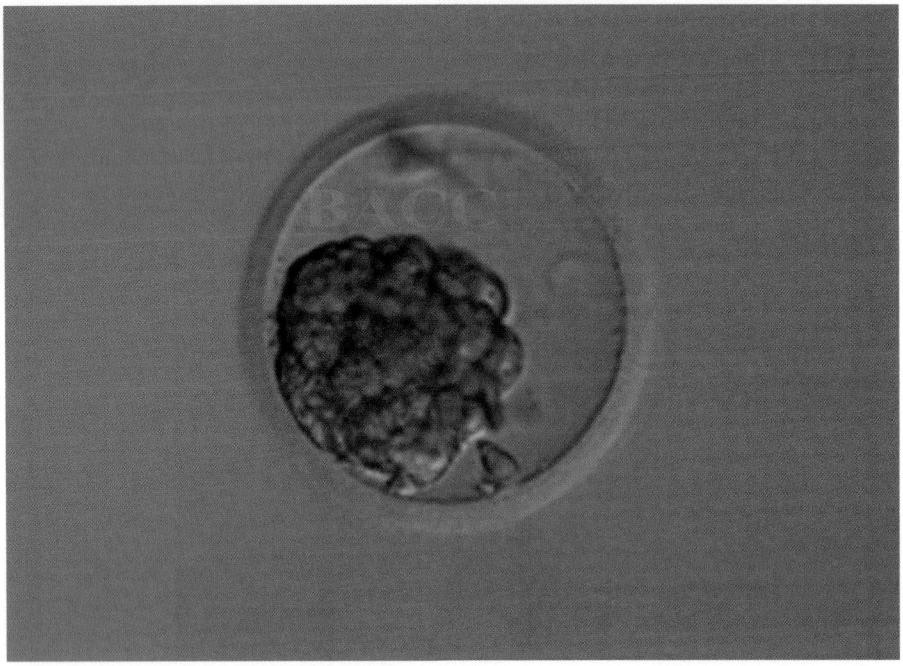

Fig. 35: Blastocyst in warming solution 2 (WS2) at 3 minutes.

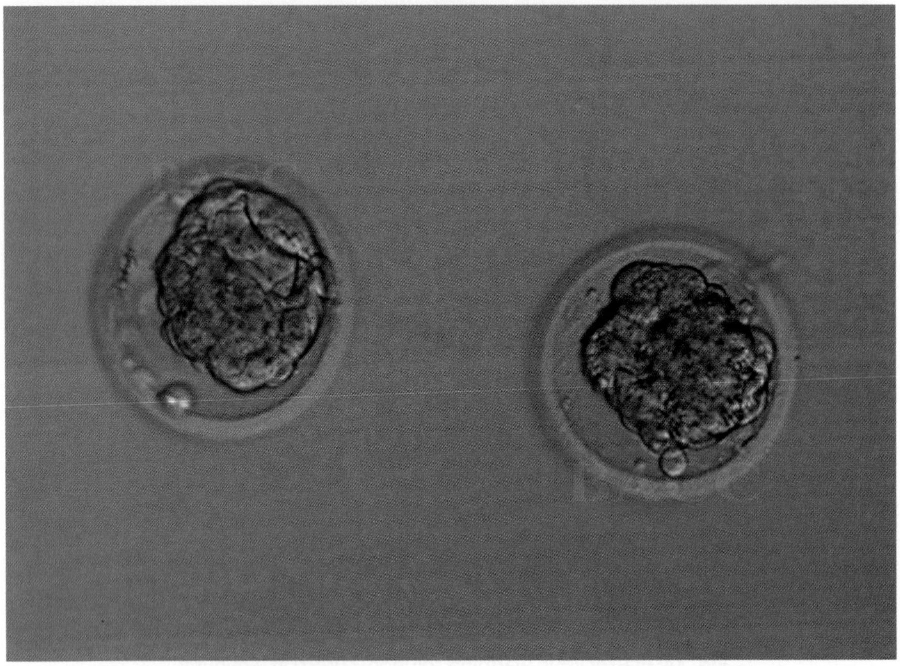

Fig. 36: Blastocyst in warming solution 3 (WS3) at 5 minutes. Note the expansion of blastocyst with in the zona. Blastocele cavity has started its appearance.

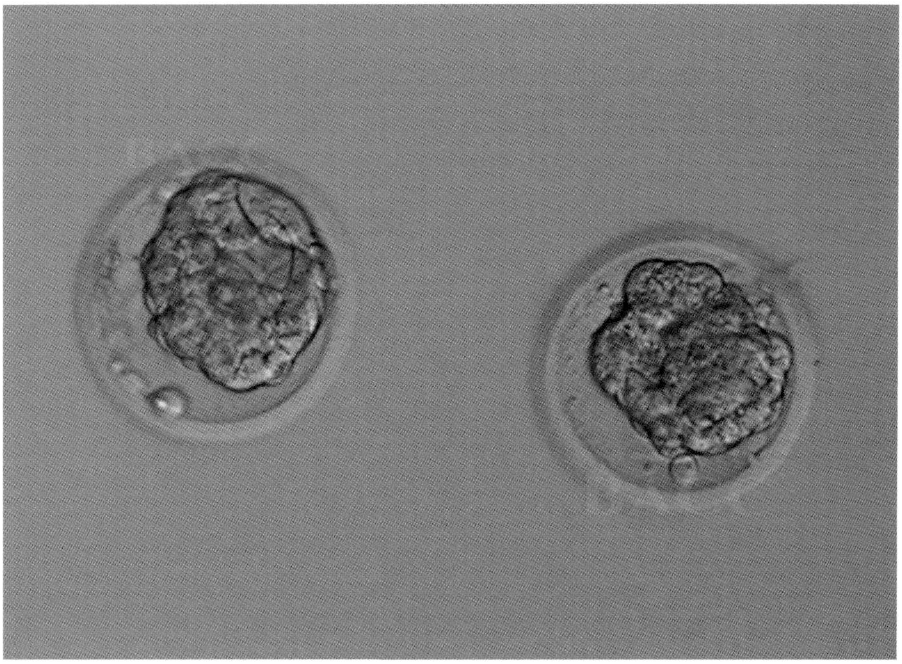

Fig. 37: Blastocyst in warming solution 3 (WS3) at 10 minutes.

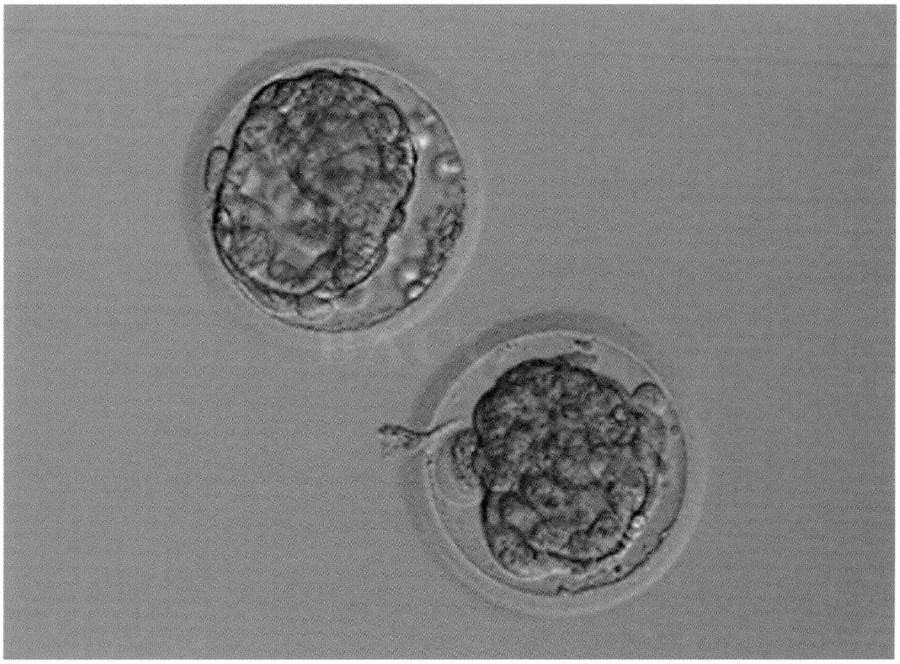

Fig. 38: Blastocyst in warming solution 3 (WS3) at 30 minutes in 200x magnification. Note fully expanded blastocysts.

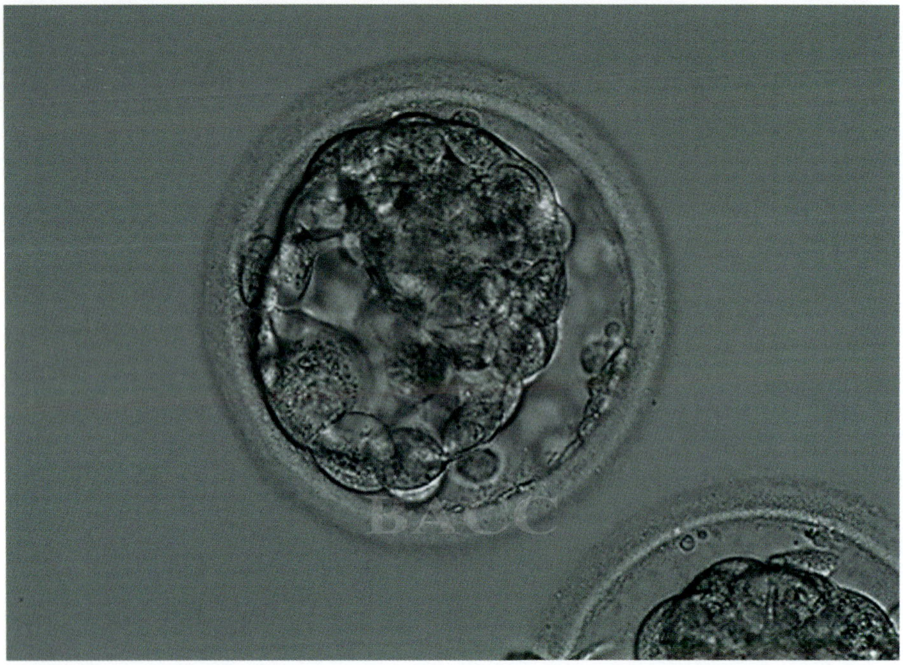

Fig. 39: Blastocyst in warming solution 3 (WS3) at 30 minutes in 400× magnification. Note the fully expanded blastocyst with distinct blastocele cavity, trophectoderm and inner cell mass (ICM).

blastocyst within the zona. Blastocele and cell types cannot be differentiated yet.

Figures 36 to 39 show blastocyst in WS3 at 5 minutes, 10 minutes and 30 minutes.

REFERENCE

1. Gardner DK, Weissman A, Howles CM, et al. Chapter 24. Textbook of Assisted Reproductive Techniques, 4th edition. London: Informa Healthcare Publisher; 2012.

CHAPTER 136

Assisted Reproductive Technology Laboratory Setting

Divyashree PS, Hemanth Kumar MA, Dileep Kumar R, Mohammed Ashraf C

ESSENTIAL EQUIPMENT OF ASSISTED REPRODUCTIVE TECHNOLOGY LABORATORY

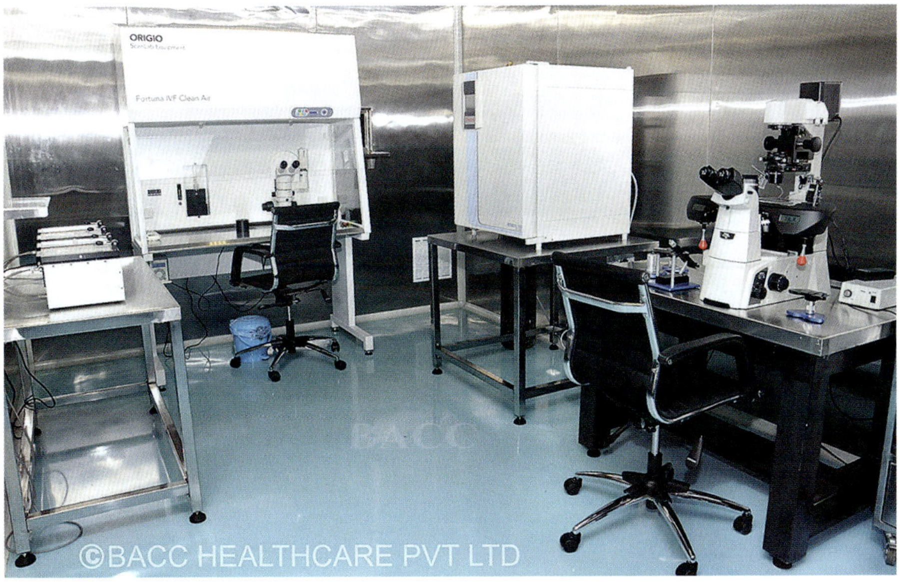

INTRODUCTION

The design, equipment and supplies of an assisted reproductive technology (ART) laboratory depend on the types of treatment offered and the workload of a particular ART clinic.

This chapter covers about:

- Essential equipment of ART laboratory
- Essential equipment for clinical procedures
- Consumables required for ART laboratory.

LAMINAR FLOW CABINETS

Laminar flow cabinets with horizontal air flow to maintain sterile environment around the gametes which are handled in vitro **(Figs. 1A and B)**.

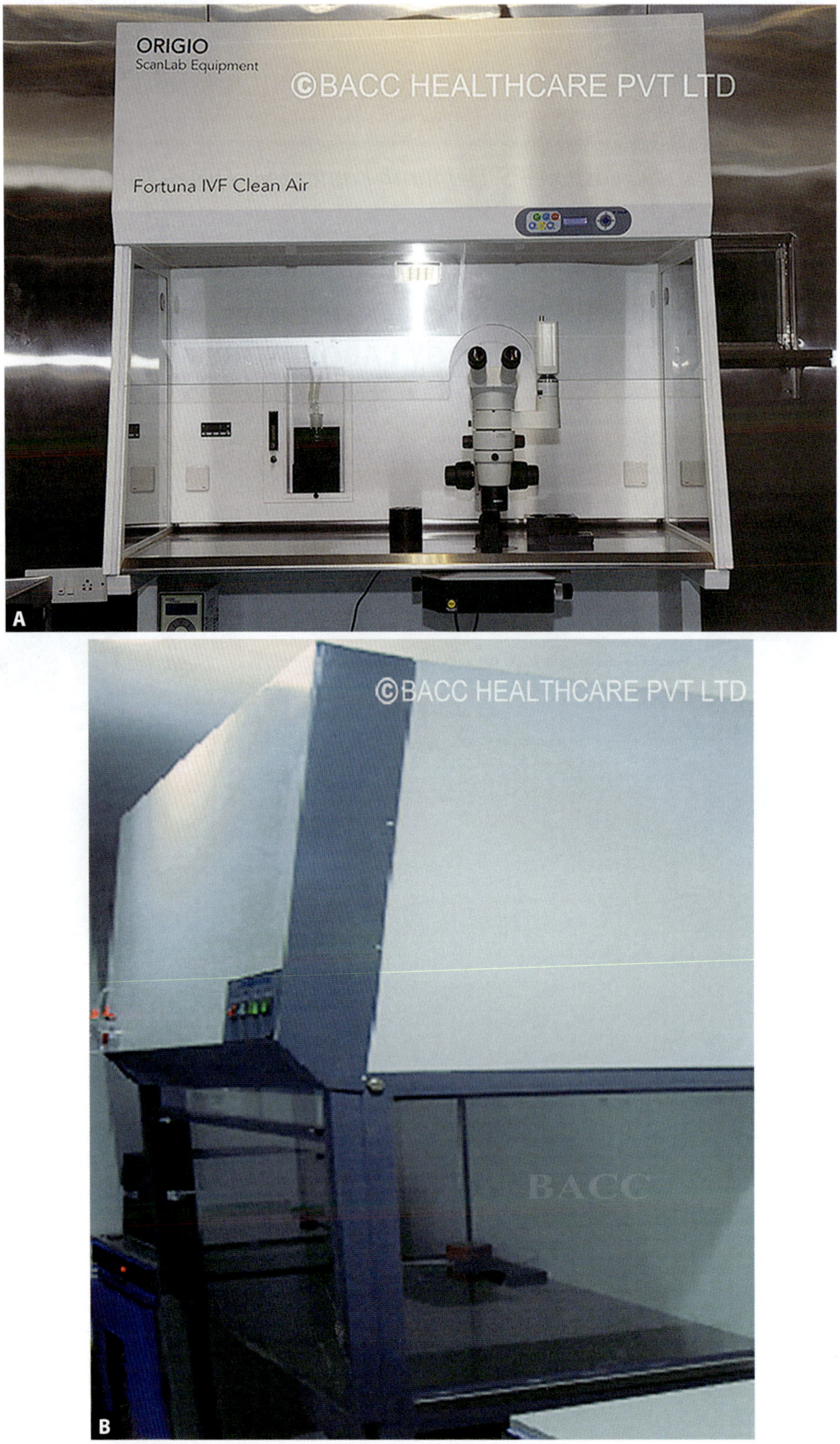

Figs. 1A and B: Laminar flow cabinets.

HEATING, VENTILATING, AND AIR-CONDITIONING

Air handling unit (AHU) should be equipped with high-efficiency particulate air (HEPA) filters for filtration of particulate matter and coda filters (activated charcoal) for the elimination of VOCs **(Figs. 2A and B)**.

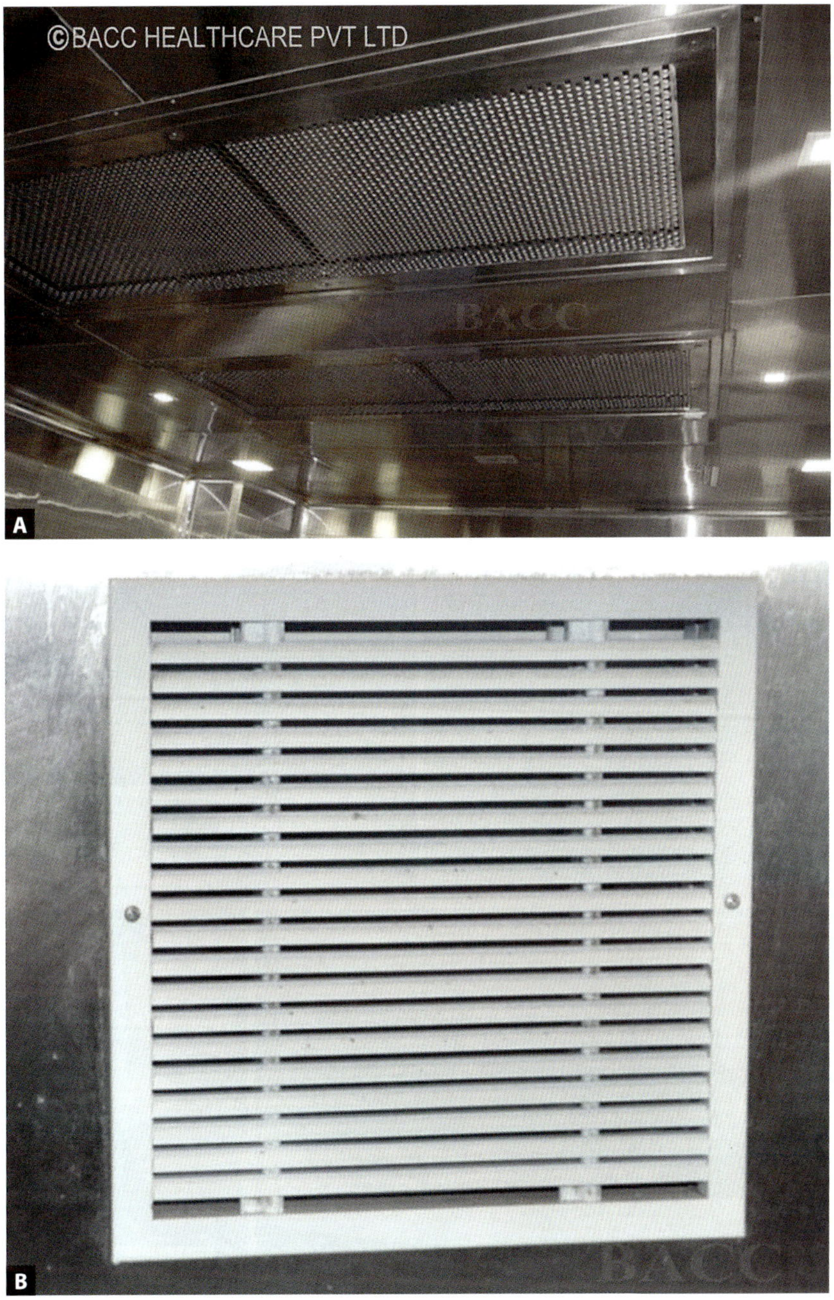

Figs. 2A and B: Air handling unit.

INCUBATORS

Types of Incubators (Figs. 3A to F)

1. *Box type incubators:* Water jacketed and air jacketed.
2. *Bench top incubators:* Cook Minc, K systems, Origio (advantage-minimal disruption of temperature and pH).
3. *Others:* Mini-incubator, portable incubator.

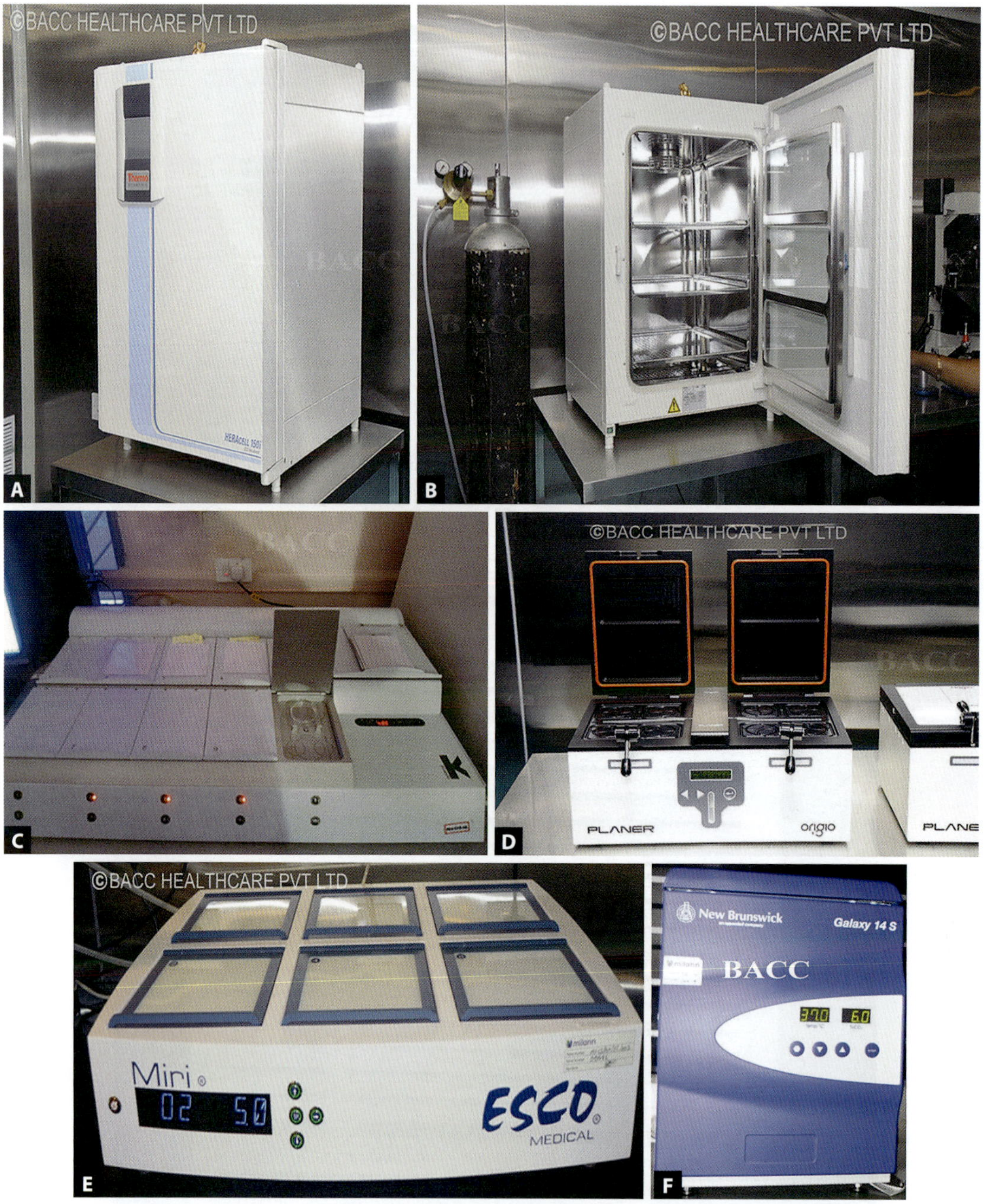

Figs. 3A to F: (A) Box type air jacketed incubator; (B) Box type air jacketed incubator (inside view) with different shelves; (C) Bench top incubator, K systems; (D) Bench top incubator, Origio; (E) Bench top incubator, ESCO; (F) Mini-box type incubator, Eppendorf.

MICROSCOPES

Compound microscope ***(Fig. 4A)***: Eye piece: 10×, objective: 10×, 20× and 40×.

Used in andrology for semen analysis and also to see post-wash count.

Dissecting/Stereozoom microscope ***(Fig. 4B)****:* Eye piece: 10×, objective: 0.7 to 1×, total magnification—10×.

Used for follicular fluid screening, and for observation of oocytes and embryos at a lower magnification.

Inverted microscope with micromanipulator ***(Fig. 4C)****:* Inverted microscope is used for intracytoplasmic sperm injection (ICSI). Two important parts of the system include the microscope and the micromanipulator.

- Inverted microscope is equipped with an eye piece of 10× and objectives of 10×, 20× and 40×.

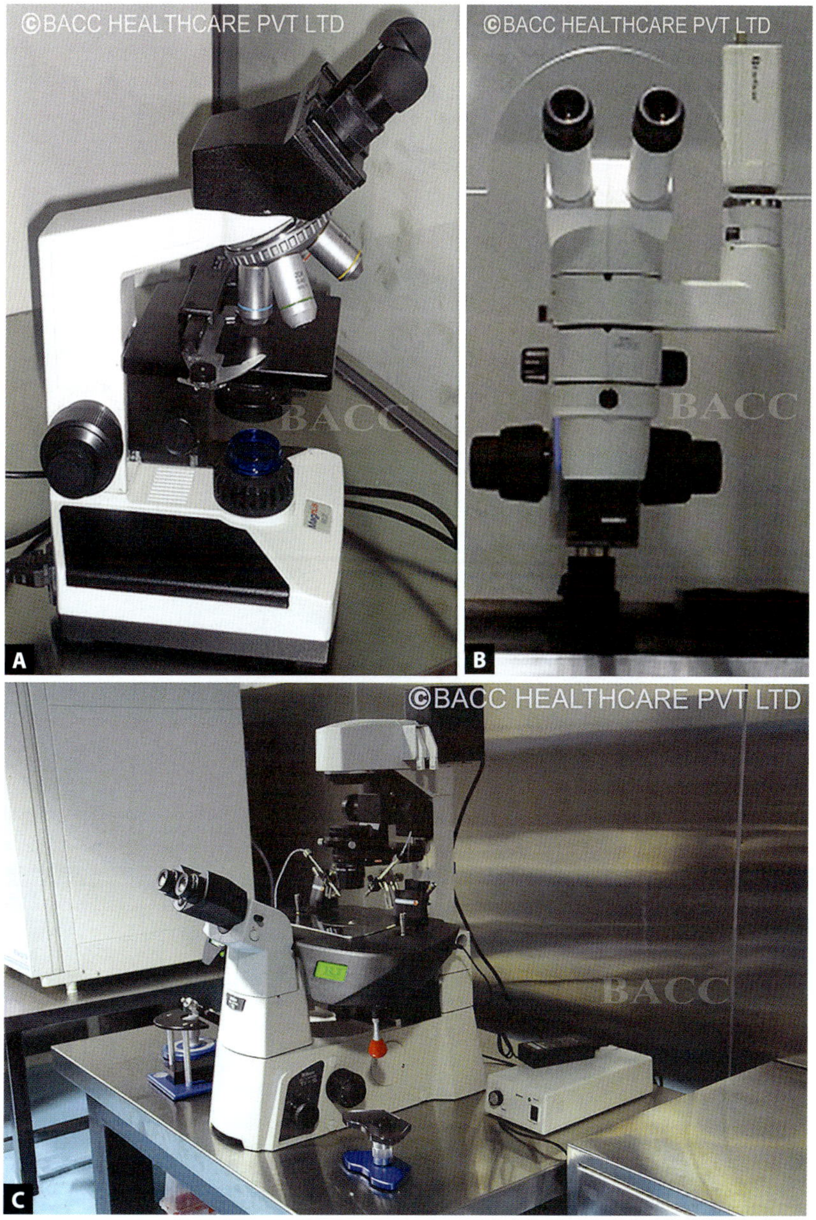

Figs. 4A to C: (A) Compound microscope; (B) Dissecting/Stereozoom microscope; (C) Inverted microscope with micromanipulator.

- Accessories used along with inverted microscope include heated stage and portal for attachment of camera.
- The micromanipulator system from research instruments (RI) is purely a mechanical system. Micromanipulator system includes microtool holders, and suction/ injection device.

Cryopreservation Equipment

Storage dewars with canisters ***(Fig. 5A)***: Storage dewars contains canisters immersed in liquid nitrogen. Canisters are containers which hold the straws in an effective and accessible manner.

Straws ***(Fig. 5B)****:* Different types of straws are available for loading the embryos after vitrification.

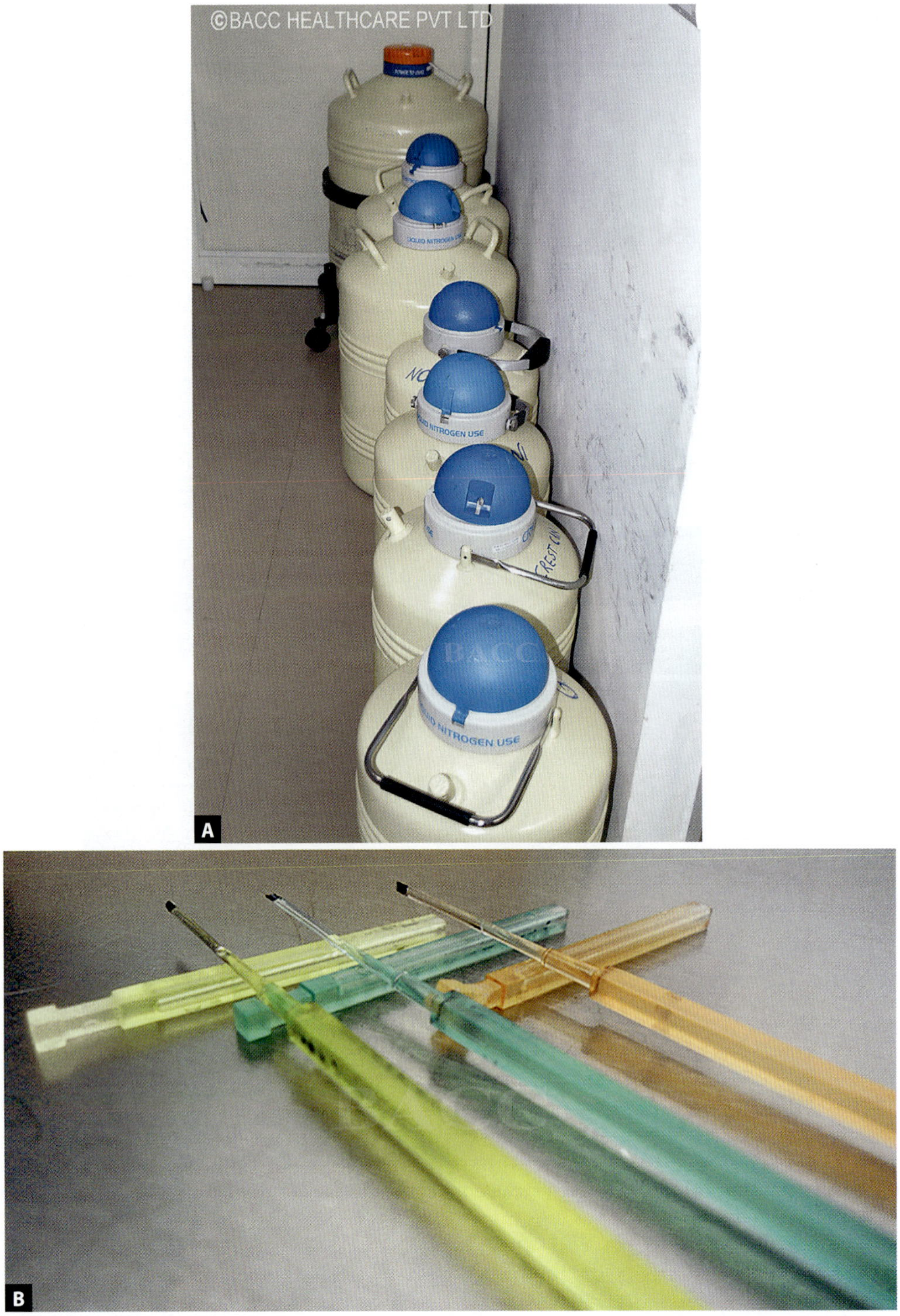

Figs. 5A and B: (A) Storage dewars with canisters; (B) Straws for embryo loading.

Centrifuge

Centrifuge is used in Andrology laboratory for semen processing for IUI/IVF/ICSI for sperm concentration **(Fig. 6)**.

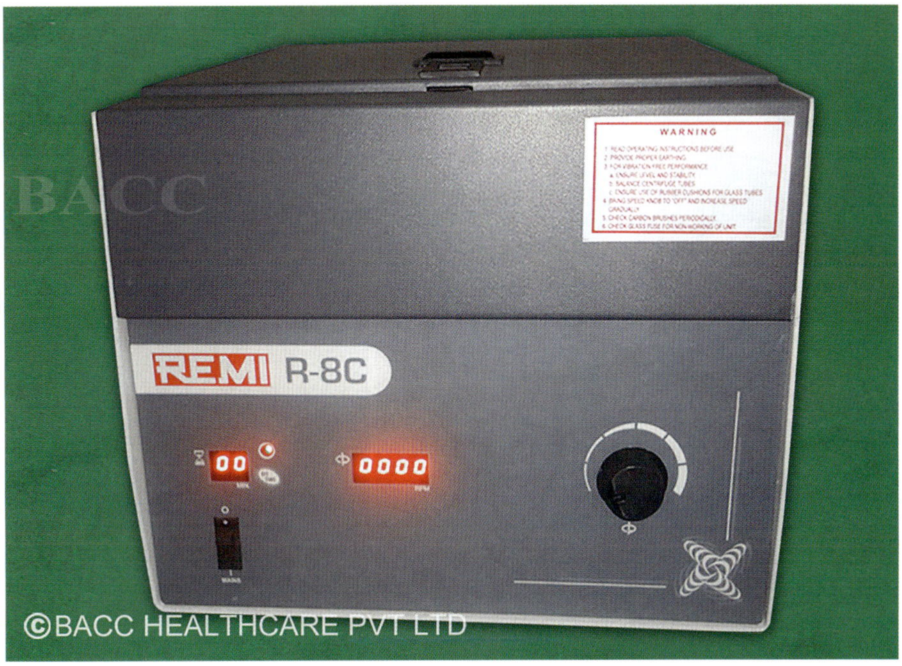

Fig. 6: Centrifuge.

Semen Analyzer

SQA-vision is an automated high resolution visual interface for assessing all semen parameters **(Fig. 7)**.

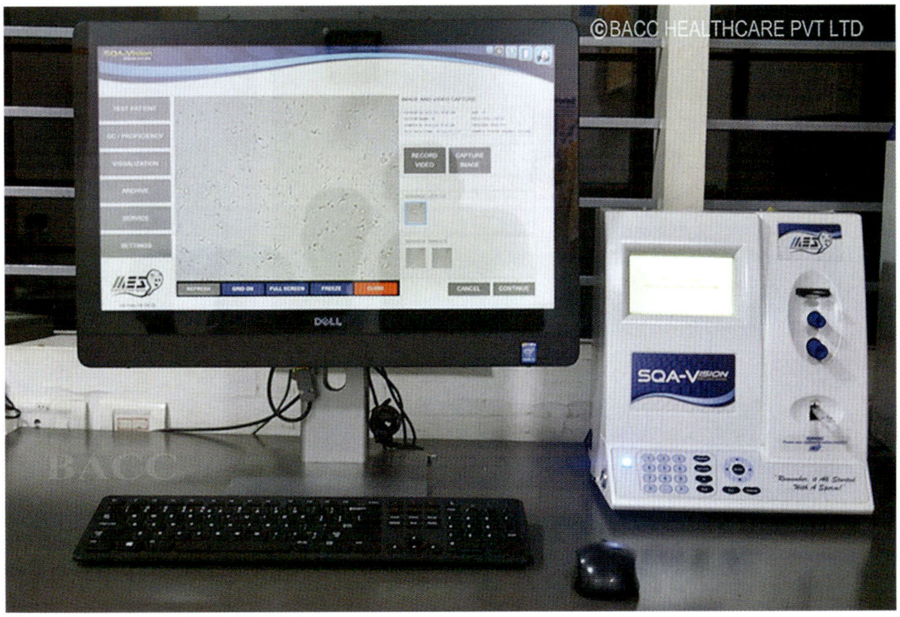

Fig. 7: SQA-vision (Automated sperm quality analyzer).

Makler Chamber

Makler chamber is used for sperm counting **(Figs. 8A and B)**.

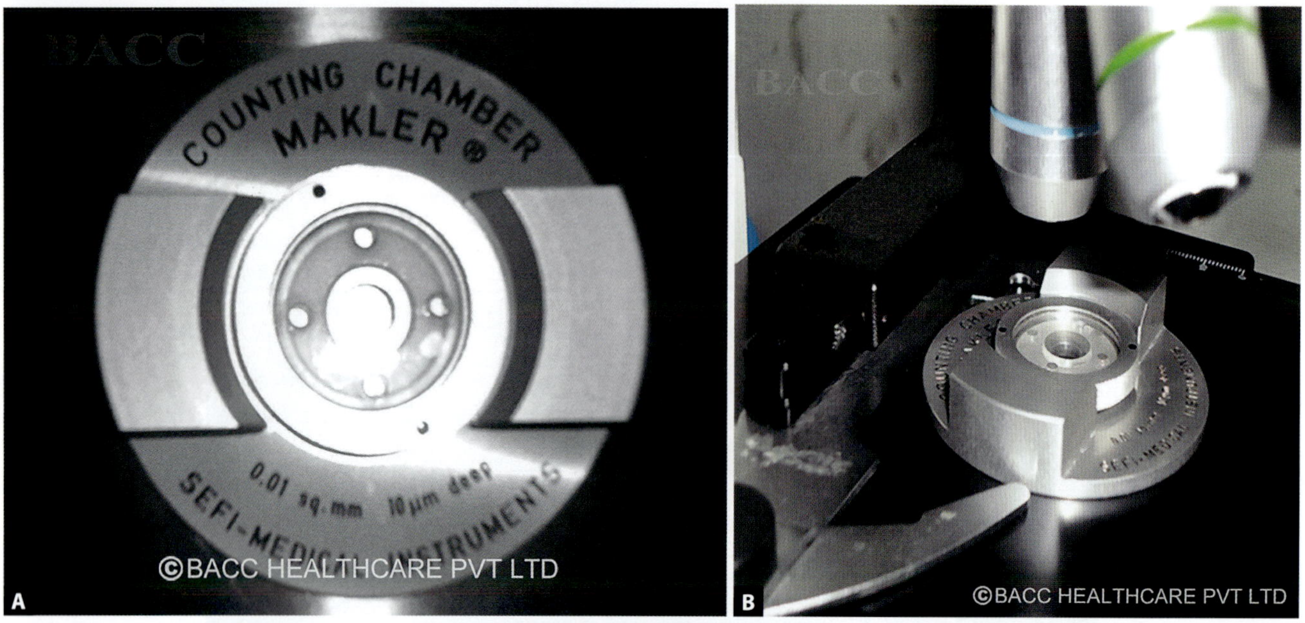

Figs. 8A and B: Makler chamber.

Test Tube Warmer

Test tube warmer maintains the temperature at 37°C, so that gametes and embryos are handled at a physiological temperature in vitro during the transition time when they are outside the incubator **(Figs. 9A and B)**.

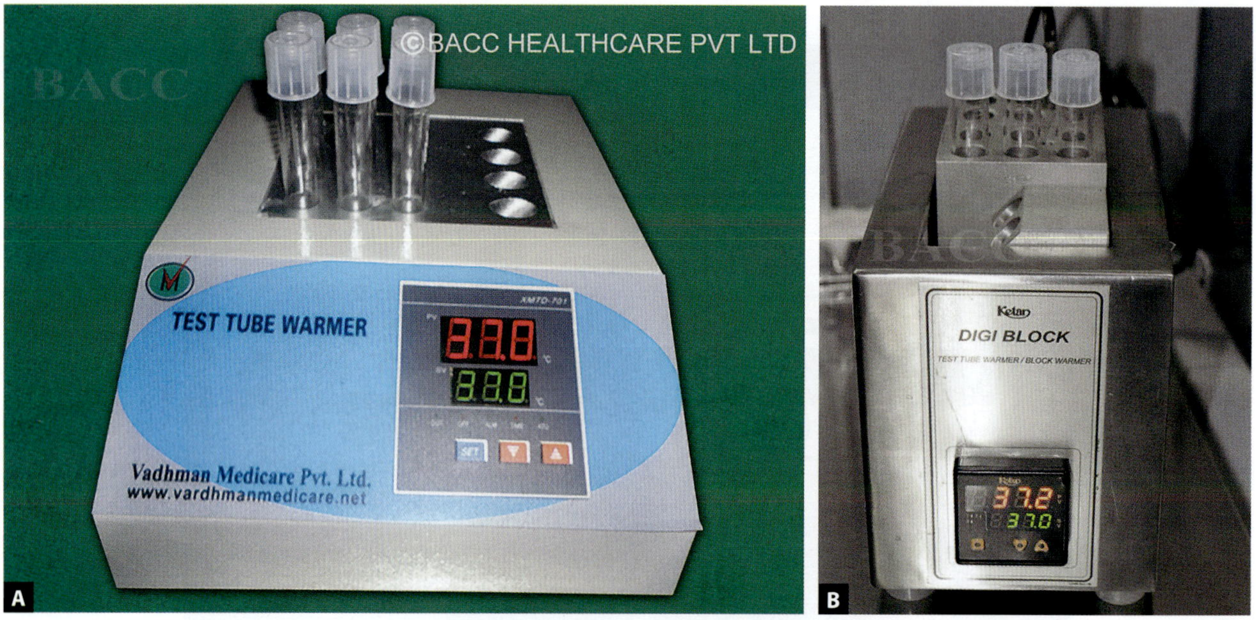

Figs. 9A and B: Test tube warmer.

Coda Tower

Coda tower **(Fig. 10)** is housed in the IVF laboratory to ensure filtration of air within the IVF laboratory. It is a purifier that reduces particulates, harmful volatile organic compounds (VOCs) and chemical airborne contaminants (CACs).

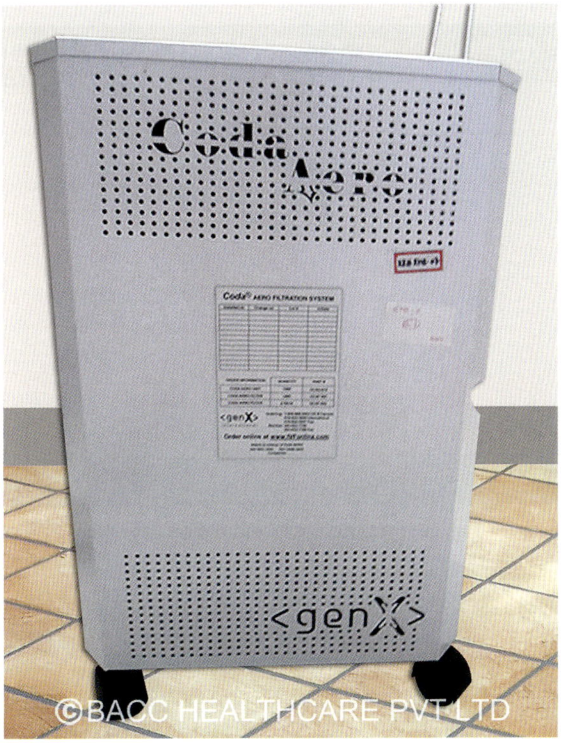

Fig. 10: Coda tower.

Coda Inline Filters

These filters improve the air quality in the incubator by reducing the VOCs. It contains a mixture of activated carbon to absorb the VOCs, aldehydes and formaldehydes from all incoming gas lines **(Fig. 11)**.

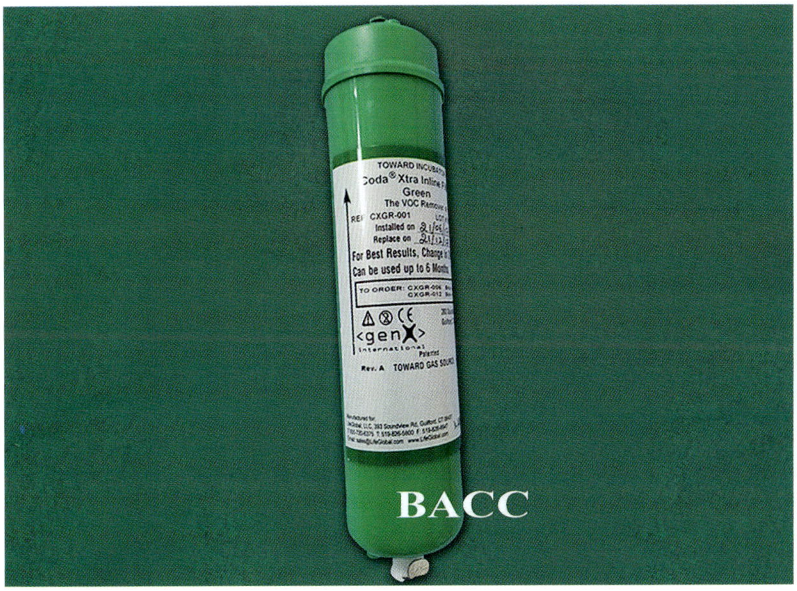

Fig. 11: Coda inline filters.

ESSENTIAL EQUIPMENT FOR CLINICAL PROCEDURES

Intrauterine Insemination Catheters

Semi-rigid catheters with open end and rounded tip should fit the curvature of the uterus **(Fig. 12)**.

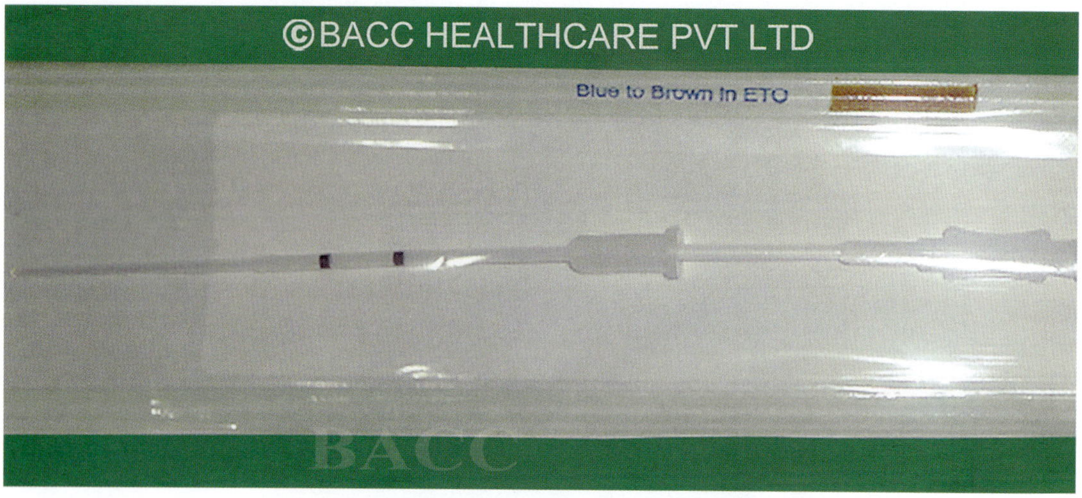

Fig. 12: Intrauterine insemination catheter.

Oocyte Aspiration Set

Oocyte aspiration set contains single or double lumen echo tip needle, connected to gas tubing, round bottom test tube and suction apparatus **(Figs. 13A and B)**.

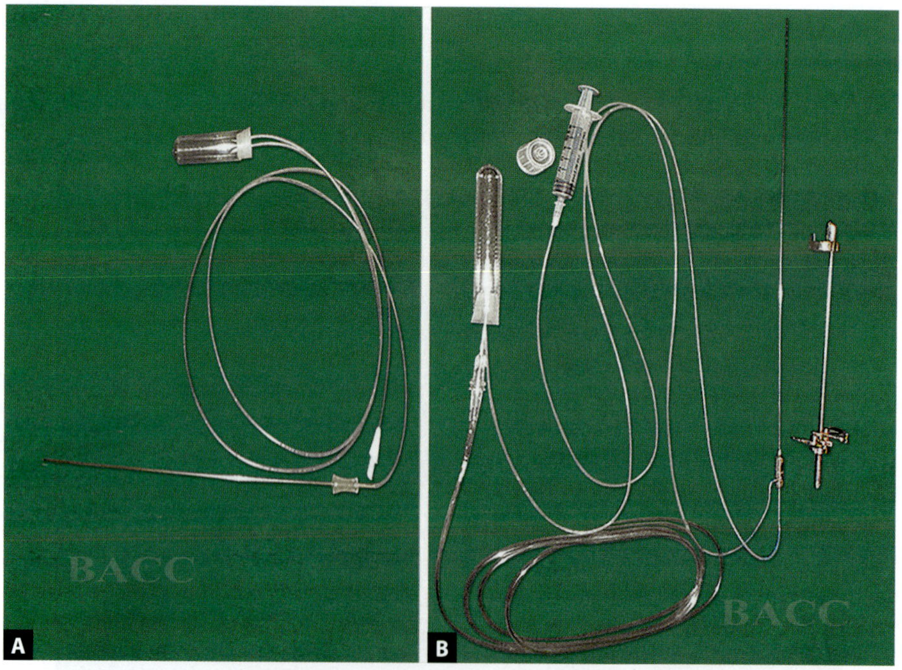

Figs. 13A and B: Oocyte aspiration set.

Embryo Transfer Catheters

There are different types of embryo transfer (ET) catheters available. Common characteristics of ET catheters include softness and flexibility. Optional characteristic include echogenicity **(Fig. 14)**.

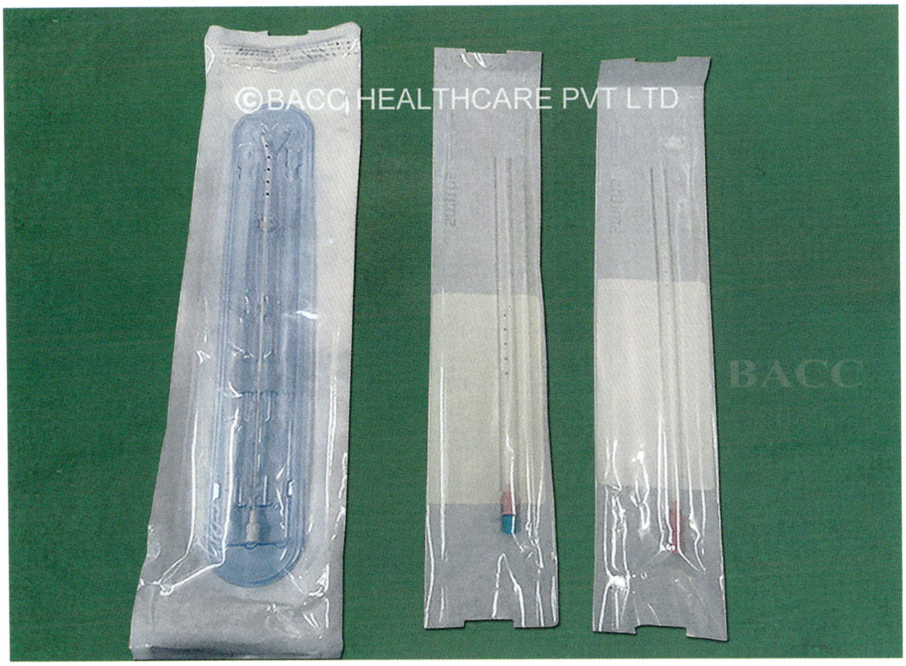

Fig. 14: Embryo transfer catheters.

Suction Pump with Foot Pedal

Suction pump with foot pedal for oocyte aspiration **(Fig. 15)**. The pressure should be set at 100 mm Hg.

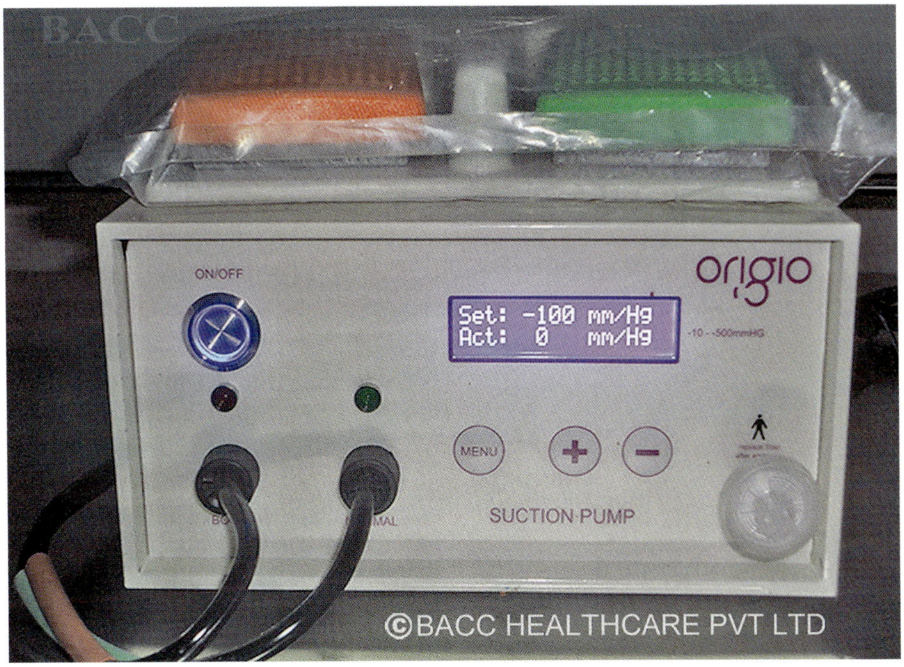

Fig. 15: Suction pump with foot pedal.

Ultrasound Machine

Ultrasound machine is used for follicular monitoring and as a guide during oocyte aspiration and embryo transfer as a guide **(Fig. 16)**.

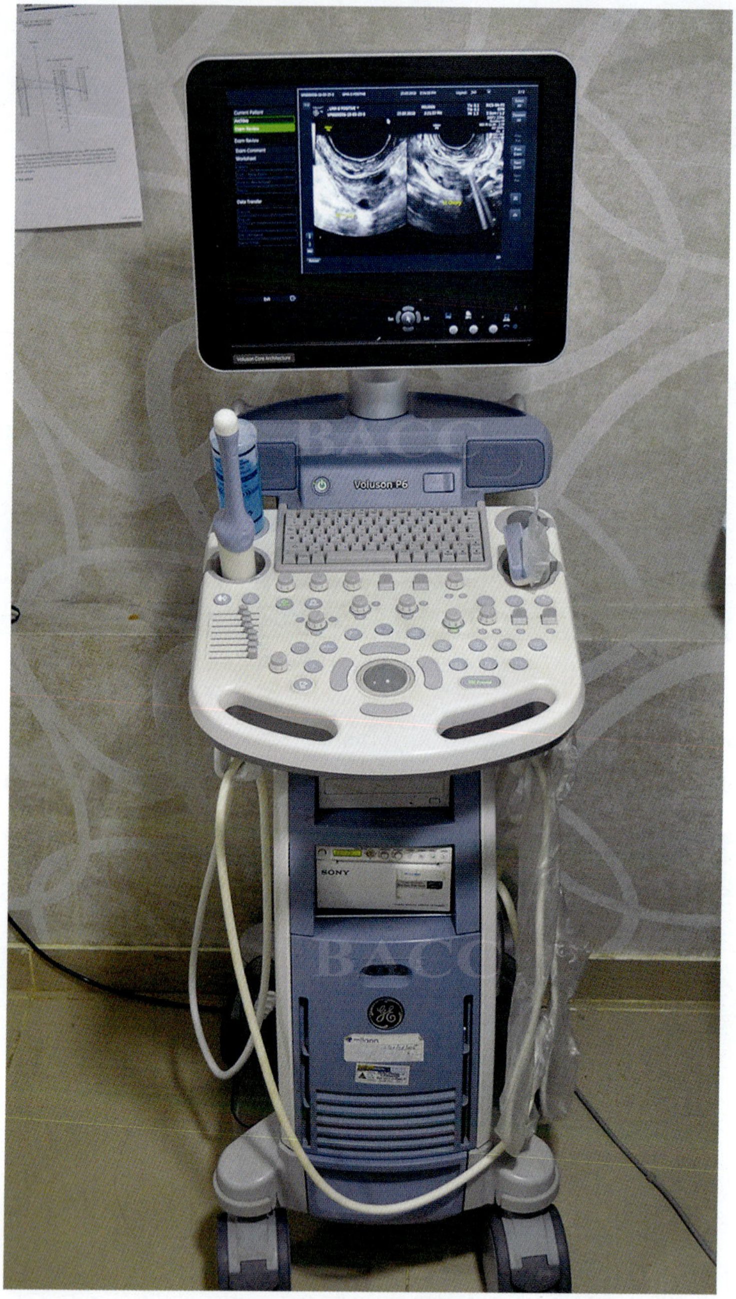

Fig. 16: Ultrasound machine.

Consumables Required for Assisted Reproductive Technology Laboratory

Plastic test tubes: Plastic tubes are of two types round bottom and conical **(Figs. 17A to C)**.

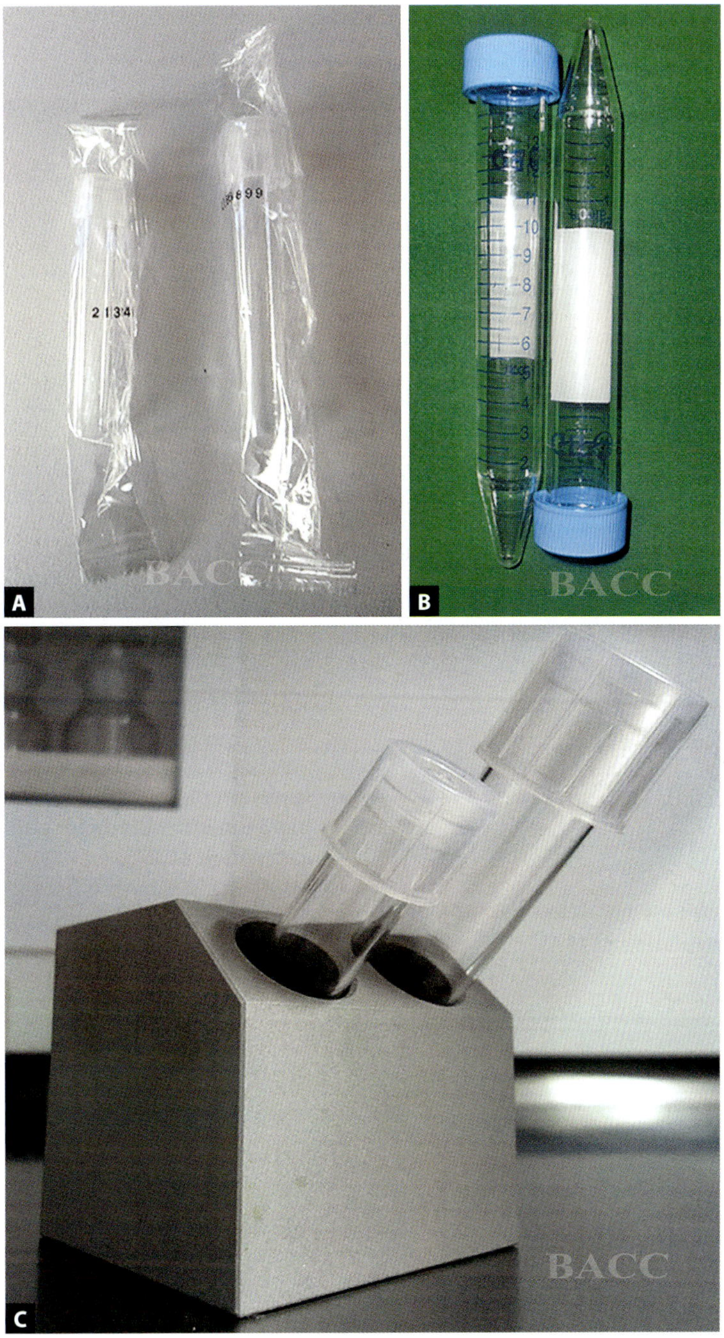

Figs. 17A to C: Plastic test tubes.

Petri Dishes

Different types of Petri dishes are as follows **(Fig. 18)**:

- *Tissue culture dish:* 60 × 15 mm, polystyrene dish used for follicular fluid screening.
- *Central well dish:* 60 × 15 mm, polystyrene, central well dish. Can be used for IVF, oocyte washing after denudation, etc.
- *Intracytoplasmic sperm injection dish:* 59× 9 mm low wall dish, with side grooves. Used for ICSI.
- *Tissue culture dish:* 35 × 10 mm, polystyrene dish used for embryo culture.

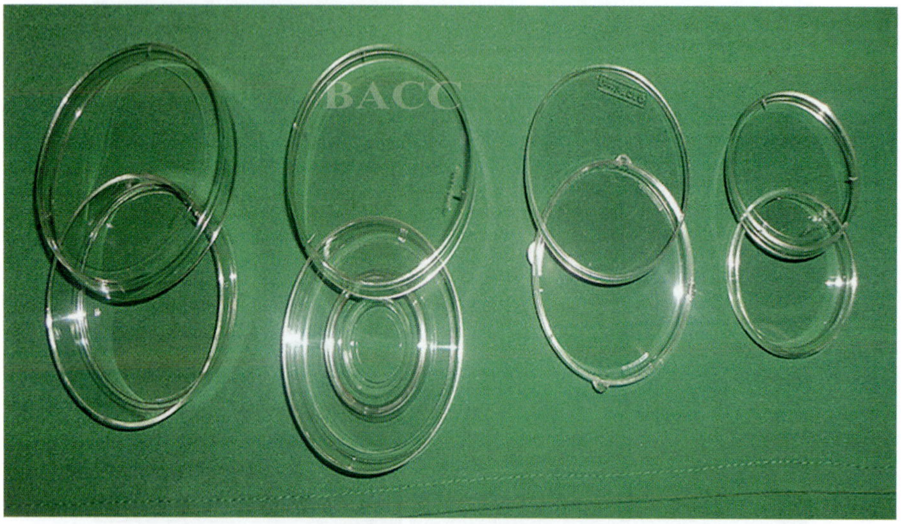

Fig. 18: Different types of Petri dishes.

Pipettes

Different types of pipettes include **(Figs. 19A to C)**:

- A 3 mL plastic pipette
- Glass pasteur pipettes
- Holding pipette to hold the oocyte. It has a diameter of 18–25 mm, and has an angulation of 35°.
- Injection pipette used for microinjection of the sperm. It has 5 µm inner diameter and 7 µm outer diameter and an angulation of 35°.
- Stripper pipettes of different diameters (140 µm, 175 µm and 275 µm) for denudation of oocyte and also for embryo handling.

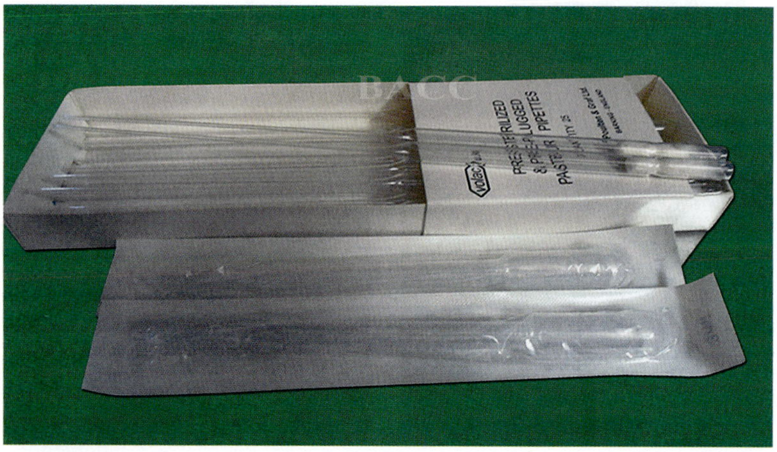

Fig. 19A: Different types of pipettes. (A) Glass Pasteur pipettes and plastic pipettes.

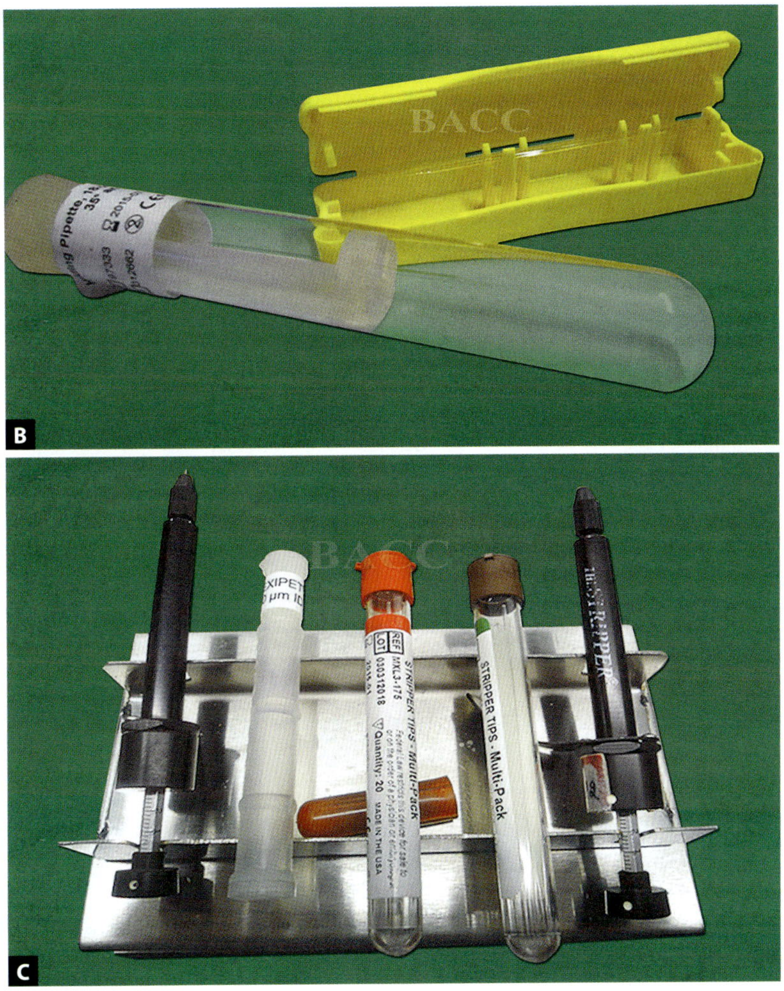

Figs. 19B and C: Different types of pipettes. (B) Holding and injection pipette used for ICSI; (C) Different types of Stripper pipettes.

Culture Medias

Different types of culture media **(Fig. 20)** required in ART laboratory are as follows:

- Flushing media
- Fertilization media
- Cleavage media
- Blastocyst media.

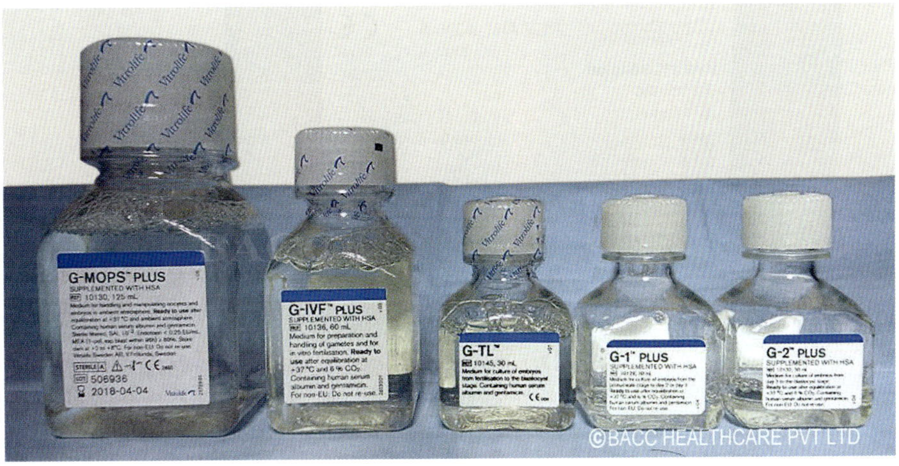

Fig. 20: Different types of culture media.

Hyaluronidase

Hyaluronidase at a concentration of 80 IU/mL is used for enzymatic dilution of cumulus mass surrounding the oocyte **(Fig. 21)**. Denudation helps in identification of oocyte maturity and oocyte abnormality and also denudation is a prerequisite for ICSI.

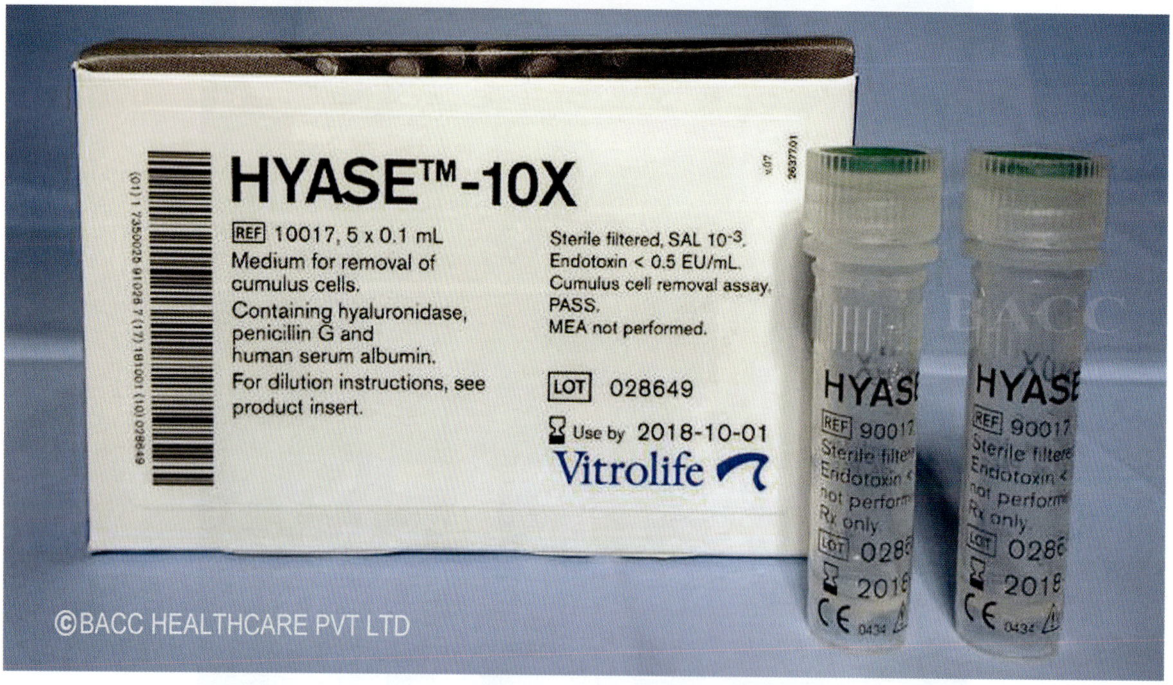

Fig. 21: Hyaluronidase.

Polyvinylpyrrolidone

Polyvinylpyrrolidone (PVP) for suspension of sperms before ICSI **(Fig. 22)**.

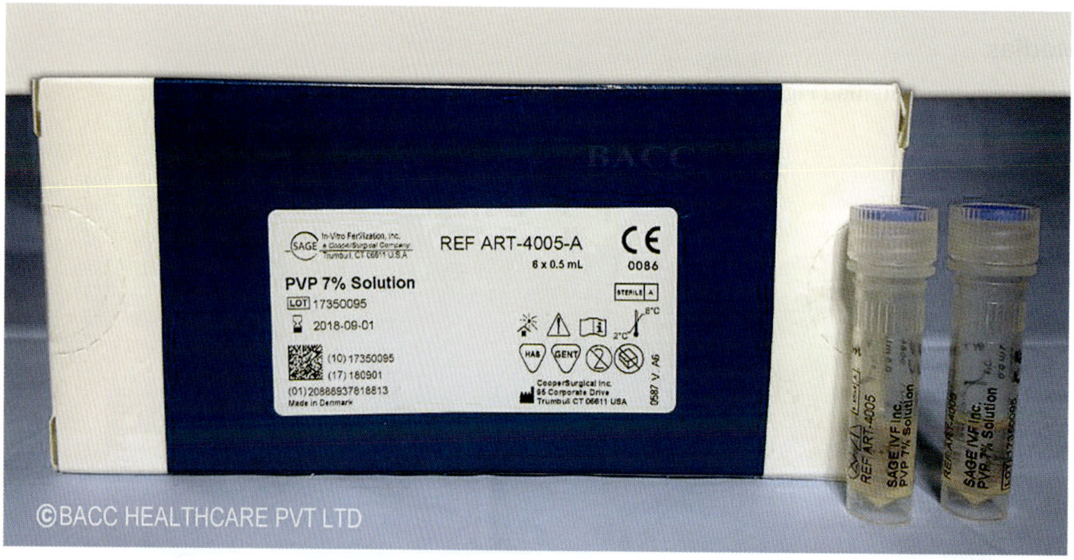

Fig. 22: Polyvinylpyrrolidone.

Mineral Oil

To overlay the culture dishes. Overlaying with mineral oil prevents evaporation of culture dots and fluctuations in temperature and pH **(Fig. 23)**.

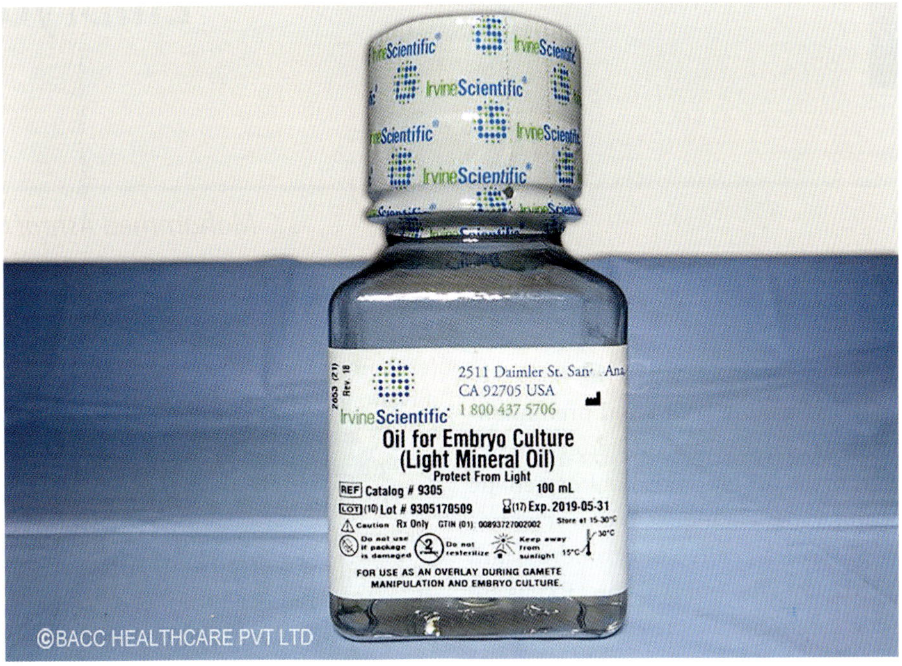

Fig. 23: Mineral oil.

CHAPTER 137

Embryo Biopsy

Mohammed Ashraf C, Anuja Kamath

INTRODUCTION

Preimplantation genetic screening (PGS) and preimplantation genetic diagnosis (PGD) are specialized techniques designed to screen embryos for chromosomal or genetic disorders. The PGS and PGD techniques are procedures requiring removal of several cells [blastomeres and trophectoderm (TE) cells] from the embryo. The TE cells are genetically evaluated to determine the presence or absence of specific chromosomal abnormalities and/or genetic diseases. After the genetic evaluation of embryos, they are selected for embryo transfer into the uterus, or frozen (cryopreserved) to be used later, to achieve pregnancy. The advantages of using PGS/PGD are to greatly reduce the risk of miscarriage or having a child with the chromosomal/ genetic problems.[1–3]

Using specially designed micromanipulation tools and microscope, an opening is created in the outer shell of the embryo (zona pellucida), and several cells are extracted. The cell(s) removed from each embryo are then subjected to PGS/PGD using various genetic analysis techniques such as polymerase chain reaction (PCR), array-comparative genetic hybridization (aCGH), or next generation sequencing (NGS).

BLASTOMERE BIOPSY (FIGS. 1A TO D)

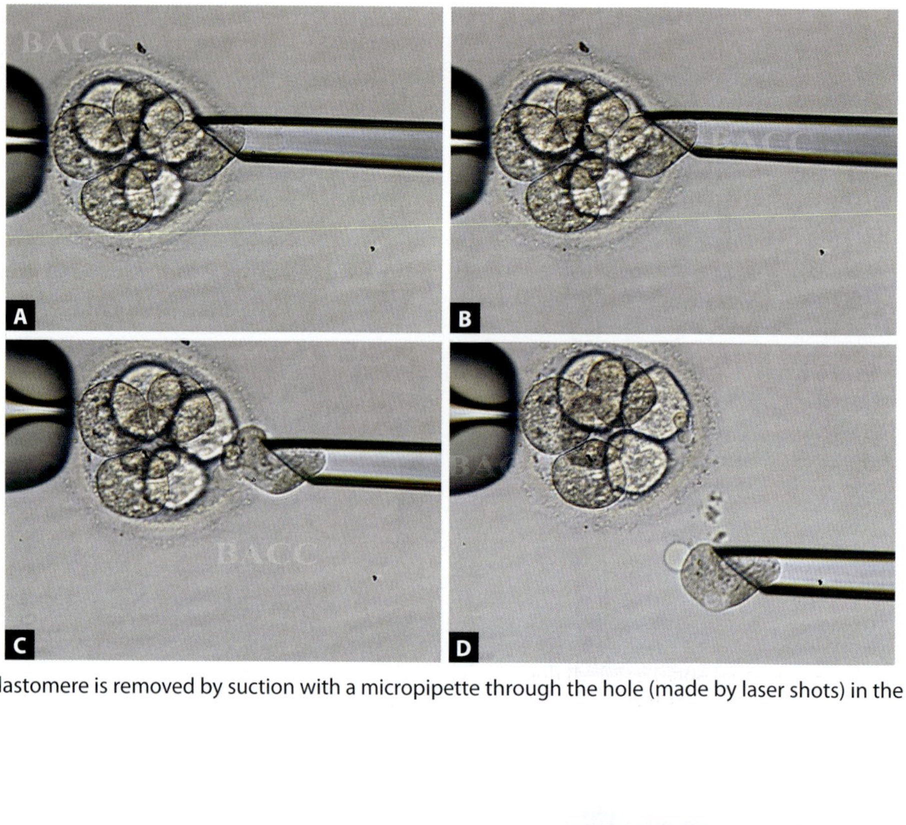

Figs. 1A to D: Blastomere is removed by suction with a micropipette through the hole (made by laser shots) in the zona pellucida.

TROPHECTODERM BIOPSY (FIGS. 2A TO H)

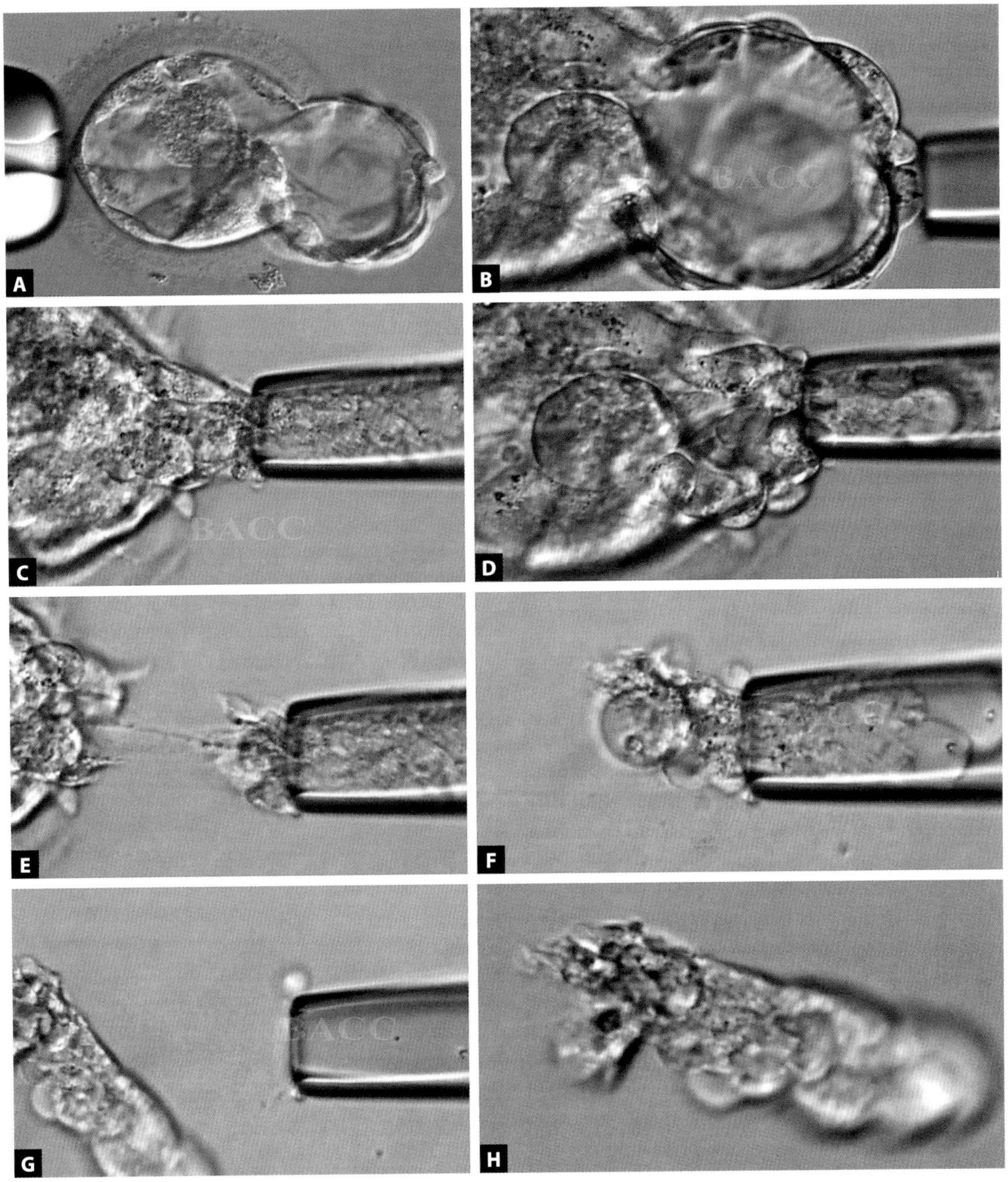

Figs. 2A to H: Involves removal of a portion of the mural trophectoderm (Trophoblast cells that is located farthest from the IMC). With trophectoderm biopsy, 5–10 TE cells can be retrieved. This approach limits the effects of mosaicism.

REFERENCES

1. Munne S, Weier HU. Simultaneous enumeration of chromosomes 13, 18, 21, X, and Y in interphase cells for preimplantation genetic diagnosis of aneuploidy. Cytogenet Cell Genet. 1996;75:263.e70.
2. Treff NR, Tao X, Ferry KM, et al. Development and validation of an accurate quantitative real-time polymerase chain reaction-based assay for human blastocyst comprehensive chromosomal aneuploidy screening. Fertil Steril. 2012; 97:819.e24.
3. Orvieto R, Gleicher N. Should preimplantation genetic screening (PGS) be implemented to routine IVF practice? J Assist Reprod Genet. 2016a;33:1445.e8.

Index

Page numbers followed by *b* refer to box, *f* refer to figure, *fc* refer to flowchart, and *t* refer to table.

A

Abbe-McIndoe procedure 1098, 1099*f*
Abdomen 913
 acute 466
 computed tomography scan of 143
 doughy feel of 466
Abdominal compartment syndrome 899
Abdominal mass 1075
 presence of 375
Aberrant phospholipase C zeta 1515
Aberrations 115
Abortion 969
 Act, regulations of 924
 incomplete 500*f*
 missed 1188
 second trimester 1188
 threatened 1188
Abruptio placenta 932, 1141
Abscess 121
Absolute uterine factor infertility 1055
Abulcasis 913
Acanthosis nigricans 531
Accessory gland infections, male 190, 314, 322, 359
Accessory sex gland 1249*t*
Acetamide 1139
Acetaminophen 575
Acetate 54
Acid
 citrate dextrose 1046
 media 1262
 peptic disease 324
 Tyrode's solution 1402, 1403*f*
Acid-fast bacillus 463, 468
Acidic alpha-glucosidase, function of 1249
Acne 369, 530
 management of 536
Acquired immunodeficiency syndrome 307, 456
Acridine 1262
 orange test 243, 1263
Acromegaly 142, 360, 363, 532
Acrosomal reaction 67, 240
Acrosome 1254, 1277, 1295
 birefringence 1437
 reaction 1343
  zona induced 1247
Acrylic dilators 1097*f*
Activated partial thromboplastin time 757
Activated volatile organic compounds 1320
Activins 21
Acupuncture 761
Acute respiratory distress syndrome 894, 1197
Adalimumab 203
Addison's disease 135
Adenohypophysis 18
Adenomyoma 495
Adenomyosis 101, 413, 426, 493, 496*f*, 843, 1035
 medical treatment of 428
 severe 954
 uterus 496*f*
Adenosine
 monophosphate 1245
 triphosphate 722, 1246, 1249
Adhesiolysis, hysteroscopic 611
Adhesion 76, 429, 572*f*
 formation, postoperative 583
 molecules 430, 1030
 scoring system 606*t*
Adhesive molecules, altered expression of 831
Adipokines 225
 function 224
 physiological role of 224
 role of 224
Adipose tissue 244*f*, 525, 1111
 endocrine function of 224
 mesenchymal stem cells 1120
Adnexa 501, 707, 1016
 anatomy of 1196, 1197*f*
Adnexal mass 467*f*
 size of 922*fc*
Adnexal tenderness 455, 466
Adnexal torsion 1196, 1197*t*, 1198, 1203
 diagnosis of 1198
 pathophysiology of 1198*fc*
 risk of 1198
 score for 1198*t*
Adoption 973
 agency 975
 domestic 974
 kind of 974
 open 974
 procedure 976
 regulations 975
 regulations of 975
 rules of 975
 types of 974
Adrenal disorders 146
Adrenal steroidogenesis pathway 108*fc*
Adrenarche 119
Adrenocorticotropic hormone 17, 107, 108, 134, 146, 147, 362, 525
 controls release of 17
Adriamycin 253, 253*t*
Adult respiratory distress syndrome 1196
Advanced air handling system 1498
Agenesis, acrosomal 1559
Agglutination 186
Air
 conditioning system 1482*f*
 exchange 1164
 handling unit 1027, 1498, 1647, 1647*f*
 injectors 1345
 jacketed incubator, box type 1648, 1648*f*
 pollution, episodes of 1498
 purification unit 1498
Air bubble
 formation 1506
 position 786
Air quality 1163, 1482, 1511
 monitor 1164*f*
Alanine 1444
Albumin 904, 1494
Alcohol 61
 consumption 1513
Aldosterone synthase 108
Alfentanil 758
Allergic skin reactions 672
Allergies 184
Alopecia 369, 530
 androgenic 530
 management of 536
 reversible 922
Alpha-fetoprotein 916
Altered sympathetic nervous system 525
Alzheimer's disease 888
Amantadine 339
Amenorrhea 130, 134, 135, 137, 138, 141, 168, 464, 549, 575, 601, 914, 1118
 classification of 130, 131*b*
 evaluation of 131
 exercise-related 170
 hypothalamic 167, 289, 664
 management of 135
 pituitary causes of primary 124
 secondary 132, 133, 134, 134*t*, 135, 1107
Amino acid 1443, 1495, 1496
 concentration of 1355
 essential 886, 1495, 1496, 1623
 metabolism 1355
 nonessential 1495, 1496
 sequence 884
 source of 1494
Aminoglutethimide 654, 669
Aminoglycoside 1495
Ammonium 1497
 ions 1497
Amnionicity 1010
Amniotic cavity 1005, 1008*f*, 1011*f*
 small 1016*f*

Amniotic fluid 1111
aspiration of 1210
Amniotic membrane 1120
Amniotic sac 1005, 1011f
Amoxicillin 1208
Amphetamines 535
Amphiregulin 1426
Ampulla 5, 913
Ampullary cells 1370
Amsel's diagnostic criteria 454
Anabolic steroid 306
abuse 360, 363
Anal sphincters, external 333
Analgesia 1325
patient-controlled 690, 761
Anastrozole 539, 654, 669
Androgen 29, 113, 150, 152, 474, 529, 691
binding protein 14, 54, 59, 328
dehydroepiandrosterone 109
dihydrotestosterone, stronger 525
evaluation of 812
excess 188, 519, 534
causes of 519
insensitivity syndrome 131, 169, 171, 308
mesterolone, modified 361
receptor 308
blocker 153
deficiency 184
resistance 360, 363
role of 30b
secreting tumor 532
supplementation 814
synthesis of 107
pathway 151
therapy 361
Androgenization, evidence of 325
Androgens, exogenous 376, 532, 691
Andrology 1233
tests 1238
Androstenedione 150, 534
peripheral aromatization of 521
Anejaculation 240, 335, 336, 355, 1515
management of 401
Anemia 931, 932
hemolytic 281
Anesthesia 757, 759, 766, 1036, 1325
drugs, safety of 761
epidural 761
resuscitation trolley 1155
techniques 758
Aneuploid 1472
cells 1416
embryos 1145, 1355, 1441, 1473
pregnancy 868
spermatozoa 1278
Aneuploidy 861, 1191, 1407, 1614
complete 878
embryonic 1327
lower incidence of 1451
origin of 861
partial 878
prediction of 1435
preimplantation genetic testing for 407, 1472
testing for 869, 879
Aneuploidy screening 861
results of 867
role of 861
Angelman syndrome 884
Angiogenesis 1021, 1030f, 1072f, 1081f
factors 1073f
Angiopoietin 1072, 1073
Angiotensin 107
Angiotensin-converting enzyme 315, 329, 345, 369, 583, 583f, 897, 1393
inhibitors 286, 292
Angiotensin-receptor blockers 292, 347
Anisotropy 1363
Anorchia 124, 305, 307
Anorexia nervosa 124
Anorgasmia
primary 339
secondary 339
Anosmia 124, 184
Anovulation 150, 167, 169, 519, 543, 668
causative factors of 171fc
causes of 168b, 170b, 171b
classification of 170fc
diagnosis of 167, 174fc
hypergonadotropic 173
hypoestrogenic 167, 664
hypogonadotropic 171
hypogonadal 167, 664
treatment of 167, 174fc
Anovulatory disorders 518
Antagonist 1128
cycle 1128
Antagonist protocol 737, 816
multiple-dose 679
protocol for 679
single dose 679
Anteflexion 6
Antenatal care 1214, 1216
Anterior pituitary venous complex 168
Anteversion 6
Antiandrogens 153, 536
Antibiotics 375, 778, 1208, 1495
intravenous 1201
use of 1495
Antibody 145
antiphosphatidylserine 833
development of 672
primary 1081
Anticancer treatment 253t
types of 253
Anticardiolipin 1020
antibodies 833
Anticholesterol medication 324
Anticoagulation 283, 284
therapy 907
Anticonvulsants 141, 324
Antidepressants 141
Antiepileptic drugs 289
impact of 289
Antiestrogens 172, 369, 666, 667
drugs 982
effects of 982
Antigen presenting cell 91
Antiglobulin reaction test, mixed 1246
Antihistamine 141, 365
Anti-Müllerian hormone 8, 24, 29, 44, 45, 49, 167, 195, 243, 250, 286, 329, 474, 475, 509, 521, 523, 524, 528, 534, 559, 560, 673, 674, 690, 700, 704, 715, 734, 735f, 736, 738, 752, 753, 793, 811, 830, 898, 905, 1039, 1075, 1093, 1129, 1143, 1324, 1394
role of 523
significance of 45
Antinuclear antibody 281, 1186
status 1186, 1188
Antioxidant 365-367, 547, 814
capacity, total 1244
therapy 814
Antiphosphatidic acid 833
Antiphosphatidylglycerol 833
Antiphosphatidylinositol 833
Antiphospholipid antibody 146, 279, 281, 833, 1188
syndrome 281-284, 284fc, 1020, 1022
Antipsychotics 141
drugs 324
Anti-Smith antibody 281
Antisperm antibody 190, 239, 243, 312
high titers of 1335
tests 1242, 1246, 1246fc
treatment of 363
Antithyroid medications 146
Antitubercular treatment 466, 468
Antral follicle
count 45, 193, 195, 243, 254, 474, 475, 559, 561, 659, 673, 674, 690, 707, 707f, 734, 738, 811, 830, 898, 905, 1035, 1129, 1223, 1231, 1324
high 473f
small 476f
Aorta 1056
Aplasia 131
Apoptosis 386
Apoptotic bodies, phagocytosis of 92f
Apoptotic spermatozoa 1279f, 1284
elimination of 1292
Applebaum's uterine scoring system 713, 713t
Arachnoid cyst 121
Arcuate uterus 418f, 491
three-dimensional ultrasound of 492f
Aromatase 131
enzyme 23
Aromatase inhibitors 172, 369, 428, 539, 654, 666, 669, 670, 742, 743, 747, 818, 901, 904, 1137
classification of 669t
generations of 654t
Array comparative genomic hybridization 865, 867, 878, 1145
Arrhenoblastoma 150
Arterial blood
flow 1199
gases 905
Arthralgia 677
Artificial insemination 965
indications for 949b, 965
posthumous 950
Artificial intelligence 263, 1250, 1319, 1330, 1466, 1467fc, 1468, 1469, 1473, 1474
application 1469, 1470
architecture 1466
recent advances of 1468
tools 1467
Artificial neural network 1474
Ascites 466, 893
Asepsis 795

Asherman's syndrome 131, 137, 432, 464, 465, 470, 601, 611, 846, 954, 1040, 1107, 1119
Asparagine 1355
Aspermia 327, 374
Aspiration
  cytoplasmic 1340
  needle 767, 1325, 1326
  pipette 1410
  pressure 546, 768
  pumps 1513
  setup 767
Aspirin 202, 844, 844*t*, 845, 901, 1022, 1108
  low-dose 813, 1108
  methods of action of 1023*fc*
  supplementation 293
  triggered lipoxins 1023
  use of 1148
Assisted ejaculation samples, preparation of 1275
Assisted hatching 429, 1401
  contraindications of 1405
  pitfalls of 1404
Assisted reproductive techniques 11, 56, 70, 161, 202, 228*b*, 272, 273*t*, 291, 365, 386, 407, 474, 571, 619, 635, 647, 690, 733, 797, 813, 843, 883, 885*b*, 887, 933, 939, 954, 970, 993, 999, 1033, 1035, 1135, 1154, 1158, 1189, 1242, 1261, 1293, 1319, 1358, 1380, 1399, 1407-1409, 1429, 1440, 1466, 1468, 1488, 1502*t*, 1525*t*, 1645
  advanced 402
  amendment rules 1159
  and surrogacy rules, timeline of 1157
  bank 956, 963, 964, 971, 1154, 1155, 1159
  bill 963, 964, 966-968, 1157
  clinic 963, 967, 1154, 1156, 1522, 1524
  complications of 891
  cycle 539, 721, 771
  failure 833
  guidelines 962
  laboratory 1481, 1645, 1657
    essential equipment of 1645
    quality management in 1161
  medical management in 1038
  practice 1154
    sex selective 943
  procedure 765
  regulation bill 959
  role of 1191
  rules 1154, 1157, 1158
  team 964
  treatment 820
  use of 950*f*
Assisted reproductive techniques act 871, 939, 968*t*, 1525, 1157-1159, 1525
  and Surrogacy (Regulation) Act 1488
Asthenospermia 374
Asthenozoospermia 188, 327, 399, 406, 620, 1237, 1257, 1279, 1444
  complete 1257
  severe 1334
Asthma 1213
Atopobium 833
  vaginae 454
Atresia 29
  follicular 29
Atretic oocyte 1360*f*
  corona cumulus 1535
Atrophy 4, 8
  endometrial 465, 1119
Attention deficit hyperactivity disorder 679
Autism 888
Autoantibody 833
  testing of 836
Autocrine substances 1459
Autoimmune 938
  diseases 252, 1429
  disorders 146, 1186
    screening for 135
    treatment of 1294
Autologous bone marrow derived stem cells, preparation of 1111
Automated volume calculation, sonography-based 708, 708*f*
Automatic fluid flow 1455
Autonomic nervous system 394
Autosomal dominant disorders 1407
Azithromycin 451, 452
Azoospermia 59, 59*t*, 211, 213, 327, 329, 354, 363, 374, 376*t*, 383, 406, 407, 949, 1275
  borderline 328
  classification of 310, 374, 374*fc*
  clinical classification of 374, 374*fc*
  diagnosis of 374
  etiology of 376, 377*t*
  evaluation 374
  factor 60, 178, 190, 212, 213*f*, 310, 377, 381, 382, 407
  hypergonadotropic 59
  hypogonadotropic 59
  management of 374, 383
  severe 329
  types of 375*t*

B

Back pain 655
Bacteria, detection of 838
Bacterial contamination 1329, 1515
  hypothesis 565, 566*f*
Bardet-Biedl syndrome 310
Bariatric procedures, types of 232*f*
Bariatric surgery 232, 536
  salient features of 232
Barker's hypothesis 223, 520, 999, 1000*f*, 1141
Bartoov criteria 1449*f*
Basal body temperature 159, 192, 705
  chart 705*f*
Basal estradiol 715
Basal follicle-stimulating hormone 560, 715
Basal ovarian volume 195
Bayle's sign 11
Bayley-Pinneau tables 127
Beak sign 501*f*
Beckwith-Wiedemann syndrome 884, 886, 1362
Behçet's syndrome 251
Benchtop incubators 1132, 1165, 1484, 1485*f*, 1498, 1648
  advantages of 1166
Bent neck sperm 187
Benzyl-alkyldimethyl chloride 1174
Beta-blockers 324
Beta-coronavirus 1212
Betadine 1174
Beta-human chorionic gonadotropin 447, 500, 794, 1201
Beta-lactam 1495
Betamethasone 1217
Beta-thalassemia 880
Bettocchi hysteroscope 595*f*
Bicarbonate
  buffered media 1337
  influx 67
  ion 67
Bicornuate uterus 414, 419, 488, 490*f*
  three-dimensional ultrasound of 489*f*
Bi-directional communication 1443
Biliopancreatic diversion 232
Biochemical pregnancy 1247, 1299, 1518
  rates 1518
Biomolecules retention 1461
Biopsy 1411
  adverse effects of 879
  device 1485
  easier, process of 1410
  endometrial 159, 193, 455, 941, 1107
  plate 1411
    preparation of 1410*f*, 1412*f*
Biotinylated deoxyuridine triphosphate 1037
Bipolar affective disorder 888]
Bipolar resectoscopic technique 425
Bipolar system 596
Bipolar tubal disease 446
Bipolar versapoint 596
Bird's nest appearance 503*f*
Birefringence 1257
  effect 1432*f*
  types of 1437
Birth
  asphyxia 931
  rates 774
Bisphenol A 528
Black-box models 1467
Bladder 1098*f*
  dissection of 1078*f*
  neck surgeries 324
Blastocele 70*f*, 881
  cavity 1568*f*, 1640, 1642*f*
Blastocentesis 866
Blastocyst 70, 829, 830, 876, 999, 1113*f*, 1140, 1146, 1175, 1182, 1310*f*, 1331, 1370-1372, 1372*f*, 1373, 1373*f*, 1374, 1375, 1414, 1444, 1450, 1463, 1586*t*, 1589, 1596*f*, 1643*f*
  applications 1473
  cell numbers 1320
  cryopreservation of 1374, 1637
  development of 1615*f*
  early 1568, 1585, 1586, 1594*f*
    hatching of 1569*f*
  evaluation of 1352, 1371
  expanded 1568, 1585, 1586, 1590
  freezing 1374
  functional 830
  glycerol for 971
  herniates 1401
  in vitrification solution 1639*f*, 1640*f*
  media 1659

microscopic analysis of 1307*f*
mid-cavitating 1587*f*
morphological evaluation of 1371
morphology of poor quality 1372, 1594
normal 1371
potential of 1371
production 1284
scoring of 1354*t*, 1472
selection of 1371, 1473
static image analysis of 1472
transfer of 1370
nine 1371
vitrification of 1140*f*, 1637
warming 1640
Blastocyst biopsy 863, 864, 877, 880, 1411, 1414, 1472
advantages of 877
exclusive 879
Blastocyst cavity 1372
fluid 1375
Blastocyst conversion 1048
rate 1524
Blastocyst culture 70, 430, 776, 998, 1370, 1371, 1376
advantages of 1375
application of 1375
Blastocyst development 1461, 1471, 1473, 1496
failure of 1376
prediction of 1471
Blastocyst embryo 1355, 1375, 1472
transfer 1352
Blastocyst formation 69, 1371, 1413, 1424
rate 1462
Blastocyst in vitro 1370
development of 1377
Blastocyst stage 1141, 1351, 1354, 1359, 1371
embryos, application of 1472
Blastocyst transfer 839, 944, 998, 1328, 1375
limitations of 1375
success of 1352
Blastomeres 1342, 1352, 1410, 1412, 1414, 1662, 1662*f*
biopsy 864, 1410, 1502, 1662
junctions of 1366
loss of 1402
shrinkage 1632*f*
Bleeding 597, 601, 1200
excessive 794
intraperitoneal 1200
Bleomycin 253
sulfate 253
Blind vagina 134
evaluation of 134*fc*
Blood
cholesterol, high 530
group 915
investigation 466, 1293
mononuclear cells, peripheral 203, 786
products 1423
profiles, basic 1186
Blood flow
endometrial 713, 1035
impairment of 386
studies 334
subendometrial 1518
Blood pressure 292, 345, 532
high 369
Blood sugar
fasting 340, 343, 1020
random 340
Blood testis barrier 58, 58*f*, 59, 364, 1393
breakdown of 313
Blood vessels 761*f*
twisting of 1199
Body fat, assessment of 222
Body mass index 61, 152, 168, 171, 184, 221, 222, 222*f*, 223, 279, 295, 325, 368, 535, 635, 673, 734, 738, 742, 758, 793, 810, 898, 927, 944, 997, 1020, 1039
high 944
Bologna convention 196
Bologna criteria, criticism of 674*fc*
Bone
demineralization of 154
loss 660
mineral density 123
pain 655
Bone marrow 1072, 1120*f*
aspiration 1121*f*
derived mesenchymal stem cells 1118*f*
Bone morphogenetic protein 24, 29, 55, 67, 523
system 1323
Borate glass 1273
Borderline abnormal semen parameters 189
Bovine herpesvirus 1394
Bovine serum albumin 1282
Bovine viral diarrhea virus 1394
Box incubator 1484
types of 1166*t*
Bradycardia, first-trimester 1016
Braille pin actuation 1456
Brain
female 8
injury, traumatic 392
Breast 120
discomfort 654
examination 325
ovarian cancer 880
size, reduced 660
tenderness 668
Breastfeeding 1217
shorter duration of 222
Breath, shortness of 1213
Breathing 1374
Breg cells 201
Broad ligament 582
fibroid 507
Bromocriptine 142
Brompheniramine maleate 365
Buccal mucosa 1099
Bulbocavernosus reflex latency 334
Bulbourethral glands 9, 12, 14
Bull's eye 1353*f*
Bupropion 231
Buserelin 680, 697

C

Cabergoline 142, 362
Cadaver dissections 1073
Cadherins 79
Cadmium 386
Caffeine consumption 1513
Cairo consensus guidelines 1488
Calcium
channel blocker 292, 313
influx 67
infusion 901, 903
ionophores 1516
ions 1245
Calorie restriction 230
Cancer 48, 576, 1407
antigen 916
childhood 1038
endometrial 552
prognosis 265
Cannula 580
Cannulation techniques 598
Capacitation 67
Carbamazepine 151
Carbohydrate 1355, 1443
metabolism 1443
Carcinoma
endometrial 532
in situ 308
Cardiac septal defects 998
Cardiopulmonary disease 1213
Cardiotocography 1217
Cardiovascular disease 234*f*, 231, 519, 523, 530*b*, 884, 886, 1189
subclinical 530
Cardiovascular system 325
Carmustine 253
Carnitine 366
Carotenoids 366
Catalase 366
Catecholamines 19
control endocrine function of 20*fc*
Catheter
removal time 785
rotation 785
types of 647, 1174
Cavity depth, estimation of 783
Cefixime 452
Cefotetan 456
Cefoxitin 455, 456
Ceftriaxone 452, 455, 456
Cell 1382
chromosomes 207
culture
medium 1411
platforms 1455
cycle 207, 207*f*
phases of 208*t*
cytoplasm 207
death 1401
activation-induced 91, 92
division 207, 861, 1354
premature 1416
stages of 1356
endometrial 1046
free nucleic acid, assay of 1414
growth factors 1121
manipulation, stereomicroscope for 1412
metabolism, number of 1278
number 1410
organelles 1320
pellet, seeding of 1029*f*
Cellular activities 1443

Cellular assessment 1358
Cellular associations 55
Cellular casts 281
Cellular damage, mechanism of 251*f*, 252*f*
Cellular hypoxia 311
Cellular metabolism, nanoparticles of 881
Centers for Disease Control and Prevention 364, 440, 440*t*
Central nervous system 121, 122, 171, 328, 759, 801
  disorders 141
  infections 121, 124
  tumors 121
  vascular malformation 121
Centrifuge 1155, 1651, 1651*f*
  machine 1155
Cephalic portion 1008*f*
Cephalosporin 1208
Cerebral edema 596
Cerebral palsy 999
Cerebral radiotherapy 170
Cerebri grafts 1076
Cervical
  agenesis 131, 414
  atresia 136
  biopsy 1041
  cultures 1041
  dilatation 775
  factor 197
    female 621
    infertility 626
  fibroids 582
  funneling 1188
  glands 1235
  lacerations 597
  lesions 492
  motion tenderness 455, 1198
  mucus 481, 482*f*, 654, 668, 706*f*, 778, 1235
    assessment 705
  myomas 426
  pregnancy 917, 924, 1014
    diagnosis of 917
Cervix 66, 465, 913
  classification of 414
  uncomplicated gonococcal infection of 452*b*
  upper 1005
Cesarean delivery 784
  greater risk of 222
Cesarean scar
  pregnancy 917, 924
  previous 913
Cesarean section, lower segment 1217
Cetrorelix 697
Charcot-Marie-tooth disease 48
Chelators 1495, 1496
Chemical depilation 153
Chemical pregnancy rates 1327
Chemical structure 667
Chemical zona 1401
Chemiluminescence 1243
Chemokines 78, 1118
Chemotaxis 1283
Chemotherapeutic agents 375
Chemotherapy 62, 121, 124, 171, 381, 1262
Chest surgery 988
Child abuse 977
Chinese hamster ovary 657, 658
Chiou classifications 387
Chi-square test 1223
Chlamydia 450, 966
  antibody test 198, 440
  infection 450
  pneumoniae 450
  trachomatis 191, 315, 364, 438, 450, 607
    antibodies 1201
Chlorine 1174
Chlorotrianisene 653
Chlortetracycline staining 1247
Cholesterol 107, 1444
  side-chain cleavage enzyme 111
Choline 1444
Choriocarcinoma 121
Choriogonadotropin receptor 25
Chorionic cavity 1005
Chorionic gonadotropin 76, 84, 86, 653, 723
  receptor 86, 520
  signaling pathways of 86*fc*
Chorionic villus sampling 125, 1004
Chromatin 1261, 1448, 1449
  compaction 1449
  condensed spermatozoa 1269, 1273
  remodeling 57
  structure 883
Chromium picolinate 548
Chromomycin 1264
Chromopertubation 441, 608
Chromosomal aberrations 1351, 1355
Chromosomal abnormalities 189, 308, 830, 1203, 1258, 1279, 1364, 1388, 1516, 1662
Chromosomal analysis 134
  biopsy materials for 1414
  methods of 863
Chromosomal disorders 998
Chromosomal inversion 880
Chromosomal mosaicism, effects of 1356
Chromosomal screening 1407
Chromosomal segment 1356
Chromosomal translocations 1093
Chromosome 47, 206, 1356, 1409, 1441, 1442, 1614
  abnormal separation of 861
  abnormalities 1384
  bacterial artificial 210, 1442
  basic structure of 206*f*
  complement of 1238
  comprehensive 1327
  deletion of 209*f*
  duplication of 209*f*
  homologous 1362
  inversion of 209*f*
  length of 878
  maternal deletion of 886
  normal 1426
  painting probes, partial 210
  set of 55
  status, assessment of 1409
  structural anomalies of 216, 381
  subunits of 206*f*
  translocations of 209*f*
Ciliary dyskinesia, primary 310, 1257
Cimetidine 62, 324
Citrate buffer 1292
Citric acid, levels of 1444
Clavulanic acid 1208
Cleavage stage biopsy 877, 1410, 1441
  advantages of 1411
  limitations of 1411
Cleavage stage embryo 862, 876, 1175, 1352, 1364, 1371, 1373-1376, 1495
  application of 1471
  evaluation of 1352
  scoring 1352*t*
Clindamycin 454, 454*b*, 455
  ovules 454
Clip applicator 580
Clomiphene 172, 539, 670*t*, 692
  isomers of 667*t*
  resistance 668, 1149
Clomiphene citrate 160, 172, 194, 245, 538, 621, 623, 643, 644, 653, 654, 667, 670, 682, 736, 738, 742, 743, 747, 818, 1107, 1137
  addition of 818
  challenge test 193, 194, 559, 561, 811
  failure 538, 654, 668, 670
Clonazepam 151
Clonidine 324
Coadjuvant therapy 283, 284
Coculture system 1496
Coda inline filters 1653, 1653*f*
Coda mini tower 1482*f*
Coda tower 1653, 1653*f*
Coenzyme
  Q 692
  Q10 548, 1223
Coital disorders 307
Coitus
  freezing of 183
  timing of 183
Cold 1213
  chain maintenance 793
Collin's knife 601*f*, 602*f*
  electrode 610*f*
Colloid 904
Colloidal microbeads 386
Colony stimulating factor 75, 81, 84, 85*f*
Combined oral contraceptive 427, 428, 571
  pill 692, 1128, 1129
Comet assay 189
Comet test 1037
Comparable biochemical pregnancy 1518
Comparative genomic hybridization 210, 865, 877, 1022, 1323, 1355, 1409, 1440, 1441, 1518
  array 1441
  microarrays 1415
Competent certification bodies, traits of 1184*b*
Competitive binding assay 1248, 1248*fc*
Complete androgen insensitivity syndrome 1094
Complete blood count 905, 1214
Complex lesions 504
Component cells, preparation of 1028
Compound microscope 1649, 1649*f*
Compound pentoxifylline 1257
Comprehensive chromosomal screening 835, 840, 867, 1407
Computational fluid dynamics simulation 1460*f*
Computed tomography scan 143, 222, 222*f*, 387

Computer-assisted
  scoring system 776
  sperm analysis 1242, 1246, 1247, 1250
Conception 239, 605, 1009
  natural 998
  products of 1020, 1024
  rate per cycle 538
Congenital adrenal hyperplasia
  late-onset 545
  nonclassical 151
Congenital anomalies 7, 222, 350, 364, 998, 1425
Congenital uterine
  abnormalities 487, 487*t*, 492
    diagnosis of 487*t*
  anomalies 101, 413, 830
    classification of 414
    management of 418*t*
Conjoint twins 929, 1404
  types of 930*f*
Conjugated equine estrogen 1137
Connective tissue
  disease, mixed 281
  growth factor 1109
Conscious sedation 758, 766
  anesthesia, monitoring of 759
Consensus scoring system 1574*t*, 1586*t*
Continuous visual analog scale 785
Contraception, methods of 924
Controlled ovarian stimulation 24, 118, 158, 257*f*, 647, 659, 659*f*, 665, 673, 674, 682, 690, 704, 733, 735*f*, 736, 737, 750, 754, 799, 810, 813, 817, 956, 896, 946, 1047, 1193, 1323, 1344, 1511
  cycles 158, 158*f*, 158*fc*, 159*b*, 162
Conventional sperm preparation techniques, limitations of 1275
Cooks catheter 779, 781*f*
Copy number variants 216
Corifollitropin alfa 1038, 1039*f*
  properties of 1038
Corifollitropin delta 1038, 1039
Corifollitropin epsilon 1038, 1039
Corona radiata cells 67, 1457
Coronavirus disease 2019 (COVID-19) 315, 329, 1212-1214, 1216, 1217, 1219*b*, 1393, 1395
  classification of severity of 1213
  clinical features of 1213
  disease 1033, 1213, 1219
  effects of 315, 1213
  home monitoring for 1216*t*
  incidence of 1212
  infection 316, 370, 685, 1035, 1213, 1214, 1219, 1393
    management of asymptomatic 1216
    management of mild 1216
    moderate 1393
    moderate to severe 1216
  management of 1217, 1217*b*, 1218*fc*
  pandemic 684, 1033, 1491
    advent of 1050
  postnatal care of 1217
  precautions for 1214*f*
  symptoms of severity of 1213
  testing 1034
    indications for 1213
  transmission of 1219
  vaccination 329, 1035, 1050, 1219
  virus 1213, 1219
Corpora cavernosal bundles 987*f*
Corporal venous occlusive disease 342
Corpus cavernosum penis 9
Corpus luteal flow 484*t*
  normal 483*f*
Corpus luteum 23, 156-158, 158*f*, 159, 502, 502*f*, 515*f*, 568, 799, 830
  Doppler of 711, 711*f*
  formation of 21, 156
  function 895
  physiology of 799*f*
  premature destruction of 23
  rescue 157
  role of 800*fc*
Cortex, adrenal 108
Cortical granules, exocytosis of 68
Corticosteroids 151, 202, 283, 284, 548, 1217
  indications for 1217
Corticotropin-releasing hormone 17, 19, 76, 84, 92, 147
  secretion 525
Corticotropin-stimulation test 545
Cough 1213
Couples intending surrogacy, eligibility criteria for 969
Cowper's glands 12
Craniopharyngioma 121, 124, 170, 306
C-reactive protein 225, 905, 1186, 1187, 1198
Creatinine 899
  clearance 899
Creutzfeldt–Jacob disease 655
Crohn's disease 252, 278, 287, 288
Crown–Rump length 1005
Cryocans 1486*f*
Cryoinjuries 1140, 1381
Cryopreservation 746, 1141, 1174, 1292, 1391, 1481, 1486, 1517, 1528, 1623
  equipment for 1155, 1650
  intraoperative 1294
  method 1174
  postoperative 1294
  preoperative 1294
  principle of 1623
  procedure 1487
  process of 1381
  system, troubleshooting 796
  technique 999, 1135, 1139, 1328
Cryopreserved tissue, management of 456
Cryoprotectants 1381, 1394, 1517, 1637
  agents 1139, 1463
  media 1634*f*
  osmotic effects of 1381
  remove 1381
  types of 1381
Cryoprotective agents
  cytotoxicity of 1388
  minimizing toxicity of 1388
  non-permeating 1388
  permeating 1388
  safety of 1388
  use of 1387
Cryostorage 1396
Cryosystems 1395
Cryptorchidism 184, 305-308, 350, 352, 360
Cryptozoospermia 327
Crystalline pellet form 361
C-type natriuretic peptide 1426
Culture media 1494, 1659
  quality control of 1490
  types of 1659, 1659*f*
  volume of 1170
Cumulus cell 30
  apoptosis 1426
  removal stress 1343
Cumulus oocyte
  complex 30, 768, 814, 856, 859, 1280
  transzonal projections, preservation of 1426
Cumulus oophorus 513*f*
  complexes 546
  mucification 724
Curvilinear path, linearity of 1250
Cushing's disease 146, 147, 360, 362
  treatment of 362
Cushing's syndrome 134, 146, 147, 152, 154, 532
  pathognomonic features of 147
Cycle pregnancy rate 645
Cyclic adenosine monophosphate 30, 47, 48, 57, 63, 86, 87, 341, 367, 722, 844, 901, 903, 1108, 1195, 1245, 1434
Cyclic guanosine monophosphate 47, 341, 367, 395*f*, 397
Cyclin dependent kinase 27
Cyclooxygenase 33
  inhibitors 49
Cyclophosphamide 62, 253, 281, 282
Cyclosporine 151
Cyproheptadine 339
Cyproterone acetate 124, 153, 536, 550
Cysts 502
  epididymal 351
  evaluation of 1036
  follicular 501
  formation of 195
  functional 705, 714
  hemorrhagic 502, 502*f*
Cystadenoma 568
Cystic dilatation, bilateral 357*f*
Cystic fibrosis 184, 190, 311, 378, 880, 1407
  transmembrane conductance regulator 185, 213, 329, 376, 406, 409
    gene 190
Cystic pattern, generalized 508, 509*f*
Cystitis, risk of 1097
Cytochromes P450 107
Cytogenetics 206
  basics of 206
Cytokines 73, 76, 80, 102, 1030, 1121
  role of 898*fc*
Cytokinesis 207, 1361
Cytomegalovirus 966
Cytoplasm 1340, 1360, 1410, 1425, 1533*f*
  color of 1351
  maturation 1434
Cytoplasmic anomalies 1470
Cytoplasmic extensions 1373
Cytoplasmic extrusion 1605
Cytoplasmic granules, exocytosis of 1421
Cytoplasmic movement 1471
Cytoplasmic organelles 1421
Cytoplasmic strings 1373, 1373*f*, 1596

Cytoplasmic vacuolation 1323
Cytosine adenine-guanine 240
Cytotoxic effects 1389
Cytotoxic therapy 251*f*, 252*f*
Cytotoxicity, risk of 1388
Cytotrophoblast 84, 90
  extravillous 88

D

Dacarbazine 253
Dalteparin 280
Danazol 427, 570
Davydov's vaginoplasty, laparoscopic 136
D-chiro-inositol 526
de Leener's classification, modified 896*t*
De Quervain's disease 145
Dead spermatozoa 1292, 1387
Death, intrauterine 1426
Decidual cast 1005
Decidual natural killer cells 1021, 1021*f*
Deep venous thrombosis 127, 279, 1197
Dehydroepiandrosterone 108, 109, 119, 146, 668, 691, 813, 814, 1095
  sulfate 134, 150, 150*f*, 172, 522, 529, 534, 545, 812
Dehydrogenases 112
Delta opioid receptor 22
Dendritic cells 88
Density gradient
  method 1253
  technique 1448
Density gradient centrifugation 1270, 1271*f*
  advantages of 1271*t*
  disadvantages of 1271*t*
Deoxyribonucleic acid 29, 35*f*, 56, 74, 189, 206*f*, 207, 239, 240, 250, 311, 314, 365, 367, 375, 386, 450, 466, 566, 655, 883, 884, 916, 920, 998, 1023, 1108, 1112, 1261, 1267, 1306, 1320, 1394, 1403, 1407, 1437, 1449, 1450, 1456, 1469, 1498, 1557, 1562
  apoptosis 386
  compaction 57
  damage 311, 386
  fragmentation index 56, 57, 228, 367, 368, 646, 1243*f*, 1562, 1562*f*, 1563*f*
Deoxyuridine triphosphate 189, 243, 1262
Dermatitis 922
Dermoids 504, 505*f*, 568
Desipramine 365
Destructive tubal surgery 446
Dexamethasone 548, 693, 1217
Dexmedetomidine 759
Dextran serum substitute 1388
Diabetes insipidus 634
Diabetes mellitus 59, 224*f*, 278, 292, 293, 340, 360, 362, 374, 529, 534, 535, 1023, 1035, 1040, 1213, 1294
  gestational 291, 523, 939, 1062, 1188
  type 1 293*f*, 294*fc*, 1039
  type 2 294*fc*, 518, 530
Diacylglycerol 48, 68
Diagnostic test performance, analysis of 1229
Diamniotic twin 927*f*, 928, 1404
Diarrhea 1213
Diazoxide 151
Dichlorodiphenyltrichloroethane 61, 62
Dichorionic-diamniotic
  placenta 928, 931*f*
  twin 1010, 1012*f*
Diencephalon 306
Dienogest 427, 428, 570*t*, 575
Diethylstilbestrol 491
Different biopsy techniques
  advantages of 864*t*
  disadvantages of 864*t*
Diffusion weighted imaging 387
Digital optoelectronic sensor 1256
Dihydrotestosterone 119, 136, 150, 229
Diiodotyrosine 143*f*
Diluent solution 1382
Dimethyl sulfoxide 255, 971, 1139, 1381, 1388
Dimethylarginine, asymmetric 527
Dimethylxanthine theophylline 1245
Directly observed treatment, short-course 463, 469
  strategy treatment 469
Disasters, natural 1491
Discoid rash 281
Disease-modifying agents 203
Distal obstruction 355
Distal seminal ducts, functional obstruction of 314
Distal tubal disease 439, 584
  causes of 439*t*
  surgery for 445
Distinct nuclear precursor bodies 1565*f*
Distorted pelvic anatomy, reconstruction of 605
Distorted uterine cavity, reconstruction of 609
Dithiothreitol 366
Dizygotic births 927
Dizygotic twins 930
Doderlein's bacillus 7
Dominant blastocyst cavity 1594*f*
Dominant follicle 540, 541, 682, 815
  atresia of 23
  growth of 46*fc*
  selection of 30, 31
Domperidone 957
Donate oocyte 967
Donepezil 151
Donor 942, 946
  cycle, legal implications of 948*t*
  embryos 1157, 1159
  factors 945
  gametes 1155, 1159
  hysterectomy 1059
  insemination 275, 382, 620
  investigations for 942*b*
  medical examination of 1156
  program 944
  selection 941
  sperm 949*b*
  surgery 1041
Donor oocyte 820, 950
  programs 1328
  use of 938
Donor semen 965
  insemination 949
  samples 1293
Dopamine 19, 20*fc*, 230, 332, 521
  agonists 142, 362, 666, 672, 903
Doppler angiogenesis 1089*f*
Dostinex 362
Double decidual sac sign 916
Double stimulation protocols 1048
Double tail sperm 187
Down syndrome 49
Doxorubicin 253
Doxycycline 451, 455, 456
Drawer incubators 1498
Drugs 1107
  administration of 260
  androgenic 691
  antiepileptic 289
  anti-hypertensive 292, 292*t*
  anti-inflammatory 49
  antipsychotics 324
  dopaminergic 142, 335
  effects of 62
Dual stimulation 818
  protocol 818*f*
Dual trigger 723, 728, 819
Dual-energy X-ray absorptiometry 222
Duchenne muscular dystrophy 48
Duct
  system 364
  transurethral resection of 12
Ductus deferens 11
Duplex protocol 683
Duplication cyst, diagnosis of 1076
Dydrogesterone 1148
Dye exclusion 186
  method 1561
Dynamic infusion cavernosography 334
Dynamic voltage scaling 1508
Dynorphin 22, 118
Dysgenesis, management of 137
Dyslipidemia 530, 532
Dysmenorrhea 426, 427
Dyspareunia 333, 427, 466
  deep 567
Dysphoria 992, 1208
Dyspnea 655
Dysregulation 521

E

Early pregnancy loss 222, 924, 1012, 1019*t*, 1185, 1322
  diagnostic of 1014
  risk of 1138
Eating disorders 158
Echocardiogram 905
Echogenic rim 1005
Ectoderm 1117
  upper 1004
Ectogenesis 1042, 1043*f*
Ectopic endometrial growth, inhibition of 575
Ectopic pregnancy 841, 913, 913*t*, 914, 915*f*, 921*fc*, 924, 1013-1015, 1201, 1202
  diagnosis of 1203, 1203*f*
  estimated 1013
  management of 447, 922*fc*, 1200*t*
  pathophysiology of 1201, 1202*fc*
  persistent 923
  prevention of 919
  risk factors for 914*fc*
  sites of 913, 1201, 1202*f*
  treatment 587
Ectopic sac 1203

Edema, peripheral 369
Eflornithine 154
Egg
  sharing 275
  transport 66
  yolk 1291
Eight cell embryo 69, 1567*f*, 1580-1582, 1620*f*, 1631*f*, 1632*f*
Ejaculates, multiple 1293
Ejaculation 13, 333, 395, 401, 1261, 1267
  failures 1515
  neuroanatomy of 397*f*
  neurophysiology of 397*f*
  painful 356
  parasympathetic outflow necessary for 398*b*
  premature 333, 335
  retarded 339
  sympathetic outflow necessary for 398*b*
Ejaculatory disorders 335
Ejaculatory disturbances 332, 334
Ejaculatory duct 11, 355, 1294
  calcification 356
  cyst 356
  dilation 357*f*
  evaluation of 355
  obstruction 12, 313, 328, 355, 376-378
  transurethral resection of 377, 378
Ejaculatory dysfunction 183, 306, 324, 392, 394, 398
Ejaculatory organ 9
Elective frozen embryo transfer 999
Elective oocyte cryopreservation 263*t*
Elective single embryo transfer 631, 871, 931, 1413
Electrocardiogram 292, 766, 905
Electrocardiography 759
Electroejaculation 337, 338, 339, 400, 402, 1294
Electrolysis 153
Electrolytes 905, 907
  imbalance 597, 893
Electron
  paramagnetic resonance 1244
  spin resonance 1244
Electronic medical record 1175, 1475
Electronic witnessing system 1486
Electrophoresis 213*f*, 1263
Electrophoretic method 1255
Electrophoretic sperm
  separation 1049
  sorting 1050
Electrospray ionization 1443
Elevated liver enzymes 922
Ellipsoid formula 1015
Embolotherapy 389
Embryo 76, 83, 87*f*, 226, 227, 834, 840, 878-880, 886, 887, 913, 992, 1005, 1007*f*, 1012, 1140, 1154, 1165, 1172, 1257, 1283, 1320, 1327, 1328, 1351, 1355, 1358, 1367, 1371, 1374, 1383, 1389, 1395, 1401, 1443, 1455, 1461, 1468*f*, 1474, 1475, 1494, 1497, 1583-1585, 1623, 1649
  abnormal 1473
  accumulation of 737
  aneuploidy rate 1323
  anomalous 1615*f*
  assessment 1440
    methods 1468
  biopsy of 1306*f*
  conditions of 1496
  cranial end of 1007*f*
  cryopreservation 256, 261, 283, 902, 982, 996, 1380, 1381, 1387, 1394, 1414, 1429, 1463, 1630
  culture of 1371, 1376
  delivery, subendometrial 775
  development of 73, 1291, 1614*f*
  donation 966, 1303
  early development of 1005*f*, 1496
  euploidy 1473
  evaluation of 835*fc*, 835*t*, 1373, 1441, 1467
  exposure of 1497
  factors 830, 834
  figure-of-eight configuration of 1404*f*
  formation, low-grade 565
  fragmentation 1516
  freezing of 727, 971, 1387
  frozen 1324, 1390
  fundus distance 783
  glue 841
  good-quality 829, 1136, 1404
  grading methods 1352, 1476
  growth, nature of 1564
  high-grade 818
  images 1367
  implantation of 429, 829, 830, 895, 1013, 1036, 1106, 1150, 1474
  injection, speed of 786
  invasion 76
  loading techniques 782, 782*f*
  manipulations of 1331, 1511
  metabolism 1444
  monitoring techniques, advanced 1466
  morphological assessment of 1358
  morphological evaluation of 1351, 1355
  nature of 1329
  number of 819, 1156, 1157, 1375, 1377
    good quality 1325
  percentage of 1171
  placement 1329
  ploidy 1328
  preimplantation genetic testing of 876
  preloading of 782
  pronuclear stage 1471
  requirement of growing 1497
  retained 785
  scoring 1570
  selling of 971
  supernumerary 1374, 1471
  three-cell 1365*f*
  time-lapse monitoring of 1050
  transfer 1141, 1630
    of multiple 1370
  transplantation 1300
  turns 1366
  two-cell 69*f*, 1566*f*, 1575, 1576
  utilization rate 830
  viability 1444, 1516
  vitrification of 737, 1140*f*, 1331, 1389, 1630
  volume of 1584*f*, 1588*f*
Embryo biopsy 877, 1145, 1394, 1408, 1409, 1662
  majority of 877
  method 877
  noninvasive methods for 1413
  protocol for 1410
Embryo culture 886, 1132, 1174, 1459, 1461
  media 1494
  systems 795, 1494
    novel 1319
Embryo development 866, 1257, 1323, 1345, 1376, 1422, 1424, 1434, 1450, 1457, 1497, 1498, 1511
  normal 1564
  stages of 1473
Embryo quality 775, 830, 839, 943, 1261, 1330, 1340, 1352, 1467, 1516
  assessment of 1414
Embryo selection 776, 1146, 1468, 1471, 1474
  methods of 1356
  tool, superior 1443
Embryo transfer 202, 307, 429, 469, 470, 510, 513, 682, 717, 742, 759, 774, 775, 778, 784-786, 789, 794, 813, 816, 839, 841, 844, 914, 1010, 1031, 1032, 1037, 1106, 1146, 1158, 1174, 1300, 1319, 1328, 1329*f*, 1376, 1416
  catheter 778, 1132, 1308*f*, 1329*f*, 1512, 1655, 1655*f*
    components of 779
    types of 778, 779*t*
  depth of 783
  difficult 784
  double 996, 1474
  factors affecting success of 775
  interval 841
  personalized 838*fc*, 1037
  procedure 788*fc*
  pump-regulated 784
  selection process for 1355
  stages of 1421
  steps of 775, 776*fc*
  stimulated cycle frozen 1137
  techniques 782, 1319
  terms of 1368
  types of 774, 1655
  ultrasound guided 841
Embryoblast 70
Embryogenesis 66, 68, 830, 885, 1368
  stage 863
Embryology 3, 8, 1297
  authority 871, 879, 942
  laboratory 1034
    complex 964
Embryonic development 883, 1498
  rate 1374
Embryonic genome 1351, 1370
  period of 1496
Embryonic implantation 76, 92
Embryonic morphology 1005
Embryonic proteome analyzation 1443
Embryonic stem cells 1043, 1116
  characteristics of 1044*f*
Embryoscope 1486, 1487*f*, 1613*f*
Emission 13, 395
  neuroanatomy of 397*f*
  neurophysiology of 397*f*
  parasympathetic outflow necessary for 398*b*
  sympathetic outflow necessary for 398*b*
Empirical therapy 368

Empty follicle syndrome 726, 794, 855, 856, 859, 1514
classification of 855, 856*t*
management of 858*fc*
risk factors for 857
Empty sella syndrome 306
Encephalitis 121, 124
Encephalocele 121
Enclomiphene 667, 682
Endocrinal disturbances 350
Endocrine 76
abnormality 1020
axis, male 328*f*
disorders 140, 148, 359, 1429
disrupting compounds 148
disturbances 284, 364
dysfunction 289
evaluation 375
factors 1020
profile 59
signals 84
strategy 844*t*
tissues, oxygen uptake of 1069*t*
Endocytotic origin 1362
Endoderm 1117
lower 1004
Endometrial breakdown 37*fc*
menstrual phase of 34, 37
phases of 34, 37
Endometrial calcification 500, 501*f*
Endometrial cavity 481*f*, 488, 491*f*, 497*f*, 794
Endometrial diseases 1117
Endometrial flow indices 714*f*
Endometrial gene expression, assessment of 1027
Endometrial gland isolation 1029*f*
Endometrial markers 159
Endometrial maturation 98*f*
abnormal 420
Endometrial microbiome metagenomic analysis 100
Endometrial microbiota 833, 838
role of 100
Endometrial micro-rejuvenation 1112, 1113
Endometrial pinopods 1402
Endometrial preparation 943, 1136, 1138, 1422
Endometrial protein, progesterone associated 82
Endometrial receptivity 97, 101, 831, 832, 837*t*, 842, 1313
analysis 429, 837, 838
array 100, 787, 1036, 1037, 1313, 1517
role of 1047
factors affecting 830, 831*f*, 834
markers of 100, 711*t*
pathology of 837*fc*
testing for 836
Endometrial receptor array 1027
Endometrial regeneration 1107, 1120
proposed mechanism of 1119
Endometrial rejuvenation 1106, 1111, 1112
cell-based therapies for 1109
methods of 1107, 1108*t*
principles of 1107
Endometrial scratch 430, 845
Endometrial synechiae 241
Endometrial thickness 708, 711, 712*t*, 713, 716, 944, 1108
Endometrial transcriptomics 100
Endometrial vascular flow indices 713
Endometrial vascularity 482*f*, 484*f*, 712*f*
Endometrial volume 713, 714*f*
Endometrioma 502, 502*f*, 503*f*, 568, 574, 1016, 1511
appearance of large 592*f*
atypical ultrasonography features of 568*t*
bilateral 251, 572
management of 591
surgical therapy of 574
typical ultrasonography features of 568*t*
Endometriosis 99, 158, 217, 241, 438, 439, 565-567, 570*t*, 572, 576, 576*t*, 580, 584, 591, 607, 668, 677, 696, 701, 834, 846, 913, 997, 1187, 1299
adolescent 575
associated infertility 1327
treatment of 572
deep infiltrating 569
diagnosis of 567
fertility index 572, 573*f*
mild 621
pathogenesis of 565, 565*fc*
recurrent 251
severe 605*f*
ultralong protocol for 683, 683*f*
Endometriotic cyst 568*t*, 574*f*
presence of 769
Endometritis 495, 497*f*
acute 495
chronic 241, 242, 413, 430, 495, 1024
Endometrium 76, 80, 82*f*, 85*f*, 87*f*, 97, 98, 225-227, 464, 480, 481*f*, 495, 512, 668, 712*f*, 841, 954, 1012, 1030, 1031*f*, 1046, 1047, 1111, 1117, 1121, 1367, 1403
assessment of 711
atrophic 470, 1111
biological functions of 35*f*
feature of mature 512
fluffy outer margin of 482*f*
growth factors 83*t*
indications of 1027
inner layers of 482*f*
multilayered 712*f*
outer margin of 482*f*
pathophysiology of thin 1107
quality of 1106
receptive 73
role of 1106
surface of 1031*f*
volume histogram of 514*f*
Endoplasmic reticulum 1360, 1363*f*
End-organ disorders, management of 136
Endorphins 22
Endosalpinx 464
infections of 450
Endoscopic procedures 1512
Endothelial cells 1021
Endothelial dysfunction 346
diagnosis of 346
Endothelial nitric oxide synthase 345
Endothelin interaction 311
Endotoxin 1292
bacterial 1171
Endotracheal intubation, indications for 1217
Endovaginal telemonitoring system, self-operated 714, 714*f*, 1036
Enkephalins 22
Enoxaparin 280
Envelop protein 1212
Enzymatic deficiencies 131, 151
Enzyme
complex 111
immunoassays 451
linked immunosorbent assay 440, 560, 715, 1244
thyroid peroxidase 143
Eosin-hematoxylin staining technique 1559*f*
Eosin–nigrosin staining 1244
Ependymoma 121
Ephedrine 365
Epidermal growth factor 23, 656, 1108, 1109, 1424, 1461
Epididymal abnormalities 351
Epididymal diameters 354
Epididymal duct 14
Epididymal maturation 57, 63
Epididymal obstruction 313, 328, 376
Epididymal sperm 1335
aspiration 13
microsurgical 379, 380, 760, 1294
Epididymis 10, 326, 352, 354*f*, 377, 1245, 1249, 1334
sperm aspiration 1305*f*
Epididymitis
acute 351
chronic 351, 353*f*
Epididymo-orchitis 351, 375, 451
Epigenetic abnormalities 1093
Epigenetic defects 1294
Epigenetic disorders 214, 1409
Epigenetic influences 884
Epigenetic modifications 883*fc*
assessment of 1441
Epilation methods 153
Epilepsy 279, 289, 290, 888
effects of 289
impact of 289
Epirubicin 253
Epithelial cells 1028, 1029*f*, 1030*f*
adhesiveness 80*f*
endometrial 80, 97
Epithelial estrogen receptor-alpha 98
Epithelial proliferation 1030
Epithelium 1111
Eppendorf micromanipulator 1508, 1509
control board of 1509*f*
Equilibration solution 1382, 1623, 1624*f*, 1626*f*, 1630, 1637
Erasure 885
Erectile dysfunction 240, 306, 324, 325, 332-334, 339, 341, 345*fc*, 346, 346*fc*, 347*fc*, 359, 392, 396, 398, 1117
assessment 343
development of 340*t*
diagnosis of 342*f*
evaluation of 396
loss of 324
management of 344, 398*fc*
treatment for 341, 342*f*
Erection 13, 333, 395
hardness score 347

neuroanatomy of 397*f*
neurophysiology of 397*f*
parasympathetic outflow necessary for 398*b*
problems 333
sympathetic outflow necessary for 398*b*
vascular process for 397*f*
Erythrocyte sedimentation rate 466, 1187
Erythromycin 375
e-Sanjeevani 1215, 1219
online outpatient department 1215*f*
Escherichia coli 312, 566
Estimated endometriosis fertility index 607
Estradiol 19, 26, 37, 84, 17, 122, 174, 194, 375, 521, 524, 669, 680, 681, 721, 743, 811, 814, 831, 844, 895, 898, 901, 905, 1129
levels 715
natural 284
stimulation of 1029
use of 1128, 1518
Estrogen 16, 22*f*, 23, 24, 25, 26, 76, 90, 98, 151, 161, 474, 479, 571, 692, 727, 802, 895, 957, 982, 1107, 1112
antagonists 653
deficiency 369
effects of 982
pretreatment 692
production 157
secretion, abnormalities of 523
supplementation, absence of 1137
support 803
synthesis of 108
Estrogen receptor 112
alpha 117
gene polymorphisms 112
polymorphism 112
Ethambutol 432, 469
Ethanesulfonic acid 1253
Ethylene
diaminetetraacetic acid 367, 1188, 1495, 1496
glycol 1381, 1388, 1623
oxide 1490
Etoposide 253
Euploid 1472
cells, development of 1416
oocytes, proportion of 1323
Euploid embryos 832, 1442
selection of 1355
transfer of 1327
Exemestane 669
Exercise 230, 535
excessive 158
programs 230
Exogenous follicle-stimulating hormone ovarian reserve test 559, 561
Exogenous gonadotropins 1420
theoretical risks of 1421
Exons, analysis of 1441
Extracellular domain 1038
Extracellular matrix 87, 528, 1046
components 54
Extracorporeal shock wave therapy 344
Extraembryonic celom 1005
Extraembryonic matrix 83, 84, 86*f*
Extraembryonic membrane 1007*f*
Extreme gonadotropin insufficiency 360
Eye
anterior chamber of 1071
piece 1433

F

Fabricate microstructures 1281
Fadrozole 654, 669
Fallopian sperm perfusion 627
value of 621, 628
Fallopian tube 3, 70*f*, 241, 438, 463, 464, 464*f*, 913, 1036, 1238, 1320, 1358
ampulla part of 1267
blocked 607
composition of 1495
inflammation of 505
ultrasound evaluation of 440
Falloposcopy 441
Falope rings 588*f*
False empty follicle syndrome 858
pathophysiology of 856
Family planning 254
recommendations for 265
Fas ligand 92
system-induced apoptosis 91
Fasciocutaneous flaps 1099
Fast growing embryo 880
Fat
distribution of 222
emulsions, intravenous 202
Fatal complications 1326
Fatigue 567
Fatty acids, polyunsaturated 1273
Fatty liver disease, nonalcoholic 532
Female genital tract 325, 1093, 1243*f*, 1261, 1276*f*, 1283
anomalies, classification of 417*f*
Female genital tuberculosis 441, 463, 464, 466, 466*b*, 467*f*, 468*f*, 470
diagnosis of 468*fc*
epidemiology of 463
symptoms in 466*b*
Female gonads, formation of 42, 42*fc*
Female infertility 191, 241, 1118
chromosomal disorders in 215
genetic of 215
Female pronucleus 1045
formation of 67
Female reproductive
cells 1394
duct, embryology of 413, 413*f*
function 23*b*
system 3, 5*f*, 16
disorders of 1117*f*
tract 1404
Female unexplained infertility, causes of 241*b*
Fentanyl 758, 760
Ferriman-Gallwey score
modified 150, 151*f*
system 152
Fertility 284, 293, 345, 986
clinics 1322
decline, causes of 176
drugs 982
use of 927
duration of previous 183
female 251, 1117
future 591
issues, types of 1117*t*
long-term 924
management 593
outcome 426, 470*t*
potential 1469
preservation of 923
rate, total 176
reduced 1261
regulation of 1040
replacement level 176
restoration 1068
sparing surgery 261
specialists, role of 178
tertiary center for 1190
treatment 245, 926, 973, 997, 1370
unexplained 158, 1273, 1327, 1335
Fertility preservation 250, 251, 254, 259*fc*, 265, 266, 286, 725, 758, 981, 991, 1387, 1394, 1429
indications of 250
interventions 254, 255*f*, 255*fc*
methods of 261*t*, 991
program 1429
recommendations for 264
Society 265
technique of 254, 256
treatments for 995
Fertilization 53, 66, 567, 757, 819, 971, 1005*f*, 1327, 1345, 1361, 1383, 1416, 1451, 1461, 1469
abnormal 1516
age 1009
analysis of 1351
assessment of 1342
confirmation of 1597
defects 240, 241
determination of 1165
failure 364, 1257, 1334, 1351, 1362, 1450
causes of 1515
in vitro 1273
in vivo 1264
issues 1515
levels of 1343
lower probability of 1341
media 1659
methods of 834
mode of 546
potential 1469
process of 67, 68*fc*, 1242, 1267, 1516
rate 227, 565, 744, 1277, 1345, 1362, 1422, 1434, 1435, 1444, 1448, 1458, 1462, 1515, 1524
higher 1327, 1347
terms of 1435
scoring for 1528
total failed 1327
Fertilized egg 1010
Fertiloscopy 443, 1036, 1036*f*
over laparoscopy, advantages of 1036
Ferulic acid 366
Fetal anomalies 996
Fetal bone, hysteroscopic removal of 603*f*
Fetal complications 289
Fetal deaths 222
Fetal demise 996
Fetal development, subsequent 1495
Fetal growth 1011
restriction 1185, 1188

- Fetal heart rate 1008, 1009f
- Fetal immune cells 201
- Fetal maternal contact 87
- Fetal origin 223, 520
- Fetal period 115
- Fetal reduction 932, 1004, 1207, 1208f, 1210, 1211
  - studies on 1210
- Fetal rejection 201
- Fetal urine production 1005
- Fetoplacental interface 1186
- Fetus 1186
  - labeling of 1012f
  - number of 1211
- Fibers, collagen 1118
- Fibroblast growth factor 29, 1072, 1073, 1109
  - basic 29
  - receptor 1072
- Fibroids 101, 492, 493, 494f, 583, 677, 1037
  - cystic degeneration of 494f
  - degenerated 583
  - endometrial 498, 499f
  - intramural 842, 843
  - multiple 954
    - small 846
  - peripheral vascularity of 494f
  - submucosal 842
  - uterus 494f, 1005
- Fibromas 503
- Fibronectin 79, 1118
- Filtration techniques 1254
- Fimbria 913
- Fimbrial agglutination 590f
- Fimbrioplasty 445, 589
- Finasteride 153, 324, 536
- Fine-needle aspiration cytology 380
- First generation tests 1355
- Fistula, risk of 1097
- Fitz-Hugh-Curtis syndrome 451, 464
- Fixed dose antagonist protocol 680f
- Flagellum 1277
- Flexible dose antagonist protocol 680f
- Flexible guidewire through catheter 598
- Flexible protocol 679
- Flow cytometry 1244
- Flow index 507, 713
- Fluid 794
  - exchange 1042
  - filled vacuoles 1545
  - level 503f
  - overload 597
  - volume 782
- Fluorescence
  - in situ hybridization 210, 309, 840, 864, 1022, 1237, 1262, 1263, 1324, 1409, 1414, 1415, 1441
  - intensity 1263
  - microscope 1263
- Fluorodeoxyglucose 466, 467f
- Fluoroscopic guided cannulation 598
- Fluorouracil 253
- Fluoxetine 151
- Flutamide 153, 536
- Folate 366
  - coenzyme 920
- Foley's catheter 499, 497, 988
- Folic acid 1188, 1189
- Folinic acid 920
- Follicle
  - aspiration 757
    - equipment 1326f
  - dominance of 43
  - fertilization of 511
  - group of 1421
  - number per ovary 508
  - premature rupture of 793
  - recruitment of 45
  - secondary 43, 45
  - selection of 43
  - stimulation 173
  - synchronization 1307
  - syndrome, early 856
  - theca cell of 156
  - ultrasound image of 1305f
- Follicle-stimulating hormone 5, 14, 22-26, 33, 46f, 59, 107, 115, 125, 144, 158f, 171, 194, 211, 229, 263, 285, 294, 306, 341, 369, 376, 406, 474, 508, 521-523, 540-542, 571, 643, 658, 666f, 671-675, 697, 721, 729, 734-737, 743, 750, 793, 800, 810-812, 830, 896, 901, 938, 1128, 1299, 1308, 1323, 1402, 1420
  - agonist 1311
  - concept of 27f
  - dose of 817
  - function of 24b
  - gate 45
  - luteal initiation of 817
  - polymorphism 25
  - receptor 25, 813, 896, 1038
    - polymorphism 528, 1038
  - role of 24fc
  - three-dimensional model structure of 1308f
  - window 45
- Follicle-to-oocyte index 817
- Follicular aspirates 904, 1423, 1515
- Follicular assessment 511
- Follicular defect 522
- Follicular development 29f
- Follicular early cessation agonist protocol 678f
- Follicular fluid 30, 566t, 725, 1173, 1444, 1514
- Follicular flushing, role of 770
- Follicular granulosa cells, luteinization of 724
- Follicular growth 708
  - assessment of 708
  - stages of 27f
- Follicular maturation 895
  - complete 1514
- Follicular maturity 479
- Follicular output rate 195, 810
- Follicular phase 26, 34
  - abnormal 158
  - early 754
- Follicular recruitment, early 477f
- Follicular ring sign 504, 504f, 1199f
- Follicular rupture 722
- Follicular stimulation 657
- Follicular volume 711
- Folliculogenesis 42, 49f, 110, 522, 665, 665f
  - abnormal 565
  - defective 524fc, 550
  - dysfunctional 857
  - early stages of 29f
  - normal 523f
  - stages of 43, 44f
- Follistatin 14, 21
  - role of 32
- Follitropin delta, use of 900
- Foot pedal 1655
- Formestane 669
- Four-axis hanging joystick oil hydraulic micromanipulator 1504f
- Four-cell embryo 69f, 217, 1463, 1555f, 1577-1579
- Fragile X
  - mental retardation gene 217
  - syndrome 131, 217, 880, 1407
- Frank dilator method 1097
- Frank Lydston implants 1067f
- Frank's vaginal dilators 136
- Free androgen index 533
- Free fatty acid 117, 224
- Free testosterone level 152, 375
- Freeze blastocysts, optimal time of 1375
- Freeze dried human spermatozoa 1502
- Freeze thaw transfer 1305
- Fresh donor oocyte 945
- Fresh embryo transfer 841, 863, 945, 1141, 1150
- Frozen embryo transfer 101, 162, 279, 284, 429, 782, 787, 800, 943, 945, 1135-1137, 1141, 1141t, 1304, 1510
  - cycles 162
  - endometrial preparation for 1136
  - indications for 1136
  - natural cycle 1136, 1137t
  - preparation methods 1136, 1136fc
- Frozen human eggs 1306
- Frozen oocytes 1310
- Frozen pelvis 464
- Frozen semen sample 646
- Frozen spermatozoa 1255
- Frozen thawed
  - oocytes, meiotic spindle of 1383
  - spermatozoa 1335
- Frozen thawed embryo transfer 944
  - cycles 1138
- Fructo-oligosaccharides 231
- Fructose 375
  - estimation 1242
  - negative azoospermia 376
- Frydman rigid catheters 779, 781f
- Fumarate hydrates 217
- Fundal endometrium 783
- Fundal myoma, initial appearance of 583f
- Fused pelvic kidney 1079f
- Fusion 413

G

- G protein-coupled receptor 22, 80
- Galacto-oligosaccharides 231
- Galactorrhea 141
- Galactose 1139
- Galactosemia 131, 135
- Gametes 830, 834, 839, 948, 1154, 1172, 1395, 1455, 1495
  - artificial 1117
  - assessment of 1440
  - donation 839, 846
    - offspring of 942

donors, screening of 941
dysfunction, severe 1243
evaluation of quality of 1351
female 886
human 1319, 1456
immature 1310
male 885
manipulations of 1331, 1511
micromanipulation of 1503
morphological evaluation of 1351
parameters, abnormal 457
transfer of 1339
use of 1157
viability of 66
Gametes intrafallopian transfer 760, 997, 1304
procedure 1305*f*
Gamma-aminobutyric acid 23, 117, 231, 521, 801
Ganirelix 697
Gardnerella vaginalis 454, 838
Gartner's duct 4
Gas chromatography 1440, 1444
Gastrectomy, vertical sleeve 232*f*
Gastric band, laparoscopic adjustable 232
Gastroesophageal reflux disease 324
Gastrulation 1004
Gay couples 982
Gelatin assay test 1247
Gender affirmation surgery 986, 990
complications of 989
criteria for 986
Gender dysphoria 980, 986, 989
Gene 76, 80
autosomal 884
editing 1046
expression 883, 1320
global profiling of 100
mutations 240
polymorphisms 214, 217
silencing 883
General anesthesia 380, 760, 765
Genetic abnormality 169, 381, 861, 871, 876, 1276
Genetic analysis 867, 877, 880
techniques 1662
Genetic anomalies 307
Genetic composition, nonreflection of 863
Genetic control 60
Genetic couple 956
Genetic defects 240, 532, 1473
Genetic diseases 1662
Genetic disorders 939, 1262, 1293, 1662
Genetic factors 1020, 1021
Genetic material 950
Genetic predisposition 927
Genetic screening 189
Genetic workup 1022, 1022*fc*
GeneXpert 441, 466
Genital chlamydial infections, treatment of uncomplicated 364*b*
Genital examination 325
Genital mycoplasmas 453
Genital organs 464
female internal 3
Genital surgeries 986, 989
Genital system 3
Genital tract
infection 306
male 1238, 1261
obstruction 191
Genital tuberculosis 464*t*, 465, 466*b*, 470
prevalence of 464, 464*t*
Genitalia
ambiguous 151
external 4, 9
male 120
normal 966
external 1094*f*
Genitofemoral nerve 10
genital branch of 9
Genitoplasty 1093
Genitourinary tract infections, male 314
Genome 1189, 1415
activation 69
amplification 1415
wide association studies 217, 520
Genomic aberrations 216
Genomic analysis 1441
Genomic hybridization
array 1441
complete 430
Genomic imprinting 884
Genomic stability 883
Gentamicin 452, 1495
sulfate 1623
Genuine empty follicle syndrome 855, 858
pathophysiology of 857
Germ cells 53, 54, 62, 308, 885, 1046
development 885
female 1420
immature 1049
male 1273
numbers 28*f*
stages of 55*fc*
tumors 121
Germ stem cells 43
Germinal vesicle 43, 251, 665, 1359*f*, 1361*f*, 1383, 1426, 1537, 1539*f*, 1540*f*
breakdown 48, 665
oocyte 1537, 1539
presence of 1470
stage 1539*f*
Gestation, period of 1010
Gestational age 914, 1004, 1016
assessment of 1009
large for 523, 549
small for 121, 287, 523*f*, 549, 946, 1142
Gestational sac 829, 1005, 1013
measurement of 1009*f*
small 1016*f*
Ghrelin 23, 117
Giant oocytes 1360*f*, 1516
Glands 1111
accessory 364
adrenal 17*f*, 522
Glandular enlargement 1030
Glass bottom dish 1335, 1345
Glass heating stage 1506
Glass pasteur pipettes 1658*f*
Glass petri dishes 1503
Glass wool
fibers 1273
filtration 1253, 1254, 1273
advantages of 1274*t*
disadvantages of 1274*t*
Glial cell derived neurotrophic factor 54
Global imprinting disorders 887
Globozoospermia 56, 1049, 1050, 1451, 1515, 1557, 1559
Glucagon-like peptide 231
receptor agonists 548
Glucocorticoids 108, 113, 154, 845, 901, 903
resistance, familial 121
supplementation 147
Glucose 1139
6-phosphate dehydrogenase 365
fasting 534
metabolism 1355
tolerance test, intravenous 525
transporter type 4 526, 528
Glucuronide 112
Glutamate 117
metabolism 1444
Glutamine 1444
Glutathione 367
depletion of 1497
Glycation end products, advanced 524
Glycerol 971, 1388
Glycerophosphocholine 1249
Glycerophosphorylcholine 14
Glycine 425, 1292, 1355
Glycodelin 76, 81, 82
concentrations 82
Glycogen 35
Glycoprotein 857
hormones 1038
high levels of 896
Glycosylphosphatidylinositol 67
Golgi
apparatus 56
complex 1360
Gonadal agenesis, management of 137
Gonadal dysgenesis 938
Gonadal function 359
Gonadal steroid feedback, regulation of 1039
Gonadal suppression 256
Gonadal tissue colonization 42
Gonadarche 116, 119
Gonadectomy 137
Gonadogenesis 53
Gonadostat theory 116
Gonadotoxic disease 1294
Gonadotoxic drugs 312
Gonadotoxins 184
Gonadotropin 20*fc*, 51, 59, 112, 116*f*, 171, 173, 246, 360, 369, 524, 622, 623, 653, 655, 660, 666, 671, 676, 690, 742, 743, 814, 815, 818, 900, 1127, 1137, 1324, 1424, 1513, 1514
agonist stimulation test 811, 812
dose, lower requirement of 814
doses of 900, 1323, 1324, 1512
embryonic chorionic 98
evolution of 656*f*
low-dose 644
mid-cycle surge of 31*t*
preparation 658*t*, 675, 675*t*
regimen 817
replacement
response, positive predictive factors of 360
therapy 360

secreting
adenoma 360, 362
tumors, treatment of 362
starting dose of 1129
stimulation 227, 1128
protocols, high dose 1324
structure of 658
surge-attenuating factor 33
therapy 360, 362, 363, 818
types of 1512
use, indications for 659
Gonadotropin-releasing hormone 14, 16-18, 19*f*, 22*f*, 31, 47, 87, 123, 144, 158*f*, 168, 194, 225, 254, 280, 294, 328, 382, 568, 581, 627, 659, 666, 679, 690, 696, 723, 725*f*, 726*fc*, 727, 729, 734, 737, 743, 793, 813, 815, 819, 855, 901, 905, 943, 981, 1038, 1127, 1130, 1135-1137, 1142, 1148, 1195, 1324, 1420, 1513
agonist 154, 154*f*, 158, 161, 282, 422, 428, 559, 569, 571*t*, 660, 660*t*, 666, 676, 678, 678*f*, 680, 681*f*, 683, 696, 698, 699, 702, 702*t*, 721, 721*f*, 723-726, 729, 735, 802, 815, 816, 818, 839, 843, 844, 900
development of 696
flare 815
preparation 676*t*
protocols 698*f*
safety of 679
stimulation test 559, 561
trigger 727, 728, 857
trigger failure 726
trigger, indications for 725
analog 542, 659, 672, 696, 701, 799, 1047
clinical uses of 698
protocol 815
use of 698
antagonist 660, 660*t*, 666, 679, 680, 681*t*, 697, 699, 699*f*, 702, 816, 818, 819, 943, 1040
cycles 751, 754
development of 697
protocol 735, 816*f*
regimens 816
dynamics 26
endogenous 696
low concentration of 170
molecule, structure of 19*f*
pulsatile secretion of 18
structure of 697*t*
therapy 360
failure of 361
trigger 725
use of 1299
Gonads 4, 9
development of 4*f*
dysgenetic 1068
embryological development of 3*f*
Gonococcal infection 451
Gonorrhea 451, 966
Goserelin 697
G-protein coupled receptor 20
Graafian follicles 26, 43, 47, 592
Graduated embryo score 1352*t*
Gram staining 452
Granular cytoplasm 1541
Granulation 1551*f*
central 1322
Granulocyte 88
colony-stimulating factor 202, 261, 431, 844, 1023, 1046, 1108, 1109, 1517
Granulosa 156, 725, 1457
lutein cells, number of 897*f*
Granulosa cell 45, 109, 522, 1119, 1323, 1329, 1421, 1430, 1434
function 521, 814, 1323
removal 877
tumor 121
Graspers 580
Graves' disease 143, 145, 146
Greater vestibular glands, infections of 8
Ground glass appearance 503*f*
Growth factors 73, 76, 80, 83, 1030, 1107, 1455
role of 32
Growth hormone 17, 119, 142, 529, 690, 813, 1047, 1118
addition of 813
receptor 813
regulates release of 17
releasing factor 813
role of 1047
Growth problems 126
Growth restriction, intrauterine 121, 931, 996, 1062
Growth spurt 119
Guanethidine 324
Guanosine triphosphate 395*f*
Gut microbiome 234
role of 223
Guttate hypomelanosis, idiopathic abnormal 143
Gynecological procedures 1127
Gynecomastia 145, 325
presence of 375
Gynetics 779, 781*f*

H

H2-receptor antagonists 324
Haemophilus influenzae 455
Hagen-Poiseuille's law 768
Hair 149
accessories 990
axillary 119, 375
classification of 149*f*
facial 375
growth 150
phases of 149, 149*f*
removal
permanent measures of 153*t*
temporary measures of 153*t*
HAIR-AN syndrome 152
Halo test 1037
Halosperm 1343
Hamartoma, hypothalamic 121
Hamster epididymis 1170
Hamster oocyte 1344
Hamster sperm motility assay 1170
Haploid cells 1363
Haptoglobin 88, 91
Hard zona 1405
Harmonic scalpel 580
Hashimoto's thyroid disease 146
Hashimoto's thyroiditis 143
Hatching blastocysts 70*f*, 74, 75*f*, 1113*f*, 1307*f*, 1367*f*, 1372*f*, 1463, 1569, 1586, 1592, 1592*f*, 1593, 1595*f*
Hawthorne effects 1224
Head
injury 124
magnetic resonance imaging of 134
Headache 654, 677, 1213
Healthcare
team 1041
workers 1035
Healthy embryo 1366
Healthy oocyte 1362
Healthy pregnancy 1186
Heart
disease, congenital 223
failure, congestive 345
rate 897
transplants 1294
Heartbeat, absent 920
Hegar's dilators 1209
Helper T-cell subsets 201
Hematocrit 894, 899, 905, 907
Hematological disorder 281
Hematoma formation 584, 923
Hematopoietic precursor cells 99
Hematopoietic stem cell 253, 1118
use of 432
Hematospermia 356
Hemizona index 1248
Hemochromatosis 360, 363
Hemoconcentration 893
Hemodialysis, intensive 286
Hemoglobin 466, 535, 1247
electrophoresis 956
glycated 956, 1020
Hemoperitoneum 907
Hemophilia 1407
A 48
Hemorrhage 422
antepartum 932, 997, 1141, 1142
Heparin 845
binding epidermal growth factor 83
Hepatitis 1394
B 942, 965
infection 1495
surface antigen 451, 942, 956
B virus 457, 458, 1156
infection 458
C 942, 965
antibody 941
virus 451, 459, 1156
Hepatoblastoma 886
Hepatocyte growth factor 1111
Hernia 376
Herniorrhaphy 184
Heterodimers 1038
Heterotopic pregnancy 913, 916, 918, 924, 1015
diagnosis of 1203
incidence of 918
Heterotopic transplantation 1429
Highly active antiretroviral therapy 456, 635
High-uterine artery resistance 475*f*
Hilus sign 568
Hirsutism 147, 149, 150, 154, 530, 536, 677
diagnosis of 150
etiology of 150, 151*f*

idiopathic abnormal 150, 532
management of 153*f*, 536
physical examination of 152*t*
scoring systems 150
treatment of 152, 153*f*
Histamine 896
Histones 214
majority of 1261
Histrelin 697
Hoffman modulation 1335
Holeaccumulation diode 1448
Home isolation, guidelines for 1216
Homeobox genes 82
Homocysteine metabolism 1189*f*
Homogeneous granular cytoplasm 1542*f*
Hormonal monitoring 704
Hormonal profile 704
Hormonal suppression 258
Hormonal tests 133
Hormone 143*f*, 375, 1107, 1455
dependent tissue 1107
discovery of 1065
effects of 289, 1027
exposure, exogenous 121
hypothalamic 17
levels of 1150
male reproductive axis of 8
role of 50*f*
sensitive cancer 256
suppression 261
therapy 571, 986
gender affirming 981, 982
treatments 997
Hormone replacement
therapy 97, 126, 134, 137, 943, 1136-1138
cycle 837
treatment 818
Host cell membranes 1393
Hot flushes 154, 654, 655, 660, 677
Human albumin 1270
Human aneuploid 1442
Human blastocysts 85*f*, 1463, 1621*f*
testing of 1312
Human body 1381
Human cell 876, 1039
cryopreservation of 1380
Human cervical mucus 1237
Human chorionic gonadotropin 23, 47, 73, 100, 121, 145, 161, 173*f*, 225, 257*f*, 307, 360, 431, 476, 540-542, 619, 656-658, 678-681, 683, 691, 698, 721, 721*f*, 724*t*, 725*f*, 726, 736, 742, 770, 792, 802, 813, 815, 817, 856, 893, 895, 897*f*, 898, 901, 915*f*, 916, 922, 1019, 1034, 1108, 1129, 1148, 1194, 1299, 1325, 1383, 1422
administration 727
dose, low 817
effects of 87*f*
injection 1046
disadvantages of 360
role of 100
trigger 857
Human clinical embryology laboratory 1489
Human embryo 90, 948, 1321, 1442, 1494, 1495, 1498, 1567*f*, 1568*f*, 1570*f*, 1572*f*, 1575*f*, 1576*f*, 1578*f*-1582*f*
coculture of 1370
culture 1455
early 1371
implantation 830
selection of 833
status of 1444
Human Embryo Research Amendment Act, regulation of 962
Human embryonic
proteome, complete 1443
stem cells 947, 1045, 1375
derivation of 1375
Human endometrium 76, 1028, 1106, 1313
components of 1119
histology of 1028*f*
Human fertility, probabilistic nature of 1236
Human fertilization 871, 879, 942
Human genome project 1207
Human immunodeficiency virus 191, 275, 393, 451, 456, 463, 635, 941, 942, 956, 965, 1141, 1156, 1254, 1334, 1394, 1515
diagnosis of 1230
infection 252, 253, 949
Human intelligence 1466
Human leukocyte
antigen 90, 99, 100, 160, 832, 876, 1021, 1022, 1187, 1407
C system 832*f*
typing 880
system 832
Human menopausal gonadotropin 138, 171, 194, 194*t*, 307, 360, 625, 643, 656, 658, 666, 674, 675, 680, 683, 737, 738, 742, 743, 751, 753, 810, 1302, 1344, 1515
disadvantages of 753
dosage of 1361
Human myometrial tissue 1041
Human oocyte 1301*f*, 1306, 1365, 1394, 1424, 1573*f*
fertilization of 1306
fertilize 1301*f*
Human ovarian steroidogenesis 109
Human phenotypes 884
Human preimplantation embryos, biopsy of 1306
Human serum albumin 1388, 1448, 1494, 1623
Human sperm 1244*f*, 1380
model 1344
survival assay 1170
Human spermatozoa 1255, 1277, 1292, 1306, 1621
selection of 1267
Human tubal fluid 842, 1253, 1269, 1305, 1494, 1623
Human uterus transplantation trial 1057, 1059
Humidity 1482
Humoral immune response 201
Huntington's disease 880, 1407
Hyaluronan binding assay 1247, 1281, 1343
Hyaluronan microdroplets 1607*f*
Hyaluronate 1495
Hyaluronic acid 430, 841, 1255, 1280, 1280*f*, 1452, 1605
binding 1280, 1280*f*
physiological method of 1255
droplet 1607*f*
selection of 1452*f*, 1608*f*
sperm selection, application of 1452
Hyaluronidase 1660, 1660*f*
dishes 1338
Hydatidiform moles, partial 1015
Hydralazine 324
Hydraulic control
system 1505
unit 1506
Hydraulic unit 1504
Hydrocele 350, 352, 352*f*
Hydrocelectomy 324, 375
Hydrocephalus 121
Hydrodynamic flow 1459
Hydrogen ion
concentration 1169
efflux of 67
Hydropelviscopy 1036
Hydrosalpinges 838
surgical management for 445*t*
treatment of 846, 847*t*
Hydrosalpinx 101, 446, 506*f*, 707, 834, 1016
bilateral 585*f*
fluid 847
initial appearance of 590*f*
management of 584, 609
specimen of 585*f*
transvaginal aspiration of 609
Hydroxychloroquine 1187
sulfate 1022
action of 1023*f*
Hydroxydaun 253
Hydroxydaunorubicin 253
Hydroxyeicosatetraenoic acid 33
Hydroxyethyl starch 904
Hydroxylase 108, 109, 111, 131
deficiency 151, 158
Hydroxymethylglutaryl coenzyme A 548
Hydroxyprogesterone 30, 534, 550
level 152
Hydroxypropyl cellulose 1388
Hydroxysteroid dehydrogenase 30, 107-111, 156
deficiency 151
type 2 98
Hyperactivation 240
motility 241
Hyperandrogenemia 474, 483, 518, 550
Hyperandrogenic insulin-resistant acanthosis nigricans syndrome 526
Hyperandrogenism 134, 134*t*, 150, 158, 518, 519, 523, 534
adrenal 525
development of 521*fc*
Hypercoagulable state 899
Hyperechoic inner endometrial margin 497*f*
Hyperechoic stroma 478*f*
Hyperglycemia 293
Hypergonadism, hypergonadotropic 188
Hyperhomocysteinemia 550, 1188, 1189, 1191
Hyperinsulinemia 225, 476, 518, 529
Hyperplasia
adrenal 151
congenital adrenal 111, 121, 131, 134, 147, 152, 170, 360, 363, 545
endometrial 131, 495, 496, 498*f*, 532

Hyperprolactinemia 135, 141, 142, 142*t*, 152, 160, 169-171, 306, 325, 360, 362
- biochemical 141
- causes of 141, 141*t*
- drug-induced asymptomatic 142
- effects of 23*b*
- medical management of 142
- presentations of 141
- treatment of 142*b*, 362

Hyperprolactinemic anovulation 167, 664
Hyperresponsiveness, adrenal 525
Hypersensitivity 669
Hypertension 278, 291, 340, 529, 530, 532, 1040, 1213
- chronic 291
- gestational 1062, 1188
- impact of 291
- pregnancy induced 929, 946, 999, 1113

Hypertensive disorders 946
Hyperthyroidism 144, 188, 362
- diagnosis of 145
- treatment of 362

Hypertonic solution 1381
Hypertrichosis 150
Hypoalbuminemia 893
Hypoechoic cystic area 1005
Hypoestrogenic environment 575
Hypoestrogenic state 677
Hypogonadism 325
- acquired hypogonadotropic 306, 307
- congenital hypogonadotropic 125, 126, 305, 306
- high pitched in 375
- hypergonadotropic 124, 168-170, 352, 375
- hypogonadal 657
- hypogonadotropic 12, 117, 124, 135, 167, 168, 170, 188, 306, 328, 359, 360, 375-377, 382, 664, 751, 754, 857, 895
- idiopathic hypogonadotropic 135
- secondary 306

Hypogonadotropic hypogonadism 12, 117, 124, 135, 167, 168, 170, 188, 306, 328, 359, 360, 375-377, 382, 664, 751, 754, 857, 895
- etiology of 382*b*
- feature of 167
- management of 138

Hypomenorrhea 144
Hypo-osmotic stress 1244*f*
Hypo-osmotic swelling 186, 1244, 1560
- test 1244, 1256, 1560, 1560*f*
  - modified 1256

Hypophysectomy 170
Hypospermatogenesis 57
Hypotaurine 366
Hypotension 899
Hypothalamic amenorrhea, primary 532
Hypothalamic dysfunction 668
Hypothalamic secretions 18
Hypothalamic-pituitary
- adrenal axis 654
- axis 18*f*, 46
- failure 664
- gonadal axis 59, 115, 140, 228, 369, axis 522
- ovarian axis 25, 25*f*, 26, 115, 130, 167, 168*f*, 226*fc*, 286, 664
  - dysfunction 282
  - ovarian dysfunction, mechanism of 284, 285*f*

Hypothalamus 16, 17*t*, 25, 224, 225, 306, 1039
- central effects on 225
- pituitary system, unique features of 140

Hypothesis, adrenal 520
Hypothyroidism 23, 124, 144, 152, 170, 188, 362
- inhibits 144
- primary 121
- subclinical 143, 1189
- treatment of 362

Hypovolemia 899
- intravascular 893

Hypoxia 385, 385, 1118
Hysterectomy 954
- abdominal 606

Hysterolaparoscopy 603
Hysterosalpingo-contrast
- sonography 197, 505
- ultrasonography 439

Hysterosalpingogram 244, 836
Hysterosalpingography 196, 242, 414, 432, 439, 442, 442*t*, 466, 467*f*, 580, 603, 608, 608*f*, 760, 966, 1020
- analgesia for 760

Hysteroscopic cannulation methods 598
Hysteroscopic resection, technique of 596
Hysteroscopic subendometrial injection 1110*f*, 1121*f*
Hysteroscopic tissue retrieval system 597
Hysteroscopy 197, 466, 582, 594, 599, 603, 837, 845, 1036, 1147
- guided tubal cannulation 442
- screening 1147

I

Ice crystal formation 1292, 1389
Idiopathic testicular failure, primary 322
Ileal pouch anal anastomosis 287
Iliac arteries, external 1059
Ilioinguinal nerve 10
Imipramine 365
Immature follicles, multiple 508
Immature human oocytes 1384
Immature oocytes 1359*f*, 1384, 1420, 1423*f*, 1514, 1516, 1537
- corona cumulus 1534
- cryopreservation 256

Immaturity, high level of 1449
Immotile 188
- cilia syndrome 325, 1244, 1335
- sperm 1256, 1515
  - cells 1273
- spermatozoa 327, 1244, 1256, 1257

Immune
- cells 1030
- dysfunction 528
- factors 898, 1405
- infertility 240, 241
- modulators 91
- protein 1187
- regulation 1185
  - pathway 1185*f*
- system 88, 201
  - peripheral 88
- tolerance 430
  - synopsis of 92*f*

Immunity
- adaptive 201
- cell-mediated 89
- innate 201

Immunofluorescence technique 1186
Immunoglobulin 79
- A 1246
- G 282
  - phospholipids units 282
- intravenous 202, 431, 804, 1023
- M 282
  - phospholipids units 282

Immunohistochemistry 1081
- tests 1081

Immunological disorder 281
Immunological factors 350, 364
Immunological milieu 1020, 1020*f*
Immunological rejection 1069
- monitoring of 1041

Immunology 201, 1073
Immunomodulators 284
Immunosuppressants 283
Immunosuppression 1041
- failure of 313

Immunotherapy
- benefits of 203
- harms of 203

Impaired glucose tolerance 527, 529, 530, 532
Imperforate hymen 124, 131, 136
Implantation 73, 73*fc*, 97, 227, 567, 819, 1004, 1039
- blastocysts regulation of 76, 83
- eccentric 75
- factors affecting 101, 101*f*
- failure of 1027
- marker proteins 430
- morphological steps of 77*t*
- preparatory phase for 34
- rate 846, 945
  - lower 1372
- timeline for 74
- types of 75*f*
- window of 74, 80, 83, 84, 97, 98, 98*b*, 1027

Implantation failure 876, 878, 1157, 1496
- causes of 836
- recurrent 100, 242, 421, 800, 804, 829, 833, 833*f*, 834*fc*, 836, 839, 843, 845, 846, 1145, 1407
- repeated 793, 868, 939, 955, 1517

Imprinting disorders 885*b*, 998
In situ hybridization 1145
In situ nick translation test 1262, 1263
In utero fetal programming 223, 520, 1189, 1189*fc*
In vitro activation 259, 820
- mechanism of 1122
- treatment 820*fc*

In vitro capillary test 1246
In vitro culture 1498
In vitro fertilization 48, 112, 170, 221, 232, 258, 282, 291, 364, 400, 446, 510, 619, 643, 668, 674*t*, 734*f*, 757, 792, 804, 813, 861, 876, 914, 959*f*, 995, 1009, 1028, 1096, 1106, 1130*t*, 1154, 1181, 1190*t*, 1202*fc*, 1253, 1293, 1319, 1330*t*, 1358, 1393, 1401, 1408, 1435, 1455, 1467, 1488, 1494, 1522, 1529, 1533, 1564, 1597, 1597*f*

culture system 795, 1320
cycle 723, 877, 943, 1512
failure 189
laboratory 795, 1164*f*, 1174, 1175, 1177, 1319, 1491, 1510, 1525
quality of 1161
lite 742
management 279, 286, 292, 295
mild 681
stimulation 681*f*, 1324
modified 1448
natural cycle 681
natural cycle 681
outcome 233, 291
procedure of 757
process of 68
program performance indicators 1182
protocols 742*t*, 743*t*
screening hysteroscopy 1147
stimulation 295
protocols 1409
technique 696, 927, 956, 1312
workstation 1167, 1483*f*
In vitro gametogenesis 1045, 1470
application of 1045
In vitro handling 1495
In vitro hatching blastocyst 1031*f*
In vitro maturation 48, 256, 545, 546, 657, 745, 886, 904, 999, 1425, 1470, 1514
advantages of 1421
aspiration 1422, 1423*f*
clinical aspects of 1421, 1425*t*
culture 1423
indications for 1421
oocytes 1420, 1424
fertilization of 1424
recent advances in 1426
safety of 1425
In vitro sensitization 1031
In vitro simplified slide test 1246*fc*
In vitro spermatogenesis 62
In vitro treatment 968
In vivo culture 1498
In vivo fertilization 1042
In vivo procedure 1043*f*
In vivo test 1245
Incision 423
Incomplete miscarriage 1012
diagnosis of 1012
Incubators 1497, 1648
cleaning of 1167, 1167*t*
disinfection of 1167*t*
latest time-lapse 1498
quality control of 1166
types of 1165*t*, 1498, 1648
Infarction 352
Infections 312, 314, 363, 450, 1261
bacterial 459
chlamydial 451*b*, 459
early 1214
genitourinary 364, 375
mild 1214
risk of 1325
Infectious chronic endometritis 100
Infertile couples 973, 1238, 1264, 1351
management of 1264
Infertile male
clinical evaluation of 323, 325
endocrinological evaluation of 322
evaluation of 322
genetic evaluation of 406
Infertility 183, 184, 201, 221, 270, 276, 305, 325, 345, 374, 385, 426, 438, 450, 456, 463, 465, 466, 531, 567, 580, 607, 733, 757, 885, 962, 970, 995, 999, 1154, 1193
anovulatory 169, 518
causes of 281, 839
correction of 887
diagnosis of 183, 191, 334
duration of 183, 316
emergencies in 1193
endometriosis associated 1327
endoscopy in 580
etiological classification of 306
etiology of 1135
evaluation of 183
female factor 411
higher rates of 221
idiopathic 1452
immunological 306
incidence of 350, 464*t*
indications for 831
male factor 621, 1322, 1451, 1469
management of 286, 538, 538*t*, 1103, 1117, 1122
pathogenesis of 465
practice 1291
problem of 973
secondary 995
treatment of 362, 1312
tubal evaluation of 196
types of 316
varicocele-mediated 385
Inflammation 314, 505
low-grade 527
Inflammatory bowel disease 224*f*, 251, 287, 288
impact of 287
safety of 288*t*t
Inflammatory disorders 351
Influenza 1394
Infrared spectroscopy 1440
Infundibulopelvic ligament 1196
Infundibulum 5
Ingram method 1097
Inhibin 21, 188, 194, 375, 715, 736, 812, 895
role of 32
In-home insemination 401
Inner cell mass 69, 74, 75*t*, 87, 863, 877, 1367, 1372, 1411, 1472, 1495, 1568*f*, 1585, 1589*f*, 1592*f*, 1593*f*, 1644*f*
formation of 74*f*
morphometry 1371
small 1371
Inner zona layer 1436
Inositol 48, 526, 547
deficiency 526*f*
deficient state 526
phosphatidyl trisphosphate 526
Inpatient management 907
Insemination
artificial 965
conventional 1327, 1343
intravaginal 401
per cycle, optimal number of 621, 628
site of 645
volume of 647
Insler scoring system, modified 706*t*
Insomnia 677
Insufflation system 580
Insulin 117, 293
action 532
disorders 188
growth factor 884
hypothesis 520, 525
resistance 227, 293, 518, 522, 525, 529
Insulin like growth factor 32, 83, 84, 118, 142, 225, 226, 294, 525, 529, 750, 1073, 1108
binding protein 32, 83, 84, 87, 92, 226, 227, 525, 529, 834
receptor 526
Insulin sensitizers 154, 666, 670
agents 172, 546, 902
Integrated platforms 1461
Integrins 78, 430
Intellectual disabilities 888
Intelligence quotient 216
Intensive care unit admission, indications of 1217
Interfere normal rhythmic uterine contractions 420
Interferon 89
Interferon-alfa 151
Interferon-gamma 88, 89, 99, 157*f*, 1021
Interleukins 80, 83, 84, 85*f*, 87, 89, 224, 225, 365, 566, 804, 896, 898, 1443
Internal iliac artery 1056, 1057, 1058, 1059
Internal quality control 1510
Internal reproductive organs, development of 3, 8
Interstitial tissue 14
Intervention fallopian sperm 628
Intra-arterial injection 1111
Intracavernosal injections 346
Intracellular calcium 80*f*
Intracellular cyclic adenosine monophosphate 123
Intracellular ice
crystals 1389
formation 1389
Intracellular osmotic equilibrium 1389
Intracytoplasmic fertilization process 1450
Intracytoplasmic morphologically selected sperm injection 1038, 1048, 1277*f*, 1278, 1447, 1447*f*, 1448, 1450, 1451, 1476, 1486, 1486*f*, 1608
clinical significance of 1450, 1450*fc*
potential indications of 1277
Intracytoplasmic sperm injection 48, 70, 112, 161, 211, 244, 307, 338, 350, 376, 386, 457, 566, 621, 643, 680, 724, 797, 819, 846, 877, 886*b*, 949, 962, 995, 1033, 1049, 1112, 1155, 1190*t*, 1237, 1254, 1277*f*, 1292, 1322, 1330, 1334*f*, 1360, 1409, 1435*f*, 1464, 1497, 1502, 1516, 1533, 1597, 1598*f*, 1602*f*, 1605
automation of 1344
cycles 716
dish 1658
preparation of 1598
failure 189, 1451
indications for 1334, 1335

- insemination 1326
- microscope 1309*f*
- procedure 796, 1341*f*
- process 1309*f*
- results 1335
- setup, location of 1335
- workstations 1336*f*

Intrafollicular androgenic concentrations 814
Intralipids 431, 1023
Intramural submucosal myoma 420
Intramuscular ovarian grafts 1071
Intraovarian flow indices 708
Intra-testicular obstruction 328
Intrauterine
- adhesions 101, 413, 597, 601, 611, 611*f*, 843, 1107
- collection, small 1013
- contraceptive device 419
- devices 1019
- fetal demises 1189
- gestations, assessment of multiple 635
- lesions 1517
- perfusion 1110
- recurrence of 602
- sac 1203
- severe 1042
- synechiae 131

Intrauterine insemination 244, 245, 275, 338, 364, 376, 400, 401, 439, 457, 480, 510, 512*f*, 591, 617, 619, 625, 627, 643, 648, 659, 704, 723, 733, 800, 962, 973, 981, 1193, 1242, 1249, 1253, 1261, 1292, 1474, 1481
- catheter 1654, 1654*f*
- cycles 162, 647, 1190, 1512
- efficacy of 635
- factors for 643*f*
- indications of 621, 644
- monitoring of 645
- number of 645
- role of 543
- safety of 635
- technique of 647
- time interval 646
- time of 645
- treatment, indications for 619

Intravaginal ejaculation latency time 335
Inversion 216
Iodide 143*f*
Iodine 143*f*, 1174
Irrigation system 580
Ischemia 306, 311
Isolation place 1216
Isoleucine 1444
Isoniazid 432, 469
Isotonic crystalloids 907
Isotretinoin 151
Isthmus 5, 446, 913
- reanastomosis 446

J

Jacob syndrome 212, 212*f*
Jacobson and Weström laparoscopic criteria 442*t*
Jain's backyard theory 582
Janus kinase-signal transducers 83
Janus kinase-stat signaling 81
Joystick, movement of 1505
Jurkovic's diagnostic criteria 917

K

K system 1166, 1484
Kallmann's syndrome 124, 126, 135, 168, 170, 214, 305, 306, 329, 360, 363, 382
- treatment of 363

Kappa opioid receptor 22
Karyokinesis 207
Karyotype 135, 170, 211*f*, 215*f*
Karyotypic aberrations 307
Karyotypic chromosomal abnormalities 189
Kato protocol 682, 682*f*
Ketamine 759
Ketoconazole 154, 324
Kidney
- cells 1370
- disease
  - chronic 284-286, 381, 1213
  - end stage 286
- disorders 1294
- single 1079*f*
- transplantation 286

Killer cell inhibitory receptor 90
Killer immunoglobulin-like receptor 832*f*, 1021
Kisspeptins 20, 117, 118, 721, 728, 729, 1039
- agonists 20
- antagonists 20
- ligand 21*f*
- neurons 117, 1039, 1040
- pathway 118*f*
- protein, structure of 20*f*
- roles of 1039
- system 117

Klebsiella pneumoniae 312
Klinefelter's syndrome 12, 60, 124, 126, 211, 211*f*, 305, 306, 309, 325, 329, 381, 407, 1299, 1310
Krebs cycle 1444
Kremer test 1246
Kretztechnik's mechanical rotary vaginal scanner 1304*f*
K-system bench top incubator 1166*f*

L

Labetalol 292
Labia minora 4
Labial arteries, posterior 1099
Labial tissue transfers 1099
Laboratory quality management program 1510
Labotect embryo transfer catheters 780, 781*f*
Lacker's model 522
Lactate 54
- dehydrogenase 14

Lactic acid 1444
Laminar airflow 1483, 1483*f*
- workstation 1168*f*

Laminar flow cabinets 1646, 1646*f*
Laminin 79
Lamotrigine 151
Lanugo 149
Laparoscopic adenomyomectomy 429
Laparoscopic ovarian drilling 524, 542, 543*f*, 545, 592, 672
- surgery 173

Laparoscopic surgery 197, 580, 594
Laparoscopic technique 924
Laparoscopic tubal
- anastomosis, indications for 587
- surgery 584

Laparoscopy 197, 244, 439, 441, 466, 568, 919, 1036, 1096
- application of 1077*f*
- complications 593
- over laparotomy, advantages of 923

Laparotomic uterus procurement 1057
Laparotomy 1059
Large nuclear vacuole 1449
- sperms 1451

Large offspring syndrome 886, 1376
L-arginine 814
Laser 595, 1486
- systems
  - number of 1404
  - types of 1403
- therapy 153
- uterine nerve ablation 607

Laser-assisted
- drilling 1403
- hatching 1410, 1618, 1620*f*, 1621*f*
- sperm selection 1257

Lasmar's classification 594
Last menstrual period 1004
Late follicular phase 754
Laurence-Moon-Biedl syndrome 124
L-carnitine 367, 548
Leiomyoma 217, 420, 433, 1016
- classification of 421
- subclassification system 495*f*

Leptin 23, 76, 85, 117, 224, 225
- resistance 526

Lesbians 980, 982
Lesions
- endometrial 492, 499
- endometriotic 572*f*
- hemorrhagic 306

Letrozole 172, 265, 283, 539, 623, 624, 653, 654, 669, 670*t*, 682*f*, 692, 818
- supplementation 682

Leucine 1355, 1444
Leucovorin 920
Leukemia 48
- acute
  - lymphocytic 253
  - myeloblastic 258
  - myeloid 253
- inhibitory factor 29, 75, 81, 84, 87, 92, 98, 432
  - low 226

Leukocyte 76, 80, 311, 1268
- detection test 1244
- removal of 1274
- specific antigens 1244
- transendothelial migration 76

Leukocytospermia 364, 1244, 1262
Leukopenia 281
Leukotriene 50
Leuprolide 282, 680, 697
- acetate 123
- depot 154

Levator ani 333
contraction 333
muscles 8
Levofloxacin 451
Levonorgestrel-releasing intrauterine device 427, 537
Leydig cell 14, 53, 111, 325, 370
function 370
secrete testosterone 14
tumor 121, 137
Leydig interstitial cells 63
Leydig producing testosterone 10
Libido 183
loss of 324, 394, 660, 677
reduced 286
Light emitting diode 1509
Light microscopy 1433
Lightheadedness 914
Limulus amoebocyte lysate test 1171
Linear catheters 598
Linear eversion cannula 197
Lipid 1112, 1320
peroxidation 365, 367, 1494
Lipophilic molecules 107
Lipopolysaccharide 451, 565, 566, 1171
Lipoprotein
high-density 157
low-density 30, 31, 157
Liquefaction 185, 375, 1291
Liquid chromatography 1440, 1444
Liquid crystal 1433
Liquid nitrogen 1139, 1292, 1382, 1395, 1490
electronic monitoring of 1172
levels 1172
sterilization 1395
use of 1382
Liraglutide 231
Lithotomy position 499
Live birth rate 228, 242, 610, 619, 787, 832, 843, 846, 864, 945*t*, 980, 1062, 1279, 1407, 1517, 1524
cumulative 263
low 1145
Live donor 1055, 1057, 1058, 1062
Live spermatozoa 188
Liver
dysfunction 669
enlargement 325
enzymes 369
failure 669
function test 905, 907
Liver disease 360, 363, 369
chronic 381, 922
treatment of 363
Living cells 1610
L-methylfolate 547
Local anesthesia 13, 380
Lomustine 253
Long antagonist protocol 1048
Long gonadotropin-releasing hormone agonist protocol 751
Longitudinal intussusception vasoepididymostomy 379, 379*f*
Loop mediated isothermal amplification 463
Loose adventitial layer 1080*f*
Lorcaserin 231
Low birth weight 121, 997, 1321
Low body mass index 898
Low fertilization 1516
group 1448
rates 1515
Löwenstein-Jensen medium 463
Lower abdominal pain 914, 923
Low-molecular-weight heparin 280, 431, 846, 1022, 1197, 1023, 1517
Lumen needle, single 767*f*, 1513
Lump, abdominal 466
Lungs 325
Lupus anticoagulant 282, 833
Luteal cell 34
changes 725
Luteal deficiency 619
Luteal follicular transition 26, 34
Luteal phase 34, 36
abnormal 158
deficiency 156, 668, 711
physiology of 156
renin activity 897
Luteal phase defect 156, 158*f*, 158*fc*, 159*b*, 484*t*, 515, 565, 664, 800
concept of 156
diagnosis of 159
pathophysiology of 158, 800, 800*fc*
treatment of 160
Luteal phase support 284, 647, 699, 727, 794, 799, 800, 803, 804, 804*t*, 898, 905
indications of 800
optimal time of 802
Luteal serum progesterone levels 159
Luteal support 727
Luteinized unruptured follicle 49, 282, 479, 502, 502*f*, 515, 705
syndrome 565
Luteinizing hormone 14, 24*t*, 35, 50, 74, 85*f*, 107, 130, 156, 170, 211, 225-229, 257*f*, 284, 294, 327, 353, 375, 427, 477, 484, 520*f*, 521-525, 550, 619, 645, 658*t*, 690, 692, 696, 704, 721, 724*t*, 734, 750, 793, 810, 812, 837, 838, 856, 896, 901, 938, 1024, 1128, 1137, 1148, 1302, 1344, 1358, 1424, 1434
activity, types of 753
beta 25
controls secretion of 17
detection kits 193
hypothesis 520
indications for 569
polymorphism 24, 25
receptor 25, 813
activating mutation of 121
role of 656, 656*t*, 739, 734, 750
secretion 23
supplementation 727
rationale of 750
surge 46, 721*f*, 722
absent 856
premature 647
use of 739, 817
window 24, 46
Luteolysis 37, 157, 1194
premature 1148
Lyase 111
Lymph nodes 467*f*
enlarged 466
Lymphatic drainage 12
Lymphatic response 1067
Lymphopenia 281
Lysine 1444
Lysosomal enzymes 1337

M

Machine learning models 1466
Macroglossia 886
Macromolecules 1495
Macrophage 88, 90, 567
colony-stimulating factor 87, 92
role of 90*fc*, 1072
Macroprolactinemia 140
Macrosomia 886, 1141
Magnetic activated cell sorting 646, 1268, 1272, 1272*f*, 1279, 1322, 1469, 1621, 1621*f*
Magnetic sperm organelle morphological examination 1277*f*
Major histocompatibility complex 88, 90, 91, 281
Makler chamber 1485, 1485*f*, 1557*f*, 1652, 1652*f*
Malar rash 281
Male factor infertility, severe 869, 1450, 1469, 1509
Male fertility 315, 1261, 1444
issues 1117
Male infertility 183, 228, 303, 305, 322, 329, 232, 355, 360*b*, 369, 390, 392, 394, 406, 624, 1557
causes of 306*b*, 322*b*, 322*t*, 359*f*
chromosomal disorders in 211
diagnosis of 329
etiopathogenesis of 305
genetic of 329
investigations for 326
medical management of 359
oxidative system 189
ultrasound in 350
unexplained 239, 240*b*
Male pelvis, innervation of 12
Male pronucleus, formation of 68
Male reproduction, hormonal circuit for 14*f*
Male reproductive
cells 1393
system 8, 16
tract 9*f*, 314, 1235
dysfunction 315*f*
Malformations, congenital 1095
Malignancy 124, 184, 1213
endometrial 495
treatment for 1294
Malleable catheter, stylet of 1329*f*
Malnutrition 124
Malondialdehyde 243, 367, 527
Mammalian genes 884
Mammalian oocyte 704, 1623
Mammalian ovary 28*f*
Mammalian phenotype 884
Manipulators, types of 1503
Marburg virus 312
Marfan syndrome 880
Marriage, nonconsummation of 332, 333
Maryland bipolar forceps 1058
Mass
abdomen 466
ectopic 915
spectrometry 1440, 1441

Mastectomy, bilateral 988, 988*f*
Master gland 140
Maternal cells contamination 881
Maternal diabetes 294
Maternal disomy 884
Maternal fetal interface 1020, 1185
Maternal genes 998
Maternal hypertension 1023
Maternal immune
  cells 201
  responses 1186
  surveillance system 1021
Maternal killer immunoglobulin 832
Maternal spindle transfer 1045
Maternal weight and height 927
Matrix metallopeptidase 1108
Matrix metalloproteinase 33, 34, 76, 80, 83, 87, 92, 99, 430, 723
Maturation arrest syndrome, histological section of 13*f*
Maturation promoting factor 48, 68
Mature follicle 43, 47
  Doppler ultrasound parameters of 480*f*
  feature of 511
  natural cycle 1323
Mature oocyte 886, 982, 1359*f*, 1533, 1537, 1597, 1610
  corona cumulus 1533
  cryopreservation 256
  number of 945
Mayer-Rokitansky-Küster-Hauser syndrome 134, 414, 418, 954, 1041, 1059, 1075, 1093-1095
  differential diagnosis of 1094, 1095*t*
  types of 1091
McCune-Albright syndrome 121, 123, 124, 884
McIndoe procedure 136
McKusick-Kaufman syndrome 1095
Mean sac diameter 1005
Mechanical trauma 1209
Media alkaline 1497
Media systems 1496, 1496*t*
Mediastinal cyst 350
Medical disorders, chronic 278
Medical gonadectomy 698
Medical hypophysectomy 698
Medical termination of pregnancy 918, 969
Medical therapy 359, 569, 570
Medroxyprogesterone acetate 124, 133, 576, 818
Meiosis 48, 55, 207
  resumption of 47, 48*f*, 722*f*, 1421
  stages of 1434
Meiotic arrest 47, 1420
Meiotic cycle 1434
Meiotic maturation, timing of 1361
Meiotic spindle 1344, 1345, 1362, 1383, 1433, 1434, 1436, 1610*f*, 1612*f*
  location of 1435
  morphology 1470
  presence of 1434
Melatonin 548
Membrane 1320
  physiology of 1381
  premature rupture of 1188
  preterm premature rupture of 1210
  region of 1364
Menarche 119
Mendelian inheritance 214
Menezo's group 1370
Meningioma 306
Meningitis 124
Menopause 51, 551
  early onset of 51
  functional 286
  premature 289
  treatment of 1068
Menorrhagia 426
Menstrual abnormalities 225
Menstrual blood 1111
  stem cells 1120
Menstrual cycle 19*f*, 24*b*, 24*t*, 26*f*, 35*f*, 37*f*, 37*t*, 38, 85*f*, 116, 117, 160, 474, 477*f*, 712*t*, 713*t*, 815, 818, 1048, 1107
  length 159
  luteal phase of 156, 159
  normal 16, 530, 664
  physiology of 16, 26
  regulation of 16
Menstrual disorder 286
  evolution of 293*f*
Menstrual disturbances 281, 530
Menstrual dysfunction, management of 537
Menstruation 7, 16, 130, 481*f*
  cessation of 38
  physiology of 130
Mental health 1035, 1208
Meperidine 758
Mesenchymal stem cell 1111, 1117, 1120
Mesoderm 1117
  layers 1117
  middle 1004
  migration 1006*f*
Mesonephric ducts 8
Mesoovarian vasculature 1070*f*
Messenger ribonucleic acid 23, 74, 117, 691, 1035, 1383, 1470
  transcripts 215
  vaccine 370
Metabolic complications 529, 601
Metabolic disorder 131
Metabolic dysfunction, risk of 530*b*
Metabolic profiles 152, 1186, 1444
Metabolic syndrome 345*fc*, 518, 530
  diagnostic criteria for 530*t*
Metabolism 520, 1118
Metabolomics 1355, 1443, 1444
Metalloproteinase, tissue inhibitors of 83
Metaphase oocyte 66*f*, 1359*f*, 1537, 1538*f*, 1611*f*, 1612*f*
Metaphase spindle organizes 1434
Metformin 231, 546, 552, 693, 902, 1149, 1150
  efficacy of 1149
  group 1149
  therapy 551
  use of 1149
Methimazole 145
Methotrexate 253, 282, 920, 924, 1201
  side effects of 921
  treatment 922
Methylation 883
Methyldopa 292, 324
Methylenetetrahydrofolate reductase 214
Methylprednisolone 1405
Metoidioplasty 988
Metronidazole 454, 455, 456
Metroplasty 600
  hysteroscopic 601
  hysteroscopy for 599
Microbiology 450, 452
Microdose flare
  protocol 678, 678*f*
  regimen 815
Microdose Lupron flare protocol 1129*t*
Microdot technique 379*f*
Microdrops systems 1456
Microfilaments, localization of 1421
Microfluidic applications 1256
Microfluidic device 1256, 1331, 1455, 1456, 1458, 1461, 1461*f*
Microfluidic sperm sorter device 1282, 1282*f*
Microfluidic systems 1331, 1458
Microimmunofluorescence 440
Microinjection 1339, 1346
  dish preparation 1337
  needle 1447
  pipettes
    alignment of 1338
    setting up of 1338
  preparation 1337
  procedure 1337
Microinjector 1507, 1597
Micromanipulation systems 1503
Micromanipulation techniques 1481
Micromanipulator 1338, 1485, 1485*f*, 1502, 1597
  research instrument 1598*f*
  system 1650
  use of 1502
Micronutrients factor 1188
Micropipettes 1506, 1507, 1597
  alignment of 1338*f*, 1599
  equilibration of 1599
Microribonucleic acids 311
Microscopes 1649
  quality control of 1168
Microscopic varicocelectomy 389, 390
Microsurgery
  evolution of 585
  laparoscopic 585
Microsurgical techniques 444
Microtools, alignment of 1505, 1507
Microtubule organization 1497
Microtubule orientation 1610
Microvascular surgery 1073
Microvilli, superficial 1374
Microvolume air cooling 1395
Midazolam 758
Mid-luteal phase 484*f*
Mid-tubal disease 438
Migration method 1253
Migration sedimentation 1253, 1270
Mineral 368
  oil 1661, 1661*f*
Minimal ovarian stimulation 737
Minimal sperm production 1299
Minimal stimulation
  demerits of 1047
  protocols 1047
Minimally invasive epididymal sperm aspiration 759
Minipuberty 115
Miscarriage 419, 876, 878, 999, 1019, 1384, 1474

anembryonic 1012, 1013*f*
causes of 227*fc*
complete 1012
diagnosis of 1013
incomplete 1012
rate 228, 538, 841, 843
clinical 868
spontaneous 867
recurrent 833, 876, 1019, 1040
repeated 955
threatened 1012, 1013*f*
Miscarried embryos 1021
Missed miscarriage 1012
diagnosis of 1012
Mitochondria 51*f*, 950, 1254, 1277, 1313, 1360
activity index test 1246
deoxyribonucleic acid 214, 406
disease 950, 1045
flagellar network 1295
function 1376
oxidoreductive enzyme 1246
replacement therapy 1045, 1046
Mitogen activated protein kinase 48, 68, 109
Mitosis 207, 1364
Mitotic chromosomal abnormalities 1327
Mitotic error 878
Mobile ovarian ligaments 1196
Mobile ovary 794
Mock embryo transfer 775
Mock transfer 775
pitfalls of 775
Modern rapid methods 463
Molar pregnancy 1015
Molecular binding 1278
Molecular failures 1376
Molecular injury 1383
Molecule 76, 79
Monitored anesthesia care 758
Monoamine oxidase inhibitors 313
Monoamniotic twin 928*f*
Monocellular nature 1381
Monochorionic placenta 928*f*, 996
Monochorionic twin 928*f*
Monochorionic-diamniotic twin 930, 1011, 1012*f*
risk of 931
Monoculture media system 1496
Monocyte 88
cerebrospinal fluid 87
chemoattractant protein 224
chemotactic peptide 566
Monofollicular ovulation 900
Monogenic defects 310
Monogenic diseases 1441
Monogenic disorders 60, 214, 876, 879, 880, 1407
Monoiodotyrosine 143*f*
Mononuclear infiltrate 1081*f*
Mono-ovulatory cycles 540
Monopolar loop electrode 596
Monozygotic pregnancies 931
Monozygotic twin 928, 930, 996, 1010, 1376, 1404, 1405
formation 1404
incidence of 1376
percentage of 996
Mood swings 654
Morcellation
advantages of 597
disadvantages of 597
hysteroscopic 425, 597
Morphokinetics embryo assessment 1456
Morphologic scoring system 504
Morphological analysis 1254, 1255
Morphological assessment 1367
Morphology 186, 1242
calculation, abnormal 1243
Morula stage 70*f*, 1113*f*
biopsy 1411
Mosaic embryos 878, 1415
management of 878
number of 1356
Mosaicism 210, 878
fragment 878
Motile human spermatozoa 1248
Motile sperm 1256, 1456
high-power light microscope micrograph of 1449*f*
organelle morphology 1448, 1608
examination 1254, 1277, 1449*t*
suspension 1448
Motile spermatozoa 1254, 1257, 1269, 1273, 1282, 1339
amount of 1269
filtration of 1274
microfluidic isolation of 1281
number of 1273, 1293
single 1448
Motility 186, 1242
activators 1245
poor 1270
progressive 188, 327, 1242
score 1170
total 188, 327
Motor function 393
Motor module unit 1508
Mouse embryo 886, 1171
assay 465, 1490
culture of 1171
Mouse oocytes, maturation of 1324
Mu opioid receptor 22
Mucin 430
Mucosal cells of fimbriae 66
Müllerian agenesis 124, 131, 136, 414, 418, 1077
Müllerian anomalies 217, 413, 416*f*, 580, 1035
etiology of 413
Müllerian aplasia 1095
psychological aspects of 1096
Müllerian developmental anomalies 413
Müllerian duct 7, 8, 60, 101, 413, 487, 599
abnormalities 487
anomalies 419
development of 1075, 1090
Müllerian inhibiting substance 59
Müllerian malformations 1076
Müllerian structures 1093
Müllerian system 413
Multicystic ovaries, enlarged 1193
Multifactorial effectors, treatment of 846
Multifetal pregnancy 926, 928, 933, 1208
reduction 933, 1208, 1210, 1211
Multifollicular ovarian stimulation 50
Multigradient freezing technique 1312
Multiphoton microscopy 381
Multiple birth
pathogenesis of 928
pregnancies 871
Multiple cleavage-stage embryos 1377
Multiple displacement amplification 864
Multiple egg bank programs 947
Multiple gestation 995, 1368, 1375
etiology of 926
pregnancies, rates of 926
Multiple micromanipulation devices 1597
Multiple pregnancy 621, 632, 996, 1010, 1012*f*, 1207, 1208, 1208*f*, 1370
rate 245, 538, 654, 1146
risk of 1370
Multiple punctures 1515
Multiple-order births 926, 933
treatment of 932
Multiple-order gestation 931, 996
Multislice computed tomography 1035
Mumps 352, 375, 381
Muscle movement, loss of 395
Muscular dystrophy 880
Mutations 310
correction of 1046
preimplantation genetic testing for 407, 409
Myalgia 677, 1213
Mycobacterial smear 466
Mycobacterium tuberculosis 432, 441
complex 463
microbiology of 463
Mycoplasma 452, 966
genitalium 364, 453
resistance testing 453*b*
hominis 838
types of 452
Myoinositol 1444
Myoma 413, 420, 423, 580, 1035
blanched look of 583*f*
classification of 594*f*
enucleation of 424*f*
extraction 423
hysteroscopic
management of 424
morcellation of 425
intramural 421
removal of 583
retrieval 424*f*
screw 580
Myomectomy 842
abdominal 606
hysteroscopic 425, 426, 594, 612, 612*f*
laparoscopic 423
open 422
surgical techniques for 422
Myometrial blood flow 713
Myometrial cysts 496*f*
Myometrial echogenicity 713
Myometrial lesions 492
Myometrial wall thickness 489*f*
Myometrium 6, 492, 493
Myopathies, idiopathic inflammatory 281
Myosalpingeal hypertrophy 438

N

N95 masks 1219
Nabothian cyst 1005

N-acetylcysteine 367
Nafarelin 697
Naltrexone 231
Nanoparticles, use of 260
Narishige micromanipulator 1504
Narishige system 1338
National Family Health Survey 176
National Health Service 983
National Institute for Health and Care Excellence 197
National Tuberculosis Elimination Program 469
Natural killer cells 90, 99, 201, 430, 832, 1020, 1021*f*, 1027, 1185, 1186, 1191
  peripheral 88, 1186
  testing of 836
Nausea 654, 655, 899, 1213
Near-infrared spectroscopy 1441
Neck 1277
Necrotic foci 1372, 1594
Necrozoospermia 188, 327, 1237
Needle aspiration biopsy 380
Needle-guided transvaginal follicle aspiration 1305
Nefazodone 339
Negative predictive value 440
Neisseria gonorrhoeae 191, 364, 450, 452, 459
Neodymium doped yttrium-aluminum-garnet 611, 1404
Neonatal care 933
Neonatal complications 931, 1207
Neonatal hypoglycemia 886
Neonatal intensive care unit 871
Neophallus, necrosis of 990*f*
Neoplasm 151, 352
  adrenal 134
Neosalpingostomy 445, 589
Neovagina 1078*f*, 1079-1081, 1081*f*, 1090*f*, 1096
  functional evaluation of 1089*f*
  nonsurgical creation of 1097
  octamer 1084*f*, 1086*f*, 1087*f*
  surgical creation of 1097
  vaginoscopic pictures of 1080*f*
Neovaginal canal 987*f*, 988*f*
  stenosis of 990*f*
Neovaginal cavity 1099*f*
  creation 1077*f*, 1096, 1098, 1098*f*
Neovaginal lining 1076
Nerve growth factor 29
Neuroblastoma 886
Neuroendocrine
  abnormalities 289
  dysfunction 520
  function 1189
Neurofibromatosis 121
Neurohormone 18
Neurohypophysis 18
Neurokinin B 20, 118
Neuroleptics 141
Neurological disorder 281
Neuronal apoptosis inhibitory protein 386
Neuropeptide kisspeptin 1039
Neuropeptide Y 19, 117
Neurophysiology 396
Neurosecretion 17
Neurotrophin signaling 1039
Neurovascular bundle 987*f*
Neurovascular pudendal thigh flap 1100*f*
Neutral alpha-glucosidase 1249
Neutropenia, severe 922
Neutrophils 1072
Newer sperm selection techniques 1048
Next-generation sequencing 833, 865-867, 878, 1037, 1327, 1355, 1407, 1415, 1440-1442, 1662
  advantages of 1327
Next-generation technology, use of 1445
Nick-end labeling assay 243
Nicotinamide adenine dinucleotide 345, 386
  phosphate 345, 365
Nifedipine 292
Nikon microscope 1504*f*, 1508*f*
Nitrates 346
Nitric oxide 32, 240, 333, 341, 345, 566
  synthase 566
Nitroblue tetrazolium test 1243
Nitrogen species, reactive 311
Nitroglycerine 346, 582
  patches 844
N-methyl-D-aspartate 117, 289
No scalpel vasectomy 12
Nocturnal penile tumescence 334
Nodules, endometriotic 567*f*
Nonadhering sperm 1255
Nonapoptotic spermatozoa 1279
Nonconsummation, signs of 333
Nonerosive arthritis 281
Nongonococcal urethritis 364
Nongonococcal-nonchlamydial infections 452
Non-in vitro maturation 769
Noninvasive preimplantation genetic testing 866, 880, 881
  limitations of 881
Nonmaleficence, principle of 1208
Nonmalignant disease 256
  treatment for 1294
Nonmotile
  sperm 1456
  spermatozoa 1256, 1282
Nonobstructive azoospermia 55, 189, 307, 352, 381, 382, 406, 407*fc*, 1050
  evaluation of 382*fc*
  types of 328*t*
Nonpolarized zygote 1364*f*
Nonpregnancy cycles 1422
Nonprogressive motility 327
Nonseptated clear cysts 501
Nonsteroidal anti-inflammatory drugs 49, 427, 568, 570, 576, 906, 1195
Nonsteroidal selective estrogen receptor modulator 538
Nontoxic gloves, use of 1174
Nontubal ectopic pregnancy 917
Nontubal ectopic pregnancy, management of 923
Nontuberculous salpingitis 450, 459
Noonan syndrome 310
Noradrenaline 333
Norepinephrine 230, 231
Norethindrone acetate 427, 571
Normal fertilization 1515
  rate 1343
Normal follicular
  development 23
  fluid 567
Normogonadotropic anovulation 170, 172
Normogonadotropic eugonadism 124
Normogonadotropic normoestrogenic anovulation 167, 664
Normogonadotropic normogonadism 168
Normospermia 374
Normozoospermia 188, 327, 1237
Normozoospermic
  donors 1283
  sample 1360
Novy's cannulation system 598*f*
Nuchal translucency scan 932, 1208
Nuclear abnormalities 1277
Nuclear assessment 1358
Nuclear chromatin decondensation test 1248
Nuclear deoxyribonucleic acid 54
Nuclear magnetic resonance 1440, 1444
Nuclear maturation 1425
  complete 1421
Nuclear precursor bodies 1571*f*, 1572*f*
Nuclear proteins, removal of 1263
Nuclear vacuoles
  pathological aspects of 1449
  small 1449
Nucleic acid amplification 441, 451
  test 453
Nucleocapsid protein 1212
Nucleoside metabolism 1444
Nucleosome 884*fc*
Nuclepore membrane filter 1274
Nucleus 1254, 1295
  paragigantocellularis 396
Nugent score 454
Nutrition, regulation of 1040
Nutritional status 325

O

Obesity 61, 121, 158, 169, 221, 224*f*, 226-228, 233, 234, 292, 360, 527, 530, 531, 550, 666
  central abdominal 531
  classification of 222
  diagnosis of 222
  effects of 225, 368*b*
  fetal origin of 223*fc*
  leading 226*fc*
  male 229
  origin of 223
  pathophysiology of 223, 227*fc*
Observational studies 1224
Obstetric complications, risk of 995
Obstetric hemorrhages 997
Obstruction 306
Obstructive azoospermia 189, 311, 355, 375, 376, 406, 408, 409*fc*
  management of 378*fc*
  treatment of 377
  types of 328*t*
Obstructive lesions 313
Obstructive sleep apnea 532
Octamer-binding transcription factor 1083*f*
Octuplets 926
Olanzapine 151
Oligoasthenospermia 213
  severe 1310
Oligoasthenoteratozoospermia 112, 310*f*, 327
  severe 307, 949, 1293, 1450, 1513
  syndrome 364

Oligoasthenozoospermia 1273
Oligohydramnios 996, 1188
Oligomenorrhea 141, 144, 147, 169, 549, 1118
Oligoovulation 150
Oligospermia 57, 213, 374
 severe 355
Oligozoopsermia 228, 309, 327, 363, 406, 407, 407*fc*, 620, 1257, 1334, 1444
 severe 329, 1293
Oligozoospermic samples 1275
Oliguria 893, 907
Omphalocele 886
Oncofertility 1048
Oncogenesis 883
Oncology 701
Ongoing pregnancy 1150
 rates 572, 744
Onion-peel appearance 582
Oocyte 283, 628, 725*f*, 820, 834, 937, 946, 1140, 1116, 1331, 1338-1340, 1343, 1358, 1360*f*, 1361, 1361*f*, 1362*f*, 1383, 1393, 1410, 1429, 1433-1435, 1457-1459, 1506, 1516, 1542*f*, 1624*f*, 1626*f*, 1628*f*, 1649
 abnormal 1322
 atresia of 45
 banking 946, 947*f*
 collection 1331
 content of 1497
 cryopreservation of 256, 261, 967, 971, 1156, 1380, 1385, 1436, 1623
 cryopreserved 997, 1140, 1311, 1312, 1435
 cumulus
  cell complex 877
  complex 1267, 1421, 1512, 1533, 1597, 1597*f*
 cytoplasmic transcriptome 1416
 cytoskeleton 1169
 decumulation 1455
 deformation 1457
 degeneration rate 1343
 denudation 1435, 1457
 developmental incompetence of 550
 droplets 1337, 1339
 dysmorphia 1306
 evaluation 1599
 exposure of 1173, 1381
 fertilizable 1135
 fertilize 1242, 1261
 good-quality 815, 1324
 holding side 1340
 identification 1423
 immature 1359*f*, 1384, 1420, 1423*f*, 1514, 1516, 1537
 injection 1337
 insemination of 1174, 1447, 1528, 1597
 intravaginal culture of 1042
 lower numbers of 1325
 manipulation 1436, 1601
 meiotic spindle structure 1323
 microinjection of 1602
 migration 1004
 model 1448
 morphological assessment of 1358
 nuclear maturity 1537
 number 813, 815, 1128, 1129, 1422, 1515
  low 1515
 pick-up 476, 682, 683, 726, 738, 793, 794, 844, 1422, 1515
 plasma membranes of 67
 poor morphology 1385
 positioning 1461
 postmature nature of 1359*f*, 1362
 quality of 1434, 1435
 recovery 1165
 retrieval of number of 1156
 second meiotic division of 67
 secondary 43, 47, 66*f*
 selection 1470
 shape of 1358
 size of 1358
 source 945
 sphere of 1381
 spindle negative 1345
 transfer of 1381
 vitrification of 947, 1311, 1383*f*, 1384, 1623
 vitrified 1380
Oocyte abnormalities 1322, 1541
 category of 1541*fc*
Oocyte activation 43, 67, 1363, 1364, 1451
 artificial 1516
 assisted 1049
 molecular mechanism of 68*f*
 spontaneous 887
Oocyte aspiration 1305
 foot pedal for 1655
 set 1654, 1654*f*
Oocyte donation 275, 937, 938, 940, 946–948, 966
 cycles 876, 943
 indications for 938
 legal status of 948
Oocyte donor 725, 943, 948, 1156, 1323
 guarantee for 1156
 programs 947
Oocyte freezing 1381
 indications for 1380
Oocyte maturation 43, 47, 1420, 1513, 1514
 in vivo 1420
 inhibitor 50
 period of 1323
 physiology of 722
 potential 1470
Oocyte maturity 1424
 assessment of 1424, 1533
Oocyte morphology 1049
 score 1470
Oocyte quality 225, 242, 830, 943, 1323, 1344, 1442, 1470
 assessment of 834
Oocyte retrieval 743, 757, 765, 766, 769, 769*b*, 770, 772, 819, 904, 946, 1127, 1138, 1156, 1173, 1302, 1325, 1395, 1513, 1528
 complications of 771
 improper timing of 856
 instruments for 766
 needle 1172*f*
 number of 997
 procedure of 1515
 rate 1422, 1524
 sets 1512
 steps of 768
 technique 1135
Oocyte sharing 947
 programs 947
Oocyte-cumulus oophorus cell contact, disruption of 724
Oogenesis 42, 49*f*, 665*f*, 1361
 stages of 42
Oogonia 42, 43
Oogonial stem cells 259, 1118, 1313
Oolemma 1340, 1603
 rupture 1340
Oophorectomy 924
Oophoritis 124
Open fine needle aspiration 379
Open system
 freezing 1140
 vitrification 1382
Open testicular biopsy 380, 1299
Open varicocele repair 388
Operative deliveries 999
Operative hysteroscopy 1147
Opiates 141
Opioids 521, 758
Optic astrocytoma 121
Optic glioma 121
Optical coherence tomography 381
Optimizing embryo transfer technique 794
Optimum estradiol window 715
Oral contraceptive 535, 678, 692, 1128
 pill 153, 529, 531, 537, 545, 548, 550, 570, 668, 692, 815, 1128-1131
Oral estradiol 987
Oral estrogen 692
Oral glucose tolerance test 525, 550
Oral ovulation induction agents 538
Oral ovulogens 653, 693
Oral pharmacotherapy 340, 341
Oral progesterone 426
Oral ulcers 281
Orchidopexy 184
Orchitis 124, 307, 312, 375
 acute 351
 chronic 351
Ordinary binocular microscope 1168
Organ
 ephemeral 1055
 perfusion 893
 regeneration, matrix for 1103
Organogenesis 413
Orgasmic disturbances 339
Original capillary tube test 1246
Original migration-sedimentation method 1270*f*
Orlistat 231, 535
Orthotopic transplant 1069
Osmolality 1169, 1497
Osmotic gradient 1388
Osmotic shock 1381
Osteopenia 369
Osteopontin 430
Osteoporosis 369, 1189
Ova, fertilization of 5
Oval mass 568
Oval sperm cells, large 1449
Ovarian abnormalities 487
Ovarian activity, re-establishment of 1429
Ovarian agenesis 1068
Ovarian aging 241, 857

Ovarian artery 1056, 1070*f*
Ovarian biopsy 561
Ovarian cancer 668
Ovarian cortex
  biopsy of 561
  freezing 1429
Ovarian cryopreservation 1068
Ovarian cycle 16, 27
Ovarian cysts 121, 654, 707, 1196, 1429, 1511
  functional 669
Ovarian Doppler assessment 561
Ovarian drilling, procedure of 593
Ovarian dysfunction 168*f*, 215
Ovarian endometrioma 574
  differential diagnosis of 568
Ovarian enlargement 1193
Ovarian failure 169, 171
  acute 1226*t*
  advanced 938
  primary 131, 217, 532
Ovarian feedback 25
Ovarian fibroma 504*f*
Ovarian follicle 896, 1071
  culture in vitro 258
  in vitro activation of 259
  transplantation 259
Ovarian fossa 568*f*
Ovarian fragmentation 820, 820*fc*
Ovarian function 24*fc*, 465, 1429
Ovarian hormones 76, 84*f*, 1193
Ovarian hyperstimulation 280, 644, 1148
  controlled 195, 283, 572, 591, 690, 742, 1299, 1420, 1541
Ovarian hyperstimulation syndrome 25, 118, 161, 173, 246, 263, 264, 278, 444, 478, 522, 621, 622, 644, 657, 669, 681, 690, 698, 704, 721, 726*fc*, 728, 729, 735*f*, 738, 742, 793, 802, 804, 893, 895, 898, 898*fc*, 900*t*, 901*t*, 903, 905*fc*, 906*b*, 907, 973, 1129, 1135, 1141, 1142, 1193-1195, 1195*t*, 1196*f*, 1323, 1409, 1420, 1512
  classification of 894*t*, 899*t*, 1193, 1193*t*
  clinical manifestations of 898
  development of 897
  hallmarks of 904
  improvement of 907
  lower risk of 900
  management of 904, 906*t*
  mild 906
  moderate 903, 906
  moderate-to-severe 999
  pathogenesis of 893, 895, 897*f*, 897*fc*
  pathophysiology of 895*fc*, 1194*f*
  prevention of 753, 903, 905*fc*, 1194*t*
  risk factors for 898, 898*t*
  risk of 745, 943, 999, 1468
  symptoms of 898
  treatment of 905*fc*
Ovarian hypothesis 520, 521
Ovarian insufficiency 1117
Ovarian lesions 501
Ovarian ligament 593*f*
Ovarian malignancy 539
Ovarian neoplasm 150
Ovarian perifollicular blood flow 1036
Ovarian pregnancy 918, 924
Ovarian regeneration, proposed mechanism of 1119
Ovarian rejuvenation 1116
Ovarian reserve 193, 559, 707
  assessment of 559
  markers of 811
  test 193, 559, 559*f*, 562, 734*f*, 809
    role of 562*t*
Ovarian response 195, 707, 1323
  abnormal 809
  markers of 673*t*
  monitoring of 1513
  prediction index 715
  test 812
  types of 674*t*
Ovarian responsiveness 225
Ovarian size 1198
Ovarian steroid hormones 996
Ovarian steroidogenesis 109, 109*fc*
Ovarian stimulating drugs 264
Ovarian stimulation 51, 263, 280*t*, 444, 619, 627*fc*, 635, 651, 690, 713, 737*t*, 738, 745, 750, 886, 957, 1193, 1294, 1322-1324, 1514
  contemporary 1324
  contraindications of 283*b*
  controlled 24, 118, 158, 257*f*, 647, 659, 659*f*, 665, 673, 674, 682, 690, 704, 733, 735*f*, 736, 737, 750, 754, 799, 810, 813, 817, 956, 896, 946, 1047, 1193, 1323, 1344, 1511
  cycles 855
  drugs for 653, 653*b*
  effects of 1323, 1324
  evolution of 742
  hormonal monitoring of 714
  monitoring of 704, 716
  protocol 50, 664
    mild 745, 1325
Ovarian stroma
  assessment of 531
  flow
    index 709*f*
    low resistance 510*f*
  vessels, vascular parameters of 478*t*
Ovarian tissue 259, 1393, 1429
  cryopreservation 257, 261, 283, 982, 992, 1421, 1429, 1430
    process of 258*f*
  transplantation 257, 1430
Ovarian torsion 1197, 1199, 1429
  diagnosis of 1199*t*
  laparoscopic picture of 1200*f*
  treatment for 1199
Ovarian transplant 1065, 1068, 1071, 1074
  indications for 1068
Ovarian transplantation, site of 1069
Ovarian trauma 1423
Ovarian tumor 121, 1076, 1196, 1197
Ovarian vascularization 531
Ovarian vasculature 1069, 1070*f*, 1071
Ovarian vein 1070*f*
  Doppler blood flow 1072*f*
Ovarian volume 195, 561, 708, 709*f*
Ovary 3-5, 87*f*, 465, 507, 707, 913, 1035, 1117
  artificial 259
  control endocrine function of 17*f*
  deep-seated 1513
  enlarged 507
  extraperitonealization of 895
  hyperstimulated 906
  in vitro activation of 1122, 1122*f*
  innervation of 5
  lies 1196
  mobility of 584
  normal 1196
  simple cyst of 501
  three-dimensional ultrasound of 510*f*
  transposition of 258
  volume calculation of 508*f*
Over radical surgery 1199
Ovulation 32, 37, 45, 49, 50*f*, 895, 1004, 1005*f*
  assessment of 534
  confirmation of 711
  evidence of 1512
  failure 538
  physiology of 655, 665
  prediction of 710
  process of 50*f*
  rate 538, 654
  studies 244
  suppression of 575
  trigger 657, 721, 722, 729
Ovulation induction 170*b*, 171*b*, 439, 524, 539, 625, 659*f*, 664, 696, 739, 813, 996, 1190, 1375
  evolution of 665
  gonadotropin for 659
  management for 666
  medical options for 172
  protocols 803
Ovulatory cycle 656*t*, 705*f*, 1037
Ovulatory dysfunction 225, 519, 567
Ovulatory function 192
  evaluation of 198
Ovulatory phase 26
Ovulatory triggers, role of 723
Ovum
  aspiration pump 1155
  pickup 567, 766, 971, 1481
Oxidation 112
  reduction potential 189, 243
Oxidative stress 239, 240, 365*fc*, 375, 385, 386, 527, 566, 1185, 1244, 1261
Oxygen
  concentration 1498
  saturation 1217
    peripheral 1216, 1217
  species, reactive 58, 239, 314, 315, 315*f*, 323, 365, 367, 386, 566, 814, 1023, 1189, 1243, 1243*f*, 1253, 1292, 1374, 1450, 1456, 1515
  tension 1168, 1169
  therapy 1217

P

Pain
  abdominal 466, 899, 914
  chronic 393
Palm Coine classification 495*f*
Palomo technique 389
Panhypopituitarism 168
Papanicolaou stain 1558*f*
Papillae, absence of 568
Papillomavirus 1394

Paracervical block 760
  injection sites 761*f*
Paracrine factors 1122
Paraganglioma, familial nonchromaffin 884
Paramesonephric ducts 8
  atrophy 8
Paraovarian cyst 501, 507
Parasympathetic penile innervation 395*f*
Paratesticular abnormalities 351
Parental chromosomes 1363
Parental karyotyping 834
Parenteral testosterone 987
Parkinson's disease 1044
Particulate air, high efficiency 1320, 1481, 1489, 1498, 1511, 1647
Pasteur pipette 1269
Paternal disomy 884
Peak systolic velocity 478, 512*f*, 709*f*
Pearson's correlation 1223
Pelvic adhesions 605, 613
Pelvic anatomy 605*f*
  reconstruction of 607
Pelvic diaphragm 7
Pelvic discomfort 668
Pelvic examination 915
Pelvic floor muscles 333
  contraction of 1090*f*
Pelvic infection 440, 1201, 1325
Pelvic inflammatory disease 438, 439, 440*t*, 444, 447, 455, 455*b*, 456*b*, 505, 506*f*, 584, 771, 913, 1028, 1201
Pelvic kidney, single 1079*f*
Pelvic pain 426, 914
  chronic 466, 567
Pelvic surgery 376
Pelvic tuberculosis 450
Pelvic ultrasound 122, 533
Pelvic vasculature 1069*f*, 1073
Penetration 76
  air, ultra-low 1164, 1489
Penicillin 1495
Penile erection, neurophysiology of normal 395*f*
Penile prosthesis 343
Penile skin 987*f*
Penile vibratory stimulation 399, 401, 402, 1515
Penis 9, 13
  innervation of 13
Pentoxifylline 844, 1257
Peptide 117
  calcitonin gene related 333
Percbiopsy 380
Percutaneous epididymal sperm aspiration 13, 354, 376, 380, 758, 1131, 1294, 1311, 1481, 1502
Percutaneous testicular
  biopsy 380
  sperm aspiration 380
Pericarditis 281
Periconceptional folic acid 295
Periconceptional period 1187
Perifollicular blood flow 710, 710*f*
Perifollicular flow, spectral Doppler of 512*f*
Peri-implantation corticosteroids 202
Perimetrium 6
Perinatal mortality 997, 999, 1141
Perinuclear theca 1339
Peritoneal factors 197, 244, 567
Peritoneal flaps
  anterior 1078*f*
  mobilization of 1078*f*
  posterior 1078*f*
Peritoneal inclusion cyst 507, 507*f*
Peritoneal metaplasia 1079
Peritoneal pregnancy, primary 918
Peritoneal stem cells, identification of 1082*f*
Peritoneum 465
  fallopian tubes 468*f*
  use of 1076
Peritonitis 439
Peritubal adhesions 567
Peritubular myoid cells 53
Perivitelline space 1353*f*, 1361, 1537, 1541, 1545
  large 1385
  small 1538*f*
Peroxisomes 1360
Persistent depressive symptoms 1208
Persistent hemoconcentration 907
Personal protection equipment 1219, 1219*b*
  steps of 1219*b*
  use of 1219, 1220
Pesticides 375
Petri dish 1459, 1508, 1658
  intracytoplasmic sperm injection 1255
  replacement of 1508
  types of 1658, 1658*f*
Phagocytosis 567
Phalloplasty 988, 989
Pharmacokinetics 667
Pharmacotherapy 340
Phenothiazine 324
Phentermine 231
Phenylalanine 1444
Phenylpropanolamine 365
Phosphatidyl myo-inositol 526
Phosphatidyl phosphate 526
Phosphatidylinositol 3-kinase 27, 28, 526
Phosphatidylserine 1254, 1255, 1279
Phosphodiesterase 47, 47*f*, 48, 335, 347, 398
  efficacy of 343*f*
  pharmacokinetic comparison 345*t*
Phospholipase 68
Phospholipid 1444
Phosphorylation 87*f*
Photons, energy of 1320
Photooxidation 1165
Photosensitivity 281
Physical microfluidic system 1459
Physiological intracytoplasmic sperm injection 1048, 1247, 1447, 1452, 1605, 1606*f*, 1607*f*
  advantages of 1452
  disadvantages of 1452
  dish 1606
Piezo-assisted drilling 1404
Piezo-intracytoplasmic sperm injection 1345, 1346*f*, 1347
Pigment epithelium derived factor 726
Pinealomas 121
Pinopodes over glands 1031*f*
Pipette 1658
  alignment 1342, 1506
  attachment of 1505*f*
  types of 1658, 1658*f*, 1659*f*
Pisum sativum agglutinin 1247
Pituitary dysfunction 668
Pituitary failure 170
Pituitary gland, anterior 1047
Pituitary gonadotropins 14, 1040
Pituitary microadenoma 121
Pituitary secretions, ovarian control of 26*fc*
Pituitary tumor 141, 382, 383
Placenta 888, 927*f*, 928*f*, 930, 1185
  accreta 997, 1141, 1391
  previa 1141
    risk of 996
Placental abruption 291
Placental dysfunction 1040
Placental examination 930
Placental tissue, development of 887
Placentation, dysfunctional 1185
Plasma
  membranes, damaged 1244
  protein A, pregnancy associated 916
  rich protein 1121
Plasminogen
  activator inhibitor 224-227
  inhibitory system 33
Plastic petri dishes 1503
Plastic pipettes 1658*f*
Plastic test tubes 1657, 1657*f*
Platelet 1109
  activation of 1109
  poor plasma 1109
Platelet derived growth factor 1072
  beta receptor 1072
Platelet rich plasma 432, 1046, 1108, 1110*f*, 1121
  autologous 1109
  preparation of 1046
Pleuritis 281
Pligoasthenoteratozoospermia, idiopathic 350
Pluripotent stem cells 259, 1116
Pneumatic injector 1336
Pneumatic syringe 1341
Pneumonitis 922
Polar body 68, 1361, 1545, 1547*f*, 1612*f*
  biopsy 862, 864, 1409
  extrusion of second 68
  first 1537
  second 1383
  size of 1351
Polarization microscopy 1432, 1434*t*
  components of 1433*f*
Poloscopy 1610
  principle of 1610
Polybrominated diphenyl ethers 61
Polychlorinated biphenyls 61
Polycystic ovarian
  disease 518, 580
  morphology 147, 478, 508, 519, 531, 531*f*
    signs of 531
Polycystic ovarian syndrome 47, 99, 124, 134, 140, 150, 158, 168-171, 192, 215, 217, 226, 289, 474, 478*t*, 508, 518, 519*t*, 520*f*, 520*t*, 522*fc*, 523*f*, 525, 528, 529*fc*, 529*t*, 530*b*, 533*t*, 535, 548, 551*t*, 552, 559, 592, 628, 653, 665, 673, 693, 723, 735, 793, 804, 831, 834, 898, 900, 999, 1020, 1137, 1311, 1328, 1420
  anovulatory 47

diagnosis of 509*t*
differential diagnosis of 532*b*
evaluation of 545
management of 137, 529, 535*t*, 545, 545*f*
pathophysiology of 549*f*
phenotypes, classification of 519*t*
screening strategy for 535*b*
society 519
Polycystic ovary 44, 169, 170, 477*f*, 507, 509*f*, 511*f*, 518, 519, 735
bilateral 593*f*
Doppler features for 507
three-dimensional volume of 511*f*
Polydeoxyribonucleotide 386
Polydimethylsiloxane 1256, 1282
use of 1456
Polydioxanone 609
Polyethylene glycol precipitation 140
Polygenic complex female infertility 217
Polyhydramnios 996
Polymerase chain reaction 407, 441, 466, 468, 941, 949, 1409, 1441, 1662
Polymers 1139
Polymorphisms 240
affecting androgen receptor 310
Polypectomy, hysteroscopic 842
Polyps 101, 495, 498, 842
endometrial 241, 242, 498*f*, 612
Polysaccharide 1452
dextran 1254
Polyspermic zygote formation 1457, 1458
Polyspermy 830
Polystyrene 1456
Polyvinyl alcohol 1495
Polyvinylpyrrolidone 1268, 1337, 1337*f*, 1506, 1607*f*, 1660, 1660*f*
Pomeroy's method 446
Poor blastocyst formation 1517
Poor embryo quality, treatment of 839
Poor fertilization rate 1343, 1424
Poor oocyte
fertilization 814
quality 241, 565, 830, 1515, 1516
treatment of 839
Poor ovarian
reserve 739, 938, 1513
responder, management of 821
response 690, 809, 810
Poor quality oocytes 939
Poor responders, prediction of 810
Porcine capacitated sperm 1458
Port closure needle 580
Portal system 18*f*
POSEIDON
classification 738, 738*t*, 820
stratification 674*f*
Positive pregnancy outcome 1443
Positive pressure 1482
Postabortion survivor syndrome 1208, 1211
Postacrosomal lamina 1254, 1277
Postacrosomal region 1437
narrow 1449
Postcoital test 198
Postejaculate urinalysis 378
Postembryo transfer 785
Postfertilization 1261, 1402
Posthuman chorionic gonadotropin 1383
Posthumous reproduction 261
Postinflammatory obstruction 311
Post-insemination 1402
Post-IVF pregnancies 1189
Postmasturbation urine 336
Postmature oocyte 1516
corona cumulus 1535
Postmortem sperm retrieval 262
Postnatal growth 884
Postpartum 933
depression 997
hemorrhage 931, 958, 997, 999
thyroiditis 146
Postpubertal status 360
Post-zygote development 1337
Potassium 899, 905
chloride 1210
hydroxide 454
Potential cycle cancellation 745
Pouch of Douglas 464, 468*f*, 515, 567*f*, 591, 592*f*, 714, 1036
Powder-free latex gloves 1132
Prader orchidometer 325*f*, 353
Prader-Willi syndrome 310, 382, 383, 884
Prazosin 324
Preantral follicle 29, 43, 45
Precocious puberty 120, 121, 122*fc*, 701
causes of 121*b*
central causes of 121
evaluation of 123*b*
familial male-limited 121, 124
peripheral 121, 123
Preconception care 295
Preconceptional weight loss 233
Prednisolone 1187
Prednisone 253
Predominant hyperechoic stroma 508
Preeclampsia 931, 939, 997, 1185
Prefreezing embryo selection 1517
Pregenetic screening 1407
Pregnancy 142, 146, 264, 455, 550, 932, 945, 971, 1039, 1186, 1198, 1322
abdominal 918
biochemical 1247, 1299, 1518
complication 222
cornual 917, 923
ectopic 841, 913, 913*t*, 914, 915*f*, 921*fc*, 924, 1013-1015, 1201, 1202
effects of 88
extrauterine 1201
failure, early 1015
fear of 333
heterotopic 913, 916, 918, 924, 1015
high-risk 1190
hormones 90
human 1305
immune
acceptance of 87
paradox of 88
immunology of 201
interstitial 917, 923, 1014
intrahepatic cholestasis of 1062
intrauterine 1013, 1203
latter half of 1214
maternal recognition of 97
presence of 1201
progresses 1185
spontaneous 946
Pregnancy loss 1019, 1211, 1445
complete 1210
early 222, 924, 1012, 1019*t*, 1185, 1322
first-trimester 158
rates 1210
recurrent 211, 228, 800, 804, 868, 955, 1019, 1020, 1020*fc*, 1020*t*, 1022, 1024, 1145, 1186, 1188, 1191, 1407
spectrum of 1019*f*
Pregnancy rate 227, 583, 587, 654, 932, 1257, 1278, 1311, 1354, 1361, 1374, 1425, 1513
clinical 101, 244, 544, 568, 787, 804, 843, 868, 1060, 1146, 1137, 1524
cumulative 733
higher 100, 774
lower 810, 1150
poor 1517
recipient 943
Pregnant mare serum gonadotropin 655, 656
Pregnenolone 107, 110–112
metabolism 110, 113
Pregranulosa cells 1420
Preimplantation embryo 861, 876, 1046, 1320, 1380, 1443, 1495
arrest of 1351
development 73, 1361
isolation 1331
Preimplantation genetic
diagnosis 725, 861, 876, 949, 960, 995, 1020, 1022, 1131, 1311, 1328, 1355, 1375, 1407, 1408, 1455, 1473, 1481, 1502, 1662
screening 430, 793, 819, 840, 861, 864*t*, 886, 995, 998, 1022, 1033, 1131, 1355, 1375, 1407, 1408, 1415, 1662
techniques 1415
testing 407, 861, 862*b*, 863*f*, 865, 867, 869, 871, 876, 879, 880, 945, 1022, 1145, 1156, 1191, 1319, 1407, 1471
limitations of 879
Preleptotene 54
Premature luteinization 713
prevention of 49
Premature ovarian
aging 241
insufficiency 126, 215, 250, 857, 938, 1116, 1118
Premature ovarian failure 124, 131-133, 146, 169, 241, 259, 282, 1116
causes of 938*b*
management of 138
Premature thelarche 120
Prematurity 996, 1023
Prenatal growth 884
Preovulatory follicle 31, 43, 47
Preovulatory period 479
Preovulatory scan 511
Pre-sperm interaction 1516
Preterm birth 1142
Preterm delivery 291, 996
Prevasectomy 252
Prevent inheritable mitochondrial disease 950*f*
Prevotella 833
Primary amenorrhea 131, 133, 134, 138, 530
hypothalamic causes of 124
Primary follicle 29, 43, 44
formation of 44*t*

Primary oocyte 43
  maintenance of 47
Primary testicular failure 306, 376, 381, 382
  etiology of 381, 381*b*
  management of 382*fc*
Primordial follicle 27, 43, 44, 44*t*, 982, 1122, 1429
  activation model 28*f*
  granulosa cells 28
Primordial germ cell 4*f*, 42, 43, 62, 885
  migration 43*f*
Procarbazine 253
Progenitor cells, staining of 1083*f*, 1084*f*, 1086*f*, 1087*f*
Progesterone 16, 19, 24, 26, 32, 33, 37, 76, 84, 98, 107, 158, 160, 201, 474, 479, 534, 727, 800-802, 804, 837, 838, 858, 957, 1148, 1232, 1329, 1387, 1425
  addition of 1112
  administration of 1137
  appearance of 1030
  biosynthesis 157
  correction of 484
  induced blocking factor 89
  intensive 803
  intrauterine system 426
  levels of 1142, 1148
  natural 284
  premature elevation of 1328
  production 156
  receptor 117, 834
  secretion of 724
  supplementation 1024, 1138
  synthesis of 23, 107
  use of 1518
Progestin 113, 427
  challenge test 133, 133*fc*
  primed ovarian stimulation protocol 683, 684*f*, 739
  therapy 537
Program performance indicators 1182*b*
Programmed cell death 5
Progression, natural 393
Progressive precocious puberty 123*b*
Proinflammatory adipokine 244*f*
Proinflammatory cytokines 157*f*
Prolactin 23, 125, 140, 375, 534, 704
  disorder 158, 532
  homeostasis 23
  secretion 23
Prolactinoma 124, 188
Proline 1444
Pronuclear stage 1565
Pronuclear transfer 1045
Pronucleus 1615
  abnormal 1573
  stage 1351
Propane sulfonic acid 1607*f*
Propanediol 1381
Propane-sulfonic acid 1169, 1512, 1623
Prophylactic antibiotics 1208
  role of 766
Prophylactic oophorectomy 1429
Prophylactic steroid, use of 1405
Propofol 759, 760
Proportional growth 1005
Propylene glycol 1139, 1381
Prostaglandins 23, 33, 50, 83, 84, 570, 895, 896, 897*fc*
  stimulate secretion of 841
Prostate 9, 12, 14
  gland 1249
  hyperplasia, benign 398, 701
  hypertrophy 12
  massage 401
  specific antigen 12, 340, 361
Prostatic cancer 696
Prostatic fluid 14
Prostatic obstruction, midline 355
Prostatic secretory ducts, simple columnar epithelium of 15
Prostatic surgery 184
Prostatitis
  acute 1246
  chronic 1246
Protamine 1261
  deficiency 1261
Proteases 54
Protein 76, 82, 1112, 1381
  kinase 47, 48, 68, 86
  signaling pathways 81
  substitutes 1496
  supplement 1495
  synthesis 1421, 1424
Protein-rich fluid, transudation of 1193
Proteinuria, persistent 281
Proteolytic enzymes 311, 1247
Proteomic analysis 432
Proteomic embryonic secretome, microarray analysis of 1443
Proteomic platform 1443
Proximal block, failed tubal cannulation for 587
Proximal tubal
  block, hysteroscopic tubal cannulation for 597
  cannulation 445
  disease
    causes of 438*t*
    surgery for 445, 584
  occlusion 584
    laparoscopic 847
  region, anatomy of 597
Prune belly syndrome 375
Pseudoephedrine 365
Pseudogestational sac 1005
Pseudohermaphroditism, male 112
Pseudo-obstruction 438
Pseudostratification predominate 35
Pseudostratified columnar epithelium 15
Psychiatric disorder 1293
Psychiatric interventions 272
Psychosis 281
Psychosocial stress 973
Psychotherapy 274
Pubarche 119
Pubertal development
  stages of 118
  tanner stages of 132*f*
Pubertal disorders, classification of 120
Pubertal growth spurt 119
Pubertal milestones 119*f*, 120*f*
Puberty 20, 115, 116, 136, 549*f*
  central precocious 117, 121, 677, 696
  constitutional delay of 124, 125
  delayed 124, 124*b*, 125*fc*
  normal variants of 120
  nutritional factors determining onset of 118
  onset of 117
  phases of onset of 115*t*
  tanner stages of 120*t*
  timing of 183
Pubic hair 120, 375
Puborectalis 333
Pudendal nerve
  innervation 395*f*
  posterior scrotal branches of 10
Pulmonary edema 596
Pulsatile secretion 115
Pulsatility index 478, 479, 713, 1035
Pulse oximetry 759
Pump generates fluid flow 1456
Pumpless arteriovenous circuit 1042
Pumpless hydrostatic pressure 1256
Pyrazinamide 432, 469
Pyrexia 1213
Pyridostigmine 813
Pyruvate 1355, 1444

Q

Qualitative data 1221
Quality assurance 1161, 1488, 1510
Quality control 1161, 1168, 1172, 1172*f*, 1319, 1488, 1489, 1498
  program, components of 1162, 1163*fc*
Quality improvement 1510
  tools 1319
Quality management 1488, 1510, 1522, 1526
  system 796, 1161, 1177*t*, 1522-1525, 1532
    benefits of 1177
    drawbacks of 1177
    structure of 1523*f*
  total 1162, 1488, 1510, 1522
Quantitative polymerase chain reaction 865, 867, 1327, 1415
Quartz glass 1273
Quasi experiments 1227
Quintuplets 926

R

Radiant corona 1533*f*
Radiation 312
  cranial 121
  stimulated emission of 295
Radioactive iodine 145
Radiofrequency electromagnetic fields 323
Radiotherapy 124, 171, 250, 306, 381
Raman spectroscopy 381, 1322, 1444
  principle 1256
Randomized controlled
  study 159
  trails 161, 202, 354, 369, 420, 469, 570, 655, 668, 691, 723, 743, 765, 770, 777, 801, 836, 839, 840, 844, 846, 1142, 1145, 1228, 1228*f*, 1313, 1355
Random-start controlled ovarian stimulation 256
Ranitidine 324
Rapamycin complex 28
Rapid freezing protocols 1623
Rashes 369

Reactive oxygen species, tests for 243, 1243
Real-time polymerase chain reaction 1415, 1441
Receiver operator characteristic curves 915*f*, 1231*f*
Recent genome-wide copy number variation 213
Receptor polymorphism 734, 857
Recipient surgery 1041
Recombinant follicle-stimulating hormone 680, 682, 738, 1308*f*, 1324
  use of 817
Recombinant gonadotropins 657
Recombinant human
  anti-Müllerian hormone 561
  chorionic gonadotropin 723, 724
  follicle stimulating hormone 656
  leutinizing hormone 656
Recombinant luteinizing hormone 217, 692, 723, 724, 727, 729, 754, 803, 858, 902
  advantages of 724*t*
  disadvantages of 724*t*
Reconstructive surgery 444
Rectal examination 326
  abnormal 364
Rectum 1098*f*
  dissection of 1078*f*
  uncomplicated gonococcal infection of 452*b*
Recurrent disease 575
Recurrent implantation failure
  etiology for 830
  management of 839*fc*
Recurrent pregnancy loss, unexplained 1022-1024
Red blood cells 1109, 1423
Reductase inhibitor 153
Reflex 395
Reflexogenic erection 396
Refractile bodies 1362, 1362*f*, 1545, 1546*f*
Regional anesthesia 760
Regulatory T cells, plasticity of 1022*f*
Relaxin 76
Remifentanil 758
Renal anomalies 1094
Renal disorder 281
Renal failure 141, 282, 1196
Renal function 1062
  test 905, 907
Renal manifestations 899
Renal perfusion 893
Renal transplant 158, 1073
  recipients 284
Renin-angiotensin-aldosterone system 146, 895
Reperfusion injury 311
Repetitive sequence-specific probes 210
Reproduction artificial intelligence 1475
Reproduction techniques, artificial 286, 1093
Reproductive ages, extremes of 158
Reproductive cells 1162, 1393
Reproductive cryopreservation, safety of 1391
Reproductive dysfunction 293
Reproductive endocrinology 105, 777
Reproductive function 294*fc*, 546
Reproductive medicine 838, 1035, 1145, 1433
  practitioners 1468
Reproductive neuroendocrinology 16
Reproductive routine 178
Reproductive system 3
  anatomy of 3
  assessment of 474
  hormonal regulation of 38
  human 474
Reproductive technology 229, 940
Reproductive tissue 1394, 1395
Reproductive tract 1496
  infections 962
  inflammation 314*fc*
  microbiome 444
Rescue intracytoplasmic sperm injection 1049, 1436
Research
  hypothesis 1078
  study design 1224*fc*
Resistance index 160, 478, 484
Respiratory compromise 907
Respiratory illness 375, 1035
Respiratory system 1212
Rete testis 14, 53
Reticulocytosis 281
Reticulum 1470
Retrieved spermatids 1050
Retrograde ejaculation 324, 335, 356, 1268
  management of 336
  medical treatment of 365
  medication for 365*t*
  samples, preparation of 1275
Retroperitoneal bleeding 1193, 1200
Reverse transcription polymerase chain reaction 329, 1393
  test 1214
Rhabdomyosarcoma 886
Rheotaxis 1283
Rhesus 921
  factor 942
  typing 915
Rheumatoid arthritis 278, 281
Rhombencephalon 1005, 1007*f*
Ribonucleic acid 57, 69, 212, 450, 883, 916, 920, 1023, 1108, 1112, 1212, 1322
Ribosomal ribonucleic acid 833
Rifampicin 469
Right rudimentary utricle 1088*f*
Ring chromosomes 209*f*, 216
Ring formation test 1030*f*
Rinse embryos 1637
Robertsonian translocation 212, 309
Robotic assisted laparoscopy 1059
  myomectomy 421
Robotic assisted uterus procurement 1058
Robotic donor surgery 1058
Robotic transplantation 1059
Rogletimide 654
Rokitansky's protuberance 504
Rokitansky's tubercle 505*f*
Root cause analysis 1491
Rosenthal effects 1225
Round cells 1292, 1456, 1457
  number 186
Round-bottom tubes 1269
Roundness index 1371
Routine semen analysis 1451
Routine tests 185
Roux-en-Y gastric bypass 232, 232*f*
Rubin's insufflation test 443
Rubin's test 443
Rubin's ultrasonographic criteria 917
Rudimentary horn 923
Rupture uterus 584

S

Sacrouterine ligaments 1058, 1059
Saline infusion
  salpingography 505
  sonography 196, 439
Salivary ferning assessment 706
Salivary secretions, electronic resistance evaluation of 706
Salpingectomy 439, 445, 584, 585*f*, 608, 847, 923, 1517
  laparoscopic 448
Salpingitis
  grading of 441
  isthmica nodosa 438, 584, 587
  laparoscopic diagnosis of 441
Salpingo-ovariolysis 445, 588
Salpingoscopy 441, 584, 587*f*
Salpingostomy 445, 608, 609, 847
Sample batch calendar 1130*t*
Sanctum sanctorum 1481
Sapporo criteria, revised 282*t*
Sarbecovirus 1212
Sarteschi classification 387, 387*t*
Scanning electron microscope 1031*f*
Schizophrenia 888
Scintigraphy 388
Scleroderma 251
Sclerosis, multiple 278
Scrotal examination 375
Scrotal hyperthermia 386
Scrotal sonography, technique of 351
Scrotal ultrasound 354, 376
  indications of 350
Scrotum 10, 375
Secnidazole 454, 454*b*
Secretion, source of 14
Secretory endometrium 483*f*
Secretory phase 34, 36
  assessment 483
Secretory scan 514
Segmental aneuploidy 878
Seizure 281
Selective estrogen receptor modulators 124, 369, 428, 653
Selective progesterone receptor modulator 426, 428
Selective salpingography 442
Selenium 366
Semen 13, 400*f*, 645, 1279*f*, 1444
  abnormal quality of 394
  abnormalities 392, 399
  analysis of 1235
  bank 1291, 1293
  extender 1291
  freezing of 971, 1292
  idiopathic abnormal 306, 364
  microscopic examination of 185, 185*t*, 186*t*, 389
  pH 185, 375
  problem 1237
  processing laboratory 963

testing 1236
viscosity, reduction of 1274
vitrification 1292
volume 185, 188, 327, 328, 376
Semen analysis 184, 243, 326, 375, 1172, 1235, 1557
abnormal 183
application of 1469
extended 189
manual 1230*f*
parameters 316
Semen collection
container 1132
room 963
Semen cryopreservation 1291, 1291*t*, 1295
indications for 1293
protocol, goal of 1295
technique, consequences of 1295
Semen donor 1293
recruitment of 1293
selection of 1293
Semen parameter 364, 646
basic 1237
Semen preparation 1172, 1484
technique 621, 630, 646
Semen quality 399, 1515
poor 399
Semen retrieval
methods 402, 402*fc*
surgical 401, 402
Semen sample 1282, 1292, 1343, 1515
preparation 1448
quarantine of 949
storage of 1155, 1292, 1293
types of 1292
Semenopathy, severe 887
Seminal abnormalities 327*t*
Seminal ejaculate 1271*f*
Seminal fluid 14*t*, 619
Seminal gland 11, 11*f*, 14
Seminal plasma 203, 400, 1249*b*, 1267, 1268, 1276*f*
evaluation of 1240*f*
free spermatozoa 1241
Seminal vesicle 8, 14, 355, 1249
absent 355, 356, 356*f*
anteroposterior diameter 376
enlargement 355
hypoplastic 356
mucosa 15
secretions 14
Seminal vesicular cyst 356
Seminal vesiculography 357
Seminal volume, low 355
Seminiferous tubule 53, 354
biopsy, single 380
cross-section of 54*f*
failure 328
Semiopen adoption 974
Sensory function
complete loss of 393
partial loss of 393
Sephadex columns 1254, 1274
Septae 568
Septal resection, hysteroscopic 1107
Septal resorption 413
Septate subseptate uterus 488
Septate uterus 414, 419, 419*f*, 490*f*, 610*f*
accurate diagnosis of 610
Septum
complete 490*f*
hysteroscopic 610*f*
partial 490*f*
resection 600*f*, 610
size of 490
Sequential culture media system 1496
Sequential embryo transfer 841
Sequential hormonal therapy 1029
Sequential protocol 542, 542*fc*
Seroconcordant couples 457
Serotonin 231, 521, 896
reuptake inhibitor, selective 231, 313, 314
Sertoli cell 10, 14, 53-55, 58*f*, 62, 370, 1393
adenomas 137
nucleus of 15
only syndrome 13*f*, 55, 310*f*
Serum
albumin 1291, 1494
anti-Nüllerian hormone 193, 560
beta-human chorionic gonadotropin 1004
dehydroepiandrosterone sulfate 134
estradiol 560, 715, 812, 1512
follicle-stimulating hormone 327, 375
glutamic pyruvic transaminase 942, 949
luteinizing hormone 715, 1514
testosterone 134, 343
Serum progesterone 192, 716, 943
levels 159, 915
measurement 244
Sessile endometrial polyp 613*f*
Severe acute respiratory syndrome coronavirus 2 315, 370, 1212*f*, 1393, 1396
effects of 1393, 1394
impact of 329
Sex chromosome 1415
abnormalities 309
aneuploidies 215
inactivation 57
Sex hormone-binding globulin 144, 152, 153, 225-227, 229, 520, 525, 529
Sex reassignment therapy 981
Sex steroids 150
Sex therapy 341
Sexual abstinence
duration of 645
period of 184
Sexual abuse 333
Sexual act, fear of 333
Sexual behavioral therapy 339
Sexual dysfunction 286, 289, 324, 324*t*, 325, 328, 329, 332, 339, 365, 396*f*
secondary 395
Sexual factors 364
Sexual identity disorders 980
Sexual problems 322
Sexual reflexes, loss of 395
Sexual response, biological basis of male 332
Sexually transmitted disease 190, 253, 440, 451, 940, 1293
treatment of 444
Sexually transmitted infection 183, 375, 444, 450, 456
Shanghai protocol 683, 683*f*
Sheehan's syndrome 135, 168, 170
Shock, cold 1271
Short menstrual cycles 158
Short stature homeobox gene 215
Shoulder pain 914
Sickle cell
anemia 1311, 1407
disease 1046
Sigmoid mucosa 1102*f*
Sigmoid vaginoplasty 1102, 1102*f*
Signal transduction pathways 86
Sildenafil 339, 343*f*, 345
citrate 844, 1108, 1515
Silicate glass 1273
Silicon master 1456
Silver-Russell syndrome 884
Simple wash method 1268
Sims' speculum 1209
Single blastocyst
stage 945
transfer 998, 1311
Single cell
analysis of 880
gel electrophoresis assay 189
Single chromosome 878
Single embryo 1141
transfer 284, 544, 832, 905, 996, 1050, 1190, 1356, 1474
cycle, selective 776
Single follicle
dominance of 46
selection of 46
Single gene
diseases 1442
disorders 217, 876, 879, 880, 1412
Single layer epithelium 1080*f*
Single nucleotide polymorphism 24, 112, 210, 865, 867, 877, 1355, 1415
arrays 865
microarrays 878, 1415
of follicle-stimulating hormone receptor gene 1038
Single-cell genomics, application of 1415
Sinus tubercle 8
Sion's test 443
Sjögren's syndrome 251, 281
Skene's glands 4
Skin 525, 1088*f*
flaps 1099
graft 989, 1098
donor scars 1099
Skull base fractures 306
Sleep apnea 228
Sleeve gastrectomy 232
Slow follicle growth 565
Slow freezing method 1139
Small intestine 1088*f*
Small supernumerary marker chromosomes 210
Smartphone apps 1250
Smell, loss of 1213
Smith's grading 711
Smooth endoplasmic reticulum 1322, 1362, 1541, 1545, 1545*f*
cluster 1545
oocytes 1322
Smooth muscle cell 340, 345
Social egg freezing 262
Social issue 1154, 1159

Society for assisted reproductive technology 898, 997
Sock, signs of 393
Sodium 899, 905
  tetradecyl sulfate 389
Soft catheters 1329
Soft hair 149
Soft protocol 738, 738*fc*
Softer cannula 1329
Solid organ transplants 1071
Somatic cell lines 1370
Somatic follicular cells 1442
Somatosensory evoked potentials 334
Somatostatin analogs 143
Sono-automatic volume calculation 508
Sonoembryology 1007, 1008
  normal 1004
Sonoendocrinology 474
Sonohysterography 498, 500*f*, 601
Sonohysterosalpingography 443
Speckle reduction imaging 474
Spent culture medium 867
Sperm 53, 58, 63, 66, 379, 725*f*, 913, 1337, 1437, 1459, 1557, 1598, 1599, 1603*f*, 1605, 1609*f*
  abnormal 187, 1270
  abnormalities 1240*f*
  acrosome 1433
  analysis 1469
  aneuploidy 1278
  antibody 1245
    detection 381
  antigens 313
  apoptotic 1049, 1255, 1622
  binding of 1363
  birefringence 1255
  capacitation 1495
  catch 1337
  cells 1268, 1270, 1275, 1282*f*
  contribution of 1517
  cryopreservation 254
  demonstration of 336
  deposition of 1341
  donation 937, 949
  droplet 1339
  evaluation, components of 1557
  extraction, surgical 357
  factor 68
  fishing dish 1337
  flow 1458
  head 1449
  health 1238
  hyperactivated motility 1469
  immaturity of 885, 1049
  immobilization 1346, 1347*f*, 1506, 1600, 1601*f*
  inactivation 567
  inlet ports 1462, 1463*f*
  intracellular 1469
  isolation 1455, 1456
  linearity coefficient 1469
  manipulation, prolonged 1451
  maturation 1449
  maturity of 1452
  metabolism 1457
  microinjection of 1502
  morphological selection of 1452
  morphology of 1261
  mucus interaction tests 1242, 1245, 1245*fc*
  nonviable 1515
  normal 1522*f*
  nucleus 1277
  number of 1236
  organellar morphology 1322
  plasma membranes of 67
  populations, motility of 1274
  proportion of 1262
  reactive 1256
  retrieval, posthumous 252, 253
  samples 1171, 1281
  screening 1461
  selection of 1253, 1279, 1437, 1452, 1469
  sorting medium 1282
  tail 1256
  trajectory 1250
  transport 66
  use of 937
  viability 1562*f*
Sperm chromatin 1339
  assessment 1261, 1264
  dispersion test 189, 243, 1037, 1262, 1263
  quality 1264
  structure assay 189, 240, 1023, 1037, 1242, 1262
Sperm concentration 186, 188, 327, 1242, 1457, 1557
  lower median 1326
Sperm count 1557
  manual 1230*f*
Sperm deformity 1243
  index 1243
Sperm deoxyribonucleic acid 239
  damage 239, 240, 243
  fragmentation 1023, 1451, 1557
    index 1248
Sperm donor
  investigations for 949*b*
  screening 949
Sperm flagella 407*fc*
  multiple morphological abnormalities of 406, 409
Sperm function 364, 567, 1238
  defects 183
  normal 1278
Sperm function tests 189*b*, 1238, 1242, 1249*t*
  classification of 1242*b*
  number of 1250
  rationale behind 1243*f*
Sperm injection 1157, 1448, 1517, 1608
  standard-intracytoplasmic 1347
Sperm membrane 1272, 1278, 1339
  potential 1469
Sperm morphology 188, 1235, 1242, 1557, 1558, 1558*f*
  abnormal 322, 1280
Sperm motility 1257, 1268, 1444, 1456, 1490, 1557
  reduce 1274
  scores 1170
Sperm number 186
  total 188, 327
Sperm oocyte
  fusion 1363, 1516
  interactions 1515
Sperm parameters 228
  isolated abnormalities of 306
Sperm penetration 67, 1363, 1458
  assay 1242, 1248
Sperm plasma membrane 1269
  fusion of 67
Sperm preparation 1275, 1528
  methods of 1253
Sperm preparation technique 1275
  advanced 1267
  future development of 1284
Sperm quality 645, 830, 1262, 1351, 1434
  analyzer, automated 1651*f*
  influence of 620, 626
  terms of 1279
Sperm retrieval technique 379, 380*fc*
  anesthesia for 13
  types of 380*t*
Sperm selection 1250, 1253, 1254, 1255, 1257, 1278*f*, 1283, 1339, 1437, 1605
  advance 1608
    strategies of 1276
  assay 1283
  chemical stimulators mediated 1257
  methods of 1280*f*, 1283*f*, 1284*f*
  microfluidic-based 1256
  sites of 1276*f*
  technique of 1280
    novel 1334
Sperm separation
  microfluidic-based 1256
  sephadex columns for 1254
Sperm survival 1490
  test 1167
Sperm suspension 1346
  aliquot of 1339
Sperm vitality 1557, 1560, 1561
  tests 1242, 1244, 1244*f*
Sperm wash 1268, 1271
  methods 456
  procedures 1396
  techniques 457
Spermatids 54, 54*f*
  immature 885
  injection, elongated 1050
Spermatocele 351
Spermatocelectomies 375
Spermatocytes, primary 15
Spermatocytogenesis 55
Spermatogenesis 53-55, 55*fc*, 57, 61, 62, 214, 282, 370, 1261
  complete arrest of 1294
  endocrine control of 59, 59*fc*
  impairment of 386
  normal 188
  stages of 54*f*, 57*f*
Spermatogenic arrest 310*f*
Spermatogonia 54, 55, 1118
  inability of 55
  stem cell 252
Spermatozoa 15, 54, 58, 628, 634, 1049, 1238, 1243-1246, 1254, 1261, 1267-1269, 1275, 1277-1279, 1283, 1284, 1284*f*, 1291, 1293-1295, 1311, 1334, 1387, 1393, 1437, 1449-1452, 1470, 1502, 1506, 1561*f*, 1605, 1622
  abnormal 1243, 1292
  apoptotic 1279*f*, 1284
  characteristics of mature 1276
  concentration 327*f*

damage of 375, 1273
dimensions of normal 1449*f*
enhancement of 1279
fertilizing ability of 1291
fragmented 1254
functional 1268, 1273
competence of 1295
globozoospermic 1451
high quality 1279
membrane of 1278
morphology of 1237
normal 1254, 1274, 1448
number of 1274, 1282
parameters 324*t*
penetrate 1245
potential of 1268
quality of 1267
safety pool of 1293
selection of 1278
types of 1277
Spermatozoon 1038, 1267, 1270, 1276, 1338
mature 1261
normal 1447
penetrates 1238
single 1275, 1447
Spermiation 55, 57
Spermiogenesis 55, 1261
Spiegelberg's ultrasonographic criteria 918
Spinal anesthesia 761
Spinal cord
injury 392, 392*f*, 393, 394, 400*f*, 401
levels of 394*f*
lesions of 396*f*
Spindle dynamics 1434
Spindle imaging 1434, 1436
Spindle near polar body 1363*f*
Spiral artery 482, 1106
flow 484*t*
Spironolactone 153, 324, 536, 982
Spleen 1071
Spontaneous abortion 215, 287, 888, 1141
rates 1262
Spontaneous luteinizing hormone surge, abolition of 677
Spontaneous ovarian hyperstimulation syndrome 896*t*
Sporadic spontaneous pregnancies 938
Standard insemination concentration 1597
Standard operating procedures 734, 797, 1173, 1489, 1510, 1522
Starvation 158
State Adoption Resource Agency 975
State Assisted Reproductive Technology and Surrogacy Board 939
Static coincubation lapses 1458
Statins 324, 548
Steelman-Pohley bioassay 1039
Stein-Leventhal syndrome 592
Stem cell 845, 1112*f*, 1116, 1117*f*, 1120
administration of 1111
based therapy 1118
components of 1118
derivation of 1121
implantation 1120*f*
laparoscopic ovarian injection of 1121*f*
marker 1081
potency 1116*f*
preparation 1120*f*
research 947, 1313
secretome 1121
therapy 1047, 1050, 1111, 1112, 1117*t*, 1120
transplantation 1120
types of 1116, 1117
Stenosis 991*f*
Stereomicroscope 1168, 1168*f*
Stereozoom microscope 1322, 1484*f*, 1649
Sterile
serological pipette 1269
technique 1172
Sterilization, reversal of 587
Steroid 110, 111, 431
abuse 382
contraception delay menopause 51
defective synthesis of 111
excretion products 112, 113*t*
hormone 73, 107
metabolism of 107, 112
synthesis 107
nucleus, hydroxylations of 112
receptors 98
resistant glomerulonephritis 251
therapy 375
Steroidogenesis 108, 110, 520
Steroidogenic acute regulatory protein 51*f*, 108, 109, 111, 156
Steroidogenic enzymes, regulation of 110
Stillbirth 291, 222, 1474
Stimulation 1129
cycle 1128
protocols 673, 943
mild 1319
test 334
Stratum
basalis 1119
compactum 34
functionalis 1119
spongiosum 34
Streptomycin 1495
Stress 158, 170
Stroma 1111
Stromal cells 1028, 1029*f*
predominate 1028
Stromal edema 1199*f*
Stromal flow index 708
Stromal ovarian blood flow 1035
Stromal peak systolic velocity 708
Structural chromosomal
abnormalities 60
rearrangements 880
Studdiford criteria 918
Subarachnoid bleeding 1060
Subchorionic hemorrhage, large 1005, 1016*f*
Subcutaneous ovarian grafts 1071
Subfertility 145, 206, 221, 531
female factor 211
male 1334
factor 210
Subinguinal microscopic varicocelectomy 389*f*
Submucous extension 421
Submucous fibroids 595
Submucous myoma 421, 425*f*, 425*t*, 596*f*, 612, 612*f*
hysteroscopic management of 424
resection of 596*f*
Suboptimal methylation 1189
Subsequent fertilization 1515
Substance abuse 323
Subzonal insemination 1306, 1334
Subzonal sperm injection 1502
Succinylcholine 758
Sucrose 1291
Suction apparatus 767, 767*f*
Suction ejection pump 333
Suction pump 1655, 1655*f*
Sulfasalazine 282, 1294
Superovulation 245, 664
gonadotropin for 659
Superoxide dismutase 338, 367, 1295
Support vector machines 776, 1467
Suppression, excessive 677
Sureview Wallace catheters 779*f*
Surgery 142
complications of 990*f*
intra-abdominal 606
signs of 1089*f*
timing of 599
Surrogacy 846, 954, 958, 959, 961, 1159
Act 968, 968*t*, 1158
altruistic 968
amendment rules 1159
arrangement, first 954
bill 960, 966, 968, 1158
clinics, registration of 961
commercial 959, 968
gestational 470, 839, 956, 960, 1055, 1103
indications for 955*f*
law, evolution in 968
legislation 958
procedure, attempts of 1157
process 955
psychological impact of 958
registry 940
rules 969, 1157
types of 954, 968
Surrogate 956, 960
babies
birth of 959*f*
born, number of 959
embryo transfer 957
gestational carriers 995
mothers, motives of 959*f*
obstetrics care of 957
pregnancy 969
prospective 956
source of 956
synchronizing cycles of 957
uterus 954
Swim-up procedure 1253
Swiss cheese appearance 496*f*
Swyer syndrome 137
Synacthen test 147
Syncope 914
Syncytiotrophoblast 88
Syndromic monogenic defects 310
Synechiae 495, 498, 499*f*, 843
Syngamy 1365*f*, 1565
Synthetic corticosteroids 1023
Synthetic kisspeptins 1039
application of 1040
Synthetic oligonucleotides 1442
Synthetic polyvinylpyrrolidone, effects of 1605
Synthetic progesterone 801

Syphilis 941, 965, 966
Systemic autoimmune diseases 281
Systemic diseases 381
Systemic lupus erythematosus 146, 251, 281-283, 283*b*, 284, 284*fc*, 1186
- effects of 283

Systemic sclerosis 281
Systolic velocity, low-peak 1203

T

T cell 88
- activity, downregulation of 88, 91
- anergy, inductions of 92*f*
- decidual 88
- regulatory 1020, 1185, 1186
- role of 89*fc*

T test, one sample 1223
Tacrolimus 203
Tadalafil 344*f*, 345
Tall stature 127
Tamoxifen 261, 265, 539, 621, 653, 654
- aromatase inhibitors, role of 256

Tandem mass spectrometry 1443
Tanner stages 120
Target tissue metabolism 112
Taxotere 253, 253*t*
Teflon tubing 1336
Temporary ovarian suspension 591
Tenderness, abdominal 1198
Teratoma, benign cystic 1197
Teratospermia 374
- severe 1049

Teratozoospermia 188, 329, 327, 1237, 1243, 1277, 1334, 1444
- index 1242, 1243

Terminal deoxynucleotidyl transferase 189, 243, 1451
- use of 1310

Terminal hairs 149
- absence of 151*f*

Tertiary sexual dysfunction 395
Test tube
- baby 1302
- warmer 1155, 1652, 1652*f*
  - stand 767

Testes 9, 10, 53, 58, 110, 307, 325, 386, 1117, 1334
- absent 350, 351*f*
- atropic 350, 351*f*
- bilateral maldescended 360
- cancer 375
- consistency of 375
- development of 53
- dysgenetic 307
- endocrinology of 14
- enlarged 350
- larger volume of 360
- Leydig cell of 110
- macroscopic structure of 10*f*
- normal 354*f*
  - histology of 15*f*
- Presence of 375
- Sertoli cell of 8
- size of 185, 328, 375
- small 350
- torsion of 307, 311, 381
- undescended 351*f*, 375
- volume of 326

Testicles, small 360
Testicular abnormalities 350
Testicular atrophy 352
Testicular biopsy 376
- new interpretation of 376*f*
- samples 1469

Testicular cancer 312, 381
- in situ 312

Testicular contribution 14
Testicular damage 282
Testicular deficiency, etiology of 307
Testicular disease, primary 307
Testicular dysfunction syndrome 308
Testicular dysgenesis syndrome 308
- components of 308*fc*

Testicular failure 377
- complete 188
- idiopathic 124
- secondary 306

Testicular feminization syndrome 124, 1076, 1094
Testicular implants 1066*f*, 1067*f*
Testicular mass, presence of 375
Testicular neoplasm 350
Testicular sensation 326
Testicular sperm 1311, 1335, 1339
- aspiration 13, 190, 255, 354, 380, 407, 758, 1128, 1131, 1481, 1502
- extraction 190, 255, 310*f*, 380, 759, 998, 1257, 1294, 1337*f*, 1481
  - microdissection 381
  - microsurgical 309, 382

Testicular spermatozoa 1268, 1275, 1294
Testicular steroidogenesis 111*fc*
Testicular tissue 352*f*
- cryopreservation 255

Testicular torsion 184, 305, 375
Testicular trauma 184, 305
Testicular tumor 307, 350
Testicular volume 351, 353
- bedside clinical assessment of 326*f*

Testosterone 11, 22*f*, 59, 60, 110, 150, 152, 188, 361, 533, 691
- action, mechanism of 361
- deficiency 341
- enanthate 361
- high intratesticular 63
- implant 361
- propionate 361
- replacement therapy 361, 382
- role of 341
- synthesis 111
- total 375, 376

Testotoxicosis, familial 121
Tetrahydrofolate 920
Thalassemia 1407
Thawing 1293
- solution 1382

Theca cell tumor 121
Theca-interstitial cells, autophagy of 1119
Thelarche 116, 119
Theophylline 1257, 1339
Therapeutic drug research 1044
Thermal injury 426
Thermography 388
Thermotaxis 1284
Thiazolidinediones 547
Thick hymen 333
Thick peritoneal grafts, technique of 1079*f*
Thick wide deep septum 600*f*
Thick zona 1502
- pellucida 1516, 1552*f*

Thin endometrium 102, 481*f*, 831, 1047, 1107
- causes of 1107
- treatment of 843, 843*fc*, 844*t*, 855*t*

Third line therapy 343
Third party reproduction 935, 937
Third space fluid collection 899
Thoracolumbar spinal ganglia 7
Three-dimensional culture system 1028
- preparation of 1028

Three-dimensional movements 1503
Three-dimensional power angiography 514*f*
Three-dimensional ultrasound 508*f*, 708
Threonine 1444
- protein kinase A 1245

Thrombocytopenia 281
Thromboembolic episodes 899
Thromboembolism 1196
Thrombophilia 832, 1020
- treatment of 843, 845*t*

Thromboprophylaxis 279
- indications of 279*b*

Thrombosis
- mechanism of 278
- occurrence of 280

Thyroglobulin 143*f*
- antibody 146

Thyroid 17*f*, 143, 145, 146, 158
- autoimmunity 146
- disease 360, 362
- disorder 143, 325, 532
  - screening for 144*b*
- dysfunction 160
- function of 143*b*
- function test 146, 704
- gland, inflammation of 145
- peroxidase 1188*t*, 1188*t*
  - antibody 144, 145, 1187
  - levels of 1187
- releasing hormone 23

Thyroiditis, subacute 145
Thyroid-stimulating hormone 17, 121, 125, 133, 144, 170, 171, 193, 534, 550, 658, 896
- regulates secretion of 17
- screening of 144*fc*

Thyrotropin releasing
- factor 17
- hormone 17, 133

Thyroxine 143*f*
Time-lapse
- imaging 841, 1354, 1613, 1617*f*
- microscopy 1146, 1467, 1613
- monitoring 1354
- system 1613*f*
- technology 1145, 1146, 1354, 1414
- video systems 1167

Tinidazole 454, 454*b*
Tinzaparin 280
Tissue 1199
- culture
  - dish 1658
  - protocol 1027
- development 884
- endometrial 1027

post biopsy 1408
stiffness 1118
typing 1040
T-lymphocytes 90
decidual 90
Tobacco pouch appearance 467*f*
Tocolysis 1208
Toluidine blue 1264
Topical eflornithine 154
Topiramate 231
Topography 425, 425*t*
Torsion 352
correction 324
Total body irradiation 253
Total fertilization failure 70, 1049, 1515
risk of 1327
Total motile sperm 646
count 620, 627, 646, 646*t*, 1343
Total ovarian
stromal area 509
volume 509
Total sperm count, lower median 1326
Touch sensation, loss of 395
Tourette syndrome 888
Toxic
damage 1381
disinfectants, use of 1489
organics 1319, 1320
Toxin, potential 1224
Traditional biopsy techniques, efficacy of 1409
Traditional monopolar resectoscope technique 424
Trakjector micromanipulators 1342, 1343*f*
Transabdominal multifetal pregnancy 1210
Transabdominal needling 1209
Transabdominal paracentesis 1195
Transabdominal scan 782, 1008
Transabdominal sonography 549
Transabdominal ultrasonography 1095
Transabdominal ultrasound 474
Transcervical aspiration 1209
Transcervical balloon cannulation 598
Transcervical embryo replacement 1329
Transcriptomics 837, 1442
Transcutaneous electrical acupoint stimulation 761
Transdermal contraceptive patch 538
Transdermal estrogen 987
Transdermal testosterone 814, 987
Transfer techniques 1203
Transferrin 54
Transforming growth factor 83, 84, 521, 522
beta 21, 29, 45, 76, 83, 84, 90, 109, 195, 810, 1072
receptor 1072
Transgender
females, hormone regimes for 987*t*
males, hormonal therapy for 987*b*
population 986
Transient blindness 596
Transient frontal headaches 677
Translocations
autosomal 212
bacterial 216
Transmembrane 1038
glucose transporter type 4 525
migration 1253, 1274
serine protease 2 1393
Transmyometrial embryo transfer 1056
Transplantation medicine 1044
Transrectal ultrasonography 191, 350, 355
technique of 356*f*
Transrectal ultrasound 376, 378
indications of 355
Transvaginal color Doppler 487, 507
Transvaginal hydrolaparoscopy 443
Transvaginal needling 1209
Transvaginal oocyte
recovery 1325
retrieval 757, 1033
sedation protocol for 759*b*
Transvaginal route 1209
Transvaginal scan 429, 1008, 1014*f*, 1513
Transvaginal sonography 193, 440, 487, 531*f*, 843, 915, 1110
Transvaginal ultrasonography 560
Transvaginal ultrasound 487, 599, 704, 837, 841, 1147
transducer 1326*f*
Transverse section duplication abnormality 488*f*
Transverse vaginal septum 131, 136, 414
Trauma 121, 312
Treponema pallidum 1156
Triangulation technique 379, 379*f*
Trichomonas 966
vaginalis 450, 453
Trichomoniasis 453, 454*b*
Tricyclic antidepressants 313, 365
Tri-gas incubator 1484
Trigger 819
shot 721
Triggering ovulation 902
alternative agents for 902
Triiodothyronine 143, 145
synthesis of 143*f*
Trilaminar pattern 36
Triphosphate 48
Triple-stain technique 1247
Triptorelin 680, 697
Trisomic cell populations 1416
Trisomy 208
Trizygotic
births 927
triplets 928
Trocar 580
Trophectoderm 74, 80, 863, 1371, 1372, 1374, 1403, 1412, 1472, 1568*f*, 1585, 1589*f*, 1591*f*, 1592*f*, 1593*f*
cells 863, 1358, 1374, 1638*f*, 1662
Trophectoderm biopsy 1312, 1410, 1441, 1663, 1663*f*
advantages of 1413
limitations of 1413
protocol for 1411
Trophoblast 1186
cell 1663*f*
extravillous 1020, 1021, 1021*f*
function, abnormal 916
invasions 1021
vesicle 1372, 1372*f*, 1594, 1594*f*
Trophoectoderm cells 880
Truncal hair 375
T-shaped uterus 420, 491, 493*f*
three-dimensional ultrasound of 493*f*
T-sign 930
Tubal abortion 923
Tubal anastomosis 587
Tubal assessment tests 440
Tubal cannulation 447
Tubal catheterization 442
Tubal damage 439
Tubal disease, bulk of 438
Tubal ectopic pregnancy 916*f*, 919*f*, 1015*t*
biomarkers of 916*t*
management of 447
Tubal factor 241, 438, 465, 1201
evaluation of 644
infertility, evaluation of 6, 439
Tubal infertility 444
management of 443
prevention of 444
surgery for 584
Tubal inflammation 507*t*
Tubal insufflation 443
test 443
Tubal lesions 487, 505
Tubal motility, altered 567
Tubal mucosa, role of 584
Tubal occlusion 587
Tubal ostia 598*f*, 601*f*, 830
Tubal ostium 420
Tubal patency 244, 441*f*, 622
tests 441
Tubal perforation 598
Tubal pregnancy 916
ectopic 7
management of 920
Tubal reanastomosis 608
Tubal reconstruction 446, 590*f*
Tubal reconstructive surgery 447, 608
Tubal repair 584
Tubal resection 445
Tubal restorative surgery 444
Tubal sterilization 439
microsurgical 447
Tubal subfertility, causes of 438
Tubal transposition 587
Tubal wall thickness 584
Tube
ampullary segment of 590*f*
anatomical distortion of 567
evaluation of 608
mobility of 584
Tubercles 468*f*
Tubercular adnexal mass 467*f*
Tuberculosis 439, 441, 463, 468, 955
endometrial 954
extrapulmonary 463
genitourinary 432
testing for 441
Tubo-ovarian
abscess 455
adhesion 580, 589*f*
anatomy 587
lesions 501
mass, bilateral 467*f*
vasculature 1070*f*
Tuboplasty 444
Tubotubal reanastomosis 585
Tubular cavity, narrow 601*f*
Tubular ectasia 351
Tubules 15

Tumor 120, 306, 312, 393
- adrenal functional 121
- benign 1197
- embryonal 886
- endometrioid 504
- epithelial 504
- intracranial 124
- malignant 1196
- necrosis factor 84, 89, 157*f*, 225, 566, 898, 1023
- necrosis factor alpha 31, 53, 83, 89, 90, 99, 201, 224, 227, 314, 430, 527, 1023
  - antagonists 1023
- subendometrial 421
- suppressor gene 29

TUNEL assay 1037
Turner syndrome 49, 124, 125, 132, 134, 137, 169, 171, 215, 215*f*, 216*f*, 250, 888, 938, 939, 939*f*, 1430
Twilight sleep 758
Twin
- discordant 929, 933
- gestation 1010
- oligohydramnios-polyhydramnios sequence 996
- pathogenesis of 929*f*, 929*t*
- peak sign 930, 1011, 1012*f*
- pregnancy 932, 1010, 1302
  - types of 1011*t*
- to-twin transfusion 927
- ultrasound labeling of 1010

Tygerberg criteria 368
Tyrode's since laser 1403
Tyrode's solution 1170
Tyrosine 1444

U

Udenafil 345
Ulcerative colitis 278, 287, 288, 1294
Ulipristal acetate 426
Ultrasonogram 244
Ultrasonography 122, 191, 291, 350, 378, 387, 414, 440, 603, 645, 677, 713, 776, 1004, 1035, 1198
- advanced 1319
- preoperative 1209

Ultrasound 100, 484, 507, 534
- advantages of 707
- elastography 787
- evaluation 152
- first-trimester 1005
- guided insemination 647
- indications of 355
- machine 1656, 1656*f*
- monitoring 707
- scan 228

Umbilical cord 1111, 1120
Umbilical vascular access 1042
Unconsciousness 393
Unexplained infertility 158, 239, 246, 621, 622, 668
- diagnosis of 239
- evaluation of 242

Upper genital tract 455
Upper vaginal absence 1075
Ureaplasma urealyticum 315, 364
Ureter, double 1079*f*
Ureteric laceration 1061
Ureteric tunnel 1057
Ureteric-vaginal fistula 1061
Urethra 987*f*, 1098*f*
- uncomplicated gonococcal infection of 452*b*

Urethral injury 990*f*, 991*f*
Urethral sphincters, external 333
Urethral stenosis 990, 991*f*
- postsurgery 991*f*

Urethral stricture 324, 989
Urethritis, risk of 1097
Urinary alkalinization, protocol for 336
Urinary human
- chorionic gonadotropin 723, 905
- menopausal gonadotropin 1299

Urinary luteinizing hormone kit 707
Urinary menotropins 656
Urinary system malformations 1095
Urinary tract
- infections 190, 400
- symptoms, lower 398

Urinary-highly purified-follicle-stimulating hormone 656
Urine
- pregnancy test 915
- samples, abnormal 190

Urogenital
- chlamydial infection 451
- infection 350, 364
- tract, distal part of 305

Uterine 5, 37*t*, 88, 1070*f*
- adenomyosis 23
- allograft 1055
- aplasia 487
- axis 6*f*
- biophysical profile 713
- bleeding, abnormal 414, 530
- contractions, excessive 1329
- endometrial cycle 34
- epithelium 1108
- fibroids 696, 701
- fundus 1071
- incision 423*f*
- infection, postoperative 597
- manipulator 580
- modulators 88
- motility 1202
- natural killer cells 88, 431, 831, 832, 1020, 1186
- pathology 831
- perforation 597
- position 775
- reconstruction 424*f*
- relaxants, role of 777
- septum 419, 609, 419, 842
- stress 1141
- surface, anterior 572*f*
- synechiae 242, 465
- tenderness 455
- transplant, first 1313
- vein 1056, 1058
- vessels 1196

Uterine abnormalities 439, 487, 831, 831*t*, 842, 1055, 1147
- acquired 492
- congenital 487, 487*t*, 492
- diagnostic modalities for 836
- effects of 1202
- treatment of 842, 842*t*

Uterine artery
- Doppler flow 713
- Doppler studies of 431
- embolization 420
- flow
  - high resistance 510*f*
  - indices 708, 709*f*
- interventions on 422

Uterine cavity 602*f*, 1007*f*, 1110*f*, 1466
- abnormal 1037
- abnormalities 241, 242
- distortion of 420
- evaluation of 244, 775
- restoration of 611

Uterine cycle 16
- stages of 35*f*, 36*f*

Uterine factor 465, 830, 834, 1020, 1202
- infertility 413, 1040

Uterine malformation 1040, 1042
- congenital 419, 419*f*

Uterine transplantation 845, 992, 1040, 1041, 1055, 1103
- ethical feasibility of 1041

Uterine tube 3, 5, 438
- innervation of 5
- parts of 5

Uterocervical length 511*f*
Uteroglobin 88, 91
Utero-ovarian
- connections 1070*f*
- ligament 1196
- veins 1060

Uterus 3, 5, 73, 464, 510, 707, 941, 1035, 1041, 1210, 1245, 1329
- acute
  - anteversion of 1518
  - retroversion of 1518
- arcuate 418*f*, 491
- arterial supply of 7
- artificial 1042
- axes of 6
- bicornuate 414, 419, 488, 490*f*
- bicorporeal 489*f*
- didelphys 414, 418, 488, 488*f*
- duplication abnormalities of 492*t*
- flexion of 6
- functioning 954
- fundus of 1198
- hypoplastic 491, 600
- innervation of 7
- large 466
- midcavity of 1329*f*
- myomectomy 580
- procurement 1058, 1059
- unicornuate 414, 418, 487, 488*f*, 587
- venous supply of 7

Uterus transplantation 1055, 1056, 1059, 1060, 1061*t*, 1062, 1062*t*, 1063, 1313
- animal research in 1055
- surgery 1313

V

Vaccination, timing of 1219
Vacuole-free sperm, selection of 1449
Vacuoles 1362, 1372, 1450, 1541, 1595
- multiple 1544*f*

Vacuum erection device 346
Vagina 3, 7, 465, 989, 1209, 1245
absent 134*fc*
anatomical relations of 1098*f*
classification of 414
innervation of 7
normal 1090*f*
Vaginal agenesis 1094*f*, 1097
causes of 1094
etiology of 1093
Vaginal atresia 1094
isolated 1095
Vaginal biopsies 1080*f*
Vaginal bleeding, abnormal 914
Vaginal canal 987
Vaginal dilators 988*f*
Vaginal dimple 1094*f*
Vaginal discharge, abnormal 466
Vaginal douching 1245
Vaginal dryness 660, 677
Vaginal egg recovery 1325*f*
Vaginal epithelium 7, 1079
Vaginal examination 915
Vaginal incubation 1042
Vaginal mold 1099*f*
Vaginal myomectomy 426
Vaginal oocyte aspiration 1305*f*
Vaginal preparation 765
Vaginal progesterone 161, 801*f*
Vaginal prolapse, risk of 1097
Vaginal reconstruction 1097
Vaginal secretions, electronic resistance evaluation of 706
Vaginal septum, longitudinal 414
Vaginal sonography 1027
Vaginal tissue 1058
Vaginal ultrasound transducer 1326*f*
Vaginal-vaginal anastomosis 1059
Vaginismus 333
Vaginitis, atrophic 154
Vaginoplasty 987, 987*f*, 1081
pictures 1088*f*
Vaginosis, bacterial 454, 455*b*
Vaginosonography 1106
Valine 1444
Valproate 289
Valsalva
absent venous reflux 353*f*
maneuver 326
Vaporizing electrode 595
use of 425
Vardenafil 345
Varicocele 184, 306, 307, 311, 322, 326, 350, 352, 354, 364, 381, 385, 387-390, 1235
classification of 184*t*
color Doppler ultrasound diagnosis of 387*t*
etiology of 385
evaluation, color Doppler for 355
grades of 184, 375, 387*t*
repair 388, 388*t*
laparoscopic 389
Varicocelectomy 324, 375
Vas ampulla 355
Vas deferens 326, 352
absence of 328
bilateral absence of 311, 408
congenital
absence of 184, 185, 305, 310, 324, 328, 350, 357, 376-378
bilateral absence of 357
obstruction 313, 328
palpation of 375
Vasa deferentia 9
Vasal agenesis 356
Vasal aspiration 339
Vascular abnormality 385
Vascular anastomosis 1071
technique of 1067*f*
Vascular connection 431
Vascular disease 345*fc*
peripheral 340
Vascular endothelial grow 844
Vascular endothelial growth factor 33, 82*f*, 83, 84, 99, 156, 431, 476, 522, 672, 710, 726, 729, 895, 896, 901, 916, 1030, 1071-1073, 1108, 1193-1195
ovarian hypersecretion of 903
production of 897*f*
Vascular ischemia 393
Vascular smooth muscles 904
Vascular stroke 1189
Vascularity flow index 507, 514
Vascularization flow index 478, 711, 713
Vasculitis 281
Vasculogenesis 1072*f*
Vasectomy 184, 253, 324, 328, 375, 376
Vasoactive intestinal
peptide 231022
polypeptide 333
Vasoactive intracorporeal drug injection 342
Vasoactive peptides 54
Vasoepididymal ductal end-to-side anastomosis 379
Vasoepididymostomy 378, 379, 1294
conventional 379*f*
Vasography 376
Vasopressin 23
injection 422*f*
Vasovasal anastomosis 378, 378*t*, 379
Vasovasostomy 379
Vecchietti
apparatus 1101*f*
operation 136, 1101*f*
procedure 1100
laparoscopic 418
Vegetal cytoplasm 1365
Vellus hairs 149
Vena cava 1056
inferior 385
Venereal disease research laboratory 941, 942
Venography 388
Venous anastomosis 1071
Venous thromboembolism 279, 280, 743
prevalence of 278
signs of 907
symptoms of 907
Venous thrombosis, risk of 1058
Verbal anesthesia 766
Veress needle 580
Vernier caliper 326*f*
Vertebral spondylosis 393
Vesicles, extracellular 881
Vesicular mole 500*f*
Vessel formation 1030*f*
Vestigial lamina 1096
Vibrational spectroscopy 1444
Vibratory stimulation 337
Vigorous sperm 1247
Villous
cytotrophoblast 87
syncytiotrophoblast 88
Vinblastine sulfate 253
Vincristine 253
Viral infections, effects of 1396
Viral markers, screening for 793
Viral screening 191
Virilization, state of 375
Virilizing adrenal
adenoma 151
carcinoma 151
Virtual organ computer-aided analysis 507, 508*f*, 510*f*, 513*f*, 708
Virus, cross-contamination of 1394
Visceral adipose tissue 526
Visceromegaly 886
Viscosity 185
treatment system 1274
Visible meiotic spindle 1434
Visual disorders 669
Visual symptoms 654
Vitality 186, 188, 327
Vitamin 368, 844*t*
B_{12} 1188, 1189
B_6 1189
D 547
deficiency 527
E 366, 844
transporters 54
Vitreous state 1389
Vitrification 1139, 1381, 1389
method 1139, 1139*f*
practical tips for 796
protocol 1390
safety of 1383
solution 1382, 1623, 1628*f*, 1629*f*, 1631*f*, 1632*f*, 1637, 1639*f*
straw, high-security 1395
techniques 1463
time schedule for 1383
Volatile organic compounds 794, 1132, 1162, 1164, 1489, 1498, 1529
Vomiting 654, 899, 1213
von Willebrand factor 278
cleaving protease 278
Vorozole 654
Vulva 465
Vulvovaginoplasty procedure 1099

W

Waist circumference 223
measurement 222, 532
Waist-hip ratio 223
Wallace surePro ultra medicals 781*f*
Wallace-Smith medicals 779
Wamstekar's classification 594
Warming protocol 1390
Washing solution 1382
Waste
disposal of 1185
products dilutants 1494

Water 1494
- jacket incubators 1166*f*, 1498

Weakness 914
Weight loss 230, 231*t*, 233, 535
- drugs for 230
- medications 230
- severe 135

Weight management 230
Wharton's jelly 1117
Whirlpool appearance 1199
Whirlpool sign 504*f*
White blood
- cell 88, 314, 894, 899, 1247
- count 455

Whole chromosome painting probes 210
Whole genome amplification 864, 1442
Wilms tumor 886, 1091
Wolffian ducts 8, 413
- system 11

Womb 5
- artificial 1042

World's first in vitro fertilization 1303*f*
Worms, bag of 184
Wound
- healing 222
- infection 989

X

X chromosome 938, 1308
X-axis movements 1508
Xenografts in vivo 1313
Xenon cold light source 580
X-linked disorders 879
X-linked genes 214
XXX syndrome 215
XYY syndrome 212

Y

Y chromosome 309, 1308, 1310
- deletions 60, 307
- microdeletion 185, 190, 212, 212*t*, 306, 309, 329, 381, 406
- specific pregnancies 1307

Yolk sac 1005, 1006*f*, 1008*f*, 1009*f*, 1011*f*, 1016
- large 1016*f*

Young's syndrome 324, 375

Z

Zeta potential method 1255, 1278
Ziehl-Neelsen staining 463
Zinc 12, 366, 548, 1248
- detection of 1249*b*

Zona
- binding assays 1242
- birefringence 1436
- breaker cells 75, 1374
- dissection, partial 1402, 1402*f*, 1502
- drilling 1402, 1403, 1502
- fasciculata 108, 109, 146
- glomerulosa 108
- hardening 1401
- lysins 1401
- reaction 67
- reticularis, central 108
- softening 1403
- thickness 1401, 1405, 1471

Zona pellucida 45, 67, 68, 70*f*, 75, 239, 567, 1308, 1340, 1348*f*, 1351, 1353*f*, 1359, 1374, 1394, 1401, 1402*f*, 1411, 1433, 1436, 1470, 1538*f*, 1552, 1552*f*, 1553*f*, 1588*f*, 1592*f*, 1593*f*, 1662, 1662*f*
- glycoprotein 68
- layers 1436*f*
- penetration of 67

Zuclomiphene 667
Zygosity 927, 933
Zygote 53, 69, 928, 971, 1175, 1311, 1353*f*, 1363, 1373, 1374, 1409, 1410, 1452, 1461, 1462*f*
- abnormal 1573*f*
- display 1364
- evaluation of 1373
- formation 68
- intra-fallopian transfer 760, 774, 842
- mice 1461
- polarized 1364*f*
- stage 878
- superior quality 1257